Complex Foot and Ankle Trauma

Complex Foot and Ankle Trauma

Editor

Robert S. Adelaar, M.D.
Professor of Surgery
Vice-Chairman, Department of Orthopaedics
Medical College of Virginia
Virginia Commonwealth University
Richmond, Virginia

Illustrations by Bob L. Shepherd, M.S.

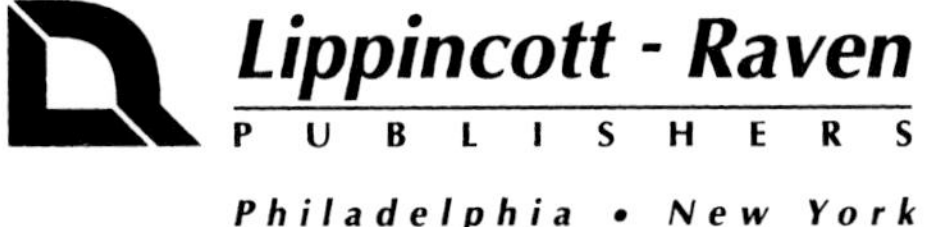

Acquisitions Editor: Danette Knopp
Developmental Editor: Stephanie Harris/Carol Field
Manufacturing Manager: Kevin Watt
Production Manager: Jodi Borgenicht
Production Editor: Jonathan Geffner
Cover Designer: Marsha Cohen
Indexer: Linda Van Pelt
Compositor: CJS Tapsco
Printer: Courier–Westford

Printed in the United States of America

9 8 7 6 5 4 3 2 1

Library of Congress Cataloging-in-Publication Data

Complex foot and ankle trauma / edited by Robert S. Adelaar;
illustrations by Bob L. Shepherd.
p. cm.
Includes index.
ISBN 0-397-51374-7
1. Foot—Wounds and injuries. 2. Ankle—Fractures. 3. Ankle—Wounds and injuries. 4. Fractures—Treatment. 5. Musculoskeletal system—Wounds and injuries. I. Adelaar, Robert S.
[DNLM: 1. Foot Injuries—therapy. 2. Ankle Injuries—therapy. 3. Dislocations—therapy. 4. Fractures—therapy. WE 880 C7365 1998]
RD563.C654 1998
617.5′85044—dc21
DNLM/DLC
for Library of Congress 98-7630
CIP

Care has been taken to confirm the accuracy of the information presented and to describe generally accepted practices. However, the authors, editor, and publisher are not responsible for errors or omissions or for any consequences from application of the information in this book and make no warranty, expressed or implied, with respect to the contents of the publication.

The authors, editor, and publisher have exerted every effort to ensure that drug selection and dosage set forth in this text are in accordance with current recommendations and practice at the time of publication. However, in view of ongoing research, changes in government regulations, and the constant flow of information relating to drug therapy and drug reactions, the reader is urged to check the package insert for each drug for any change in indications and dosage and for added warnings and precautions. This is particularly important when the recommended agent is a new or infrequently employed drug.

Some drugs and medical devices presented in this publication have Food and Drug Administration (FDA) clearance for limited use in restricted research settings. It is the responsibility of the health care provider to ascertain the FDA status of each drug or device planned for use in their clinical practice.

There are many sources of inspiration and guidance to whom I have looked over the past twenty years at the Medical College of Virginia at Virginia Commonwealth University. This book is dedicated to the orthopaedic residents, fellow attendings, and other house staff officers who have helped me develop expertise and experience in treating disorders of the foot and ankle. The orthopaedic residents have kept me sharp with their challenging questions. My immediate family of Carol, Kim, and Stephen certainly deserve a lot of credit for their personal sacrifices over the years that have allowed me to devote an inordinate amount of time to my practice. I apologize for all of those times they have had to ask, ''Where is Bob?'' Finally, this book is devoted to my roots, Robert Fulton and Magdelena, who have instilled a high work ethic and ethical values that I have attempted to follow.

Contents

Contributing Authors ix

Preface xi

Acknowledgments xii

1. Clinical Biomechanics of the Ankle Syndesmosis. . . . 1
Robert S. Adelaar

2. Complex Ankle Fracture Dislocations with Syndesmotic Diastasis 9
James B. Stiehl

3. Fractures of the Posterior Malleolus. 21
James B. Carr

4. Open Fractures of the Ankle Joint. 31
James B. Stiehl

5. Historical Review of the Treatment of Syndesmotic Ankle Injuries. 39
Thomas V. DiStefano, John A. Cardea, and Robert S. Adelaar

6. The Pilon Fracture 45
James B. Carr

7. Complex Fractures of the Talus 65
Robert S. Adelaar

8. Occult Injuries of the Talus 95
Robert S. Adelaar

9. **Subtalar Dislocations** 109
Michael J. Brennan

10. **Intraarticular Calcaneal Fractures: A Basic Science Update with Clinical Correlations** 115
James B. Carr

11. **Long-Term Results of Treatment of Displaced Intraarticular Calcaneal Fractures** 127
Roy Sanders

12. **Calcaneal Malunions and Their Treatment** 137
Roy Sanders

13. **Fractures of the Navicular and Cuboid** 145
Michael M. Romash

14. **Treatment of Tarsometatarsal Injuries** 161
Robert S. Adelaar

15. **Management of Crush and Soft Tissue Injuries of the Foot** 175
Mark S. Myerson

16. **Compartment Syndromes of the Foot** 191
Mark S. Myerson

17. **Treatment of Complex Forefoot Injuries** 205
William M. Granberry and Michael J. Shereff

18. **Fractures of the Proximal Fifth Metatarsal** 217
Alan S. Tuckman, Samuel S. Fleming, John G. Seiler III, and Lamar L. Fleming

19. **Athletic Injuries of the Great Toe MTP Joint** 231
Michael W. Bowman

20. **Guidelines for Soft Tissue Coverage of Complex Foot and Ankle Injuries** 257
L. Scott Levin

Subject Index 269

Contributing Authors

Robert S. Adelaar, M.D.
Professor of Surgery, Vice-Chairman, Department of Orthopaedics, Medical College of Virginia/Virginia Commonwealth University, Box 980153, MCV Station, Richmond, Virginia 23298

Michael W. Bowman, M.D.
Clinical Assistant Professor, Department of Orthopaedic Surgery, University of Pittsburgh Medical Center, 5820 Centre Avenue, Pittsburgh, Pennsylvania 15206-3753; Assistant Professor, Department of Orthopaedic Surgery, Allegheny University of Health Sciences, Pittsburgh, Pennsylvania 15212

Michael J. Brennan, M.D.
Orthopaedic Consultant, Arizona State University, 2222 East Highland Avenue, Suite 425, Phoenix, Arizona 85016

John A. Cardea, M.D.
Professor and Chair, Department of Orthopaedic Surgery, Medical College of Virginia/Virginia Commonwealth University, Box 980153, MCV Station, Richmond, Virginia 23298

James B. Carr, M.D.
Associate Professor, Department of Orthopaedic Surgery, Medical College of Virginia, MCV Station, Box 980153, Richmond, Virginia 23298; Department of Orthopaedic Surgery, MCV Hospitals, 401 North 12th Street, Richmond, Virginia 23298

Thomas V. DiStefano, M.D., M.S.
Sports Medicine Fellow, Department of Orthopaedics, Tulane School of Medicine, 1430 Tulane Avenue, New Orleans, Louisiana 70112

Lamar L. Fleming, M.D.
Professor, Department of Orthopaedics, Emory University, 1365 Clifton Road Northeast, Atlanta, Georgia 30322; Chairman, Department of Orthopaedics, Emory University Hospital, 1364 Clifton Road Northeast, Atlanta, Georgia 30322

Samuel S. Fleming, M.D.
Clinical Faculty, Department of Orthopaedics, Emory University, 1364 Clifton Road Northeast, Atlanta, Georgia, 30322; Department of Orthopaedics, Kennestone Hospital, 677 Church Street, Marietta, Georgia 30060

William M. Granberry, M.D.
Assistant Clinical Professor, Department of Orthopaedic Surgery, Baylor College of Medicine, One Baylor Plaza, Houston, Texas 77030; Chief, Section of Foot and Ankle Surgery, St. Lukes Episcopal Hospital, 6720 Bertner Street, Houston, Texas 77030

L. Scott Levin, M.D.
Associate Professor, Department of Orthopaedic and Plastic Surgery, Chief—Division of Plastic, Reconstructive, Maxillofacial, and Oral Surgery—Duke University Medical Center, Trent Drive, 134 Baker House, Durham, North Carolina 27710

Mark S. Myerson, M.D.
Director, Foot and Ankle Services, The Union Memorial Hospital, 3333 North Calvert Street, Baltimore, Maryland 21218

Michael M. Romash, M.D.
Clinical Assistant Professor, Department of Surgery, Uniformed Services, University of the Health Sciences, 4301 Jones Bridge Road, Bethesda, Maryland 20814; Department of Surgery, Chesapeake General Hospital, 736 North Battlefield Boulevard, Chesapeake, Virginia 23320

Roy Sanders, M.D.
Professor of Clinical Orthopaedics, Department of Surgery, Division of Orthopaedics, University of South Florida, 12901 Bruce B. Downs Boulevard, Tampa, Florida 33612; Chief, Department of Orthopaedics, Tampa General Hospital, 4 Columbia Drive, Suite 710, Tampa, Florida 33606

John G. Seiler III, M.D.
Clinical Associate Professor, Department of Orthopaedic Surgery, Emory University, 69 Butler Street Southeast, Atlanta, Georgia 30309; Department of Orthopaedic Surgery, Piedmont Hospital, 1938 Peachtree Street, Suite 603, Atlanta, Georgia 30309

Michael J. Shereff, M.D.
Associate Clinical Professor, Department of Orthopaedic Surgery, Medical University of South Carolina, 171 Ashley Avenue, Charleston, South Carolina 29425; Director, Orthopaedic Foot and Ankle Center, Orthopaedic Specialists of Charleston, 2093 Henry Tecklenburg Drive, Charleston, South Carolina 29414

James B. Stiehl, M.D.
Clinical Associate Professor, Department of Orthopaedics, Medical College of Wisconsin, 8700 West Wisconsin Avenue, Milwaukee, Wisconsin 53226; Attending Surgeon, Department of Orthopaedics, Columbia Hospital, 2015 East Newport Avenue, #703, Milwaukee, Wisconsin 53211

Alan S. Tuckman, M.D.
116 Slade Avenue, Baltimore, Maryland 21208

Preface

This book represents a gathering of the minds of this country's top foot and ankle trauma specialists. I have collected a broad spectrum of faculty members who have had long tenures in the treatment of foot and ankle trauma disorders. It is my intention to present a group of individuals who will give the reader a realistic view of the treatment options, and their outcomes, for various traumatic disorders relating to the foot and ankle. Because the foot and ankle complex is affected by such unbelievable forces during normal gait, it does not tolerate articular or soft-tissue injury very well. Therefore, injuries that particularly involve weight-bearing structures need to be treated in a manner that will still allow that part to function in the future. Convalescence from foot and ankle injuries, as we will see, is prolonged; therefore, if you attempt open techniques, your patients should expect a relatively longer convalescent period as compared with other areas of the body. I thank the authors for their diligence and wisdom and hope that the reader will enjoy the text, which is geared toward those in the medical field who deal with foot and ankle trauma.

Robert S. Adelaar, M.D.

Acknowledgments

I wish to acknowledge my secretarial staff who over the years have juggled a busy clinical practice with my academic pursuits. Their dedication to their work and high aptitude for medical affairs have certainly made my life easier. I also wish to acknowledge the work of our medical illustrator, Mr. Robert Shepherd.

Complex Foot and Ankle Trauma,
edited by Robert S. Adelaar,
Lippincott–Raven Publishers, Philadelphia © 1999.

1

Clinical Biomechanics of the Ankle Syndesmosis

Robert S. Adelaar

Ankle fractures with diastasis are the most common complex foot and ankle traumas that one encounters. In a recent study from the Hannover (Germany) Medical School, approximately two-thirds of the complex injuries to the foot and ankle involved the ankle (1) (Fig. 1). The lateral ankle structures are very important in the normal dynamics of ankle motion and stability. The ankle will have peak loads up to four times body weight, with the tibial plafond holding 80% to 90% of the weight. The fibula itself accounts for approximately 15% of the total load. The ankle with its cartilaginous surfaces is quite stable in the loaded position (2). The range of motion of the ankle in the loaded position is 32 to 45 degrees; in the unloaded position it goes from 12 to 56 degrees. Several motions around the ankle allow increased motion, such as the deep deltoid contribution to internal rotation of the talus from 4 to 8 degrees during plantar flexion. The fibula also moves during ankle motion. When it is loaded, there is external rotation of a few degrees and movement in the posterior and lateral direction.

The syndesmosis is composed of four structures: the interosseous ligament, the anterior tibiofibular ligament, the posterior tibiofibular ligament, and the transverse tibiofibular ligament (Fig. 2). In hydraulic cadaver testing, the percentage resistance to a few millimeters of diastasis was distributed in the following manner: anterior tibiofibular ligament 35%, interosseous ligament 22%, and posterior tibiofibular ligament 43% (3). The syndesmotic ligament plays a dynamic role in ankle biomechanics. Close (4) has stated that the syndesmosis permits ankle mortise flexibility because of the

R. S. Adelaar: Department of Orthopaedics, Medical College of Virginia/Virginia Commonwealth University, Richmond, Virginia 23298.

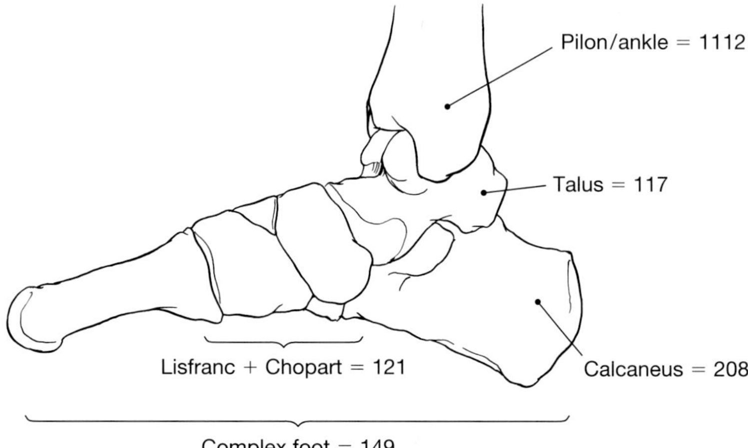

Figure 1. In a study of 149 cases of complex injuries to the foot and ankle, approximately two-thirds of the injuries involved the ankle. (From ref. 1, with permission.)

elasticity of the ligaments, which allows the intermalleolar distance to change and facilitates tibial and fibular rotation. Vukicevic et al. (5) thought that the interosseous membrane was important because it balances the loading of the foot through the fibula. The syndesmosis widens normally with weight bearing as well as when the foot goes from full plantar flexion to dorsiflexion. The interosseous membrane can accommodate these changes and up to 120% of its length before failure. Therefore, the object in treatment of ruptures of this complex injury is to restore the anatomy of the lateral syndesmosis and allow protective stress during the healing.

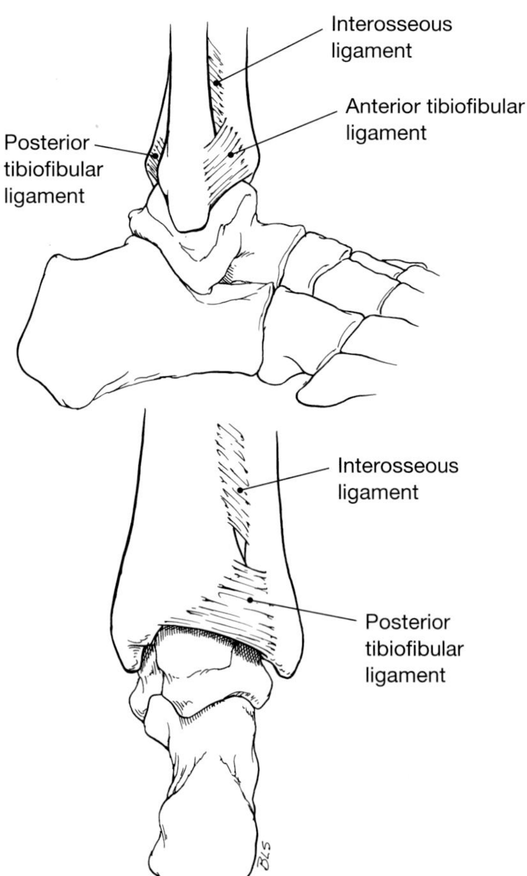

Figure 2. The syndesmosis is composed of four structures.

As we will see in the following section, the deltoid ligament provides stability to the syndesmosis. The normal deltoid ligament is composed of a superficial component consisting of the tibionavicular and tibiocalcaneal portions (Fig. 3). The deep deltoid is a short, broad ligament from the tibia to the talus near the deltoid artery with its important contribution to circulation of the body of the talus (6).

The deep deltoid is important for resisting the forces that would externally rotate the talus. In cadaver studies we have shown that the superficial tibiocalcaneal portion of the deltoid ligament is the critical component to providing physiologic contact stresses in the ankle. When the tibiocalcaneal was sectioned, the contact area significantly decreased, elevating the peak pressures and shifting the centroid in a lateral direction on the talus (7). This alters the theory that the deep deltoid was the important stabilizer of the medial side of the ankle and that reconstruction of it would be critical to the maintenance of medial stability. The superficial ligament complex originates from the anterior colliculus of the tibia, and the deep deltoid originates from the posterior colliculus.

When one analyzes the biomechanical syndesmosis data in the literature and the need for transsyndesmotic fixation of the distal tibial fibular joint in unstable ankle injuries, there is much controversy. Classification terminology in ankle fractures is important. Two major classifications are utilized, the Danis–Weber–AO and the Lauge-Hansen (Fig. 4). The Danis–Weber classifies fractures as to the location of the fibula and the components of the ankle that have been injured. Ankle fractures that are unstable with diastasis are usually classified as Danis–Weber C injuries. The Lauge-Hansen classification was developed to describe cadaver fracture patterns. The first part of the terminology refers to the foot position when the forces start, and the second refers to the major force that is transmitted to the foot. In the supination external injury,

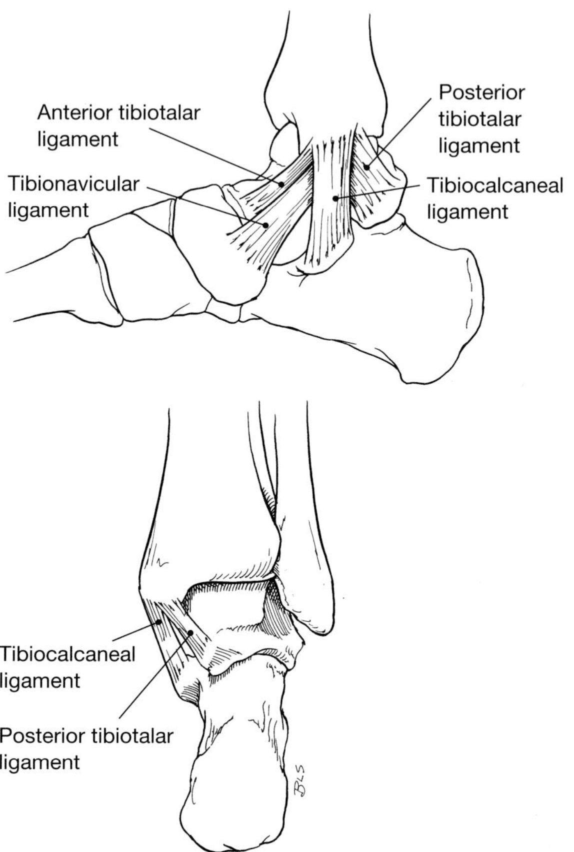

Figure 3. The components of the superficial deltoid ligament.

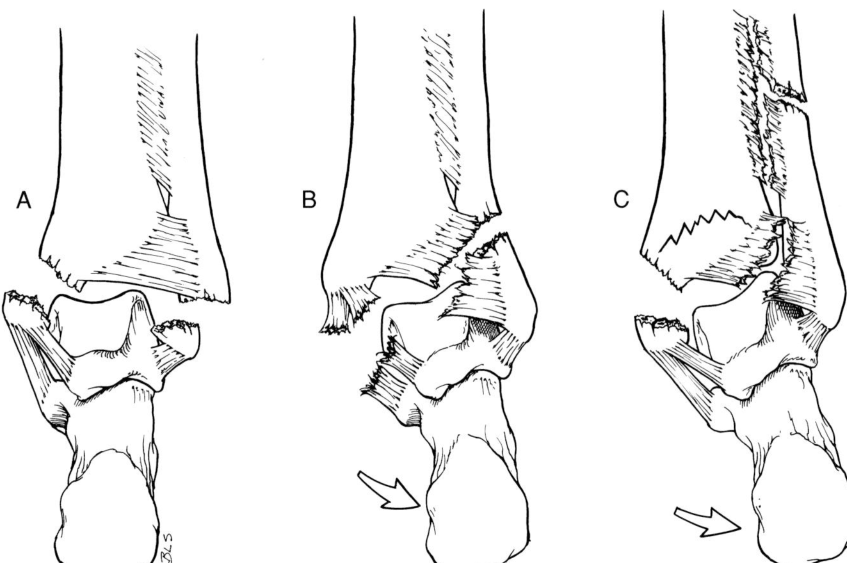

Figure 4. Davis–Weber–AO classification of ankle fractures.

the foot (Fig. 5A) is held in supination and is subjected to external rotation forces. This is the most common type of unstable ankle injury (60%) and involves injury first to the lateral structure starting with the anterior tibiofibular ligament, the remainder of the syndesmosis, fibula, posterior malleolus, and finally the medial bone structures or deltoid. Another common mechanism is the pronation external rotation injury (15%), in which the pronated foot is subjected to external rotation forces. The mechanics of the injury are forces that start on the medial side, causing a deltoid avulsion or medial malleolar fracture and then proceed to the anterior tibiofibular ligament and syndesmosis, the fibula, and finally the posterior malleolar area. The pattern of fibular fracture is distinctive; in the supination injury there is usually a long spiral with some comminution; in the pronation injury the fibula has a short oblique fracture above the mortise.

Syndesmotic diastasis may be difficult to determine by radiographic criteria due to variation in rotation and anatomy of peroneal grove and tibial tubercle (8). Some authors have reported an intraobserver variability of 1 mm in the radiographic measurement of syndesmotic widening (9). In our laboratory direct strain transducer measurements of tibial fibular diastasis demonstrates that radiographic analysis is a rather crude measure of the spread of the syndesmosis; therefore the results that depend on x-ray criteria alone should be suspect (8). The x-ray criteria that are available consist of the clear space at a point 1 cm proximal to the ankle consisting of the distance between the lateral posterior tibia and the medial posterior fibula (Fig. 6) (10). A space less than 6 mm is felt to be appropriate. A cartilage clear space of less than 2 mm in the loaded ankle and up to 4 mm in the unloaded ankle is appropriate, and the symmetry between the medial and lateral area is important (2). The tibiotalar angle is about 83 degrees plus or minus 4 degrees; a greater than 5-degree change in this angle or change in the length of the fibula would be important parameters of x-ray evidence of instability (11). The posterior tibiofibular clear space seems to be the most accurate x-ray indicator in our hands; this space seems to increase with lateral shift of the fibula and internal rotation of the fibula and to decrease when the fibula externally rotates (10).

The syndesmotic biomechanical and clinical data available to us make it difficult to make a decision as to how and when to treat the unstable syndesmosis. Stability of the ankle is provided by bone architecture and certainly increases with weight bearing due to the cartilage (2). Yablon et al. (12) felt that the lateral malleolus with its associated ligaments was key in stabilizing the ankle in both cadaver and clinical studies. He concluded that sectioning of the deltoid ligament did not result in instability unless the

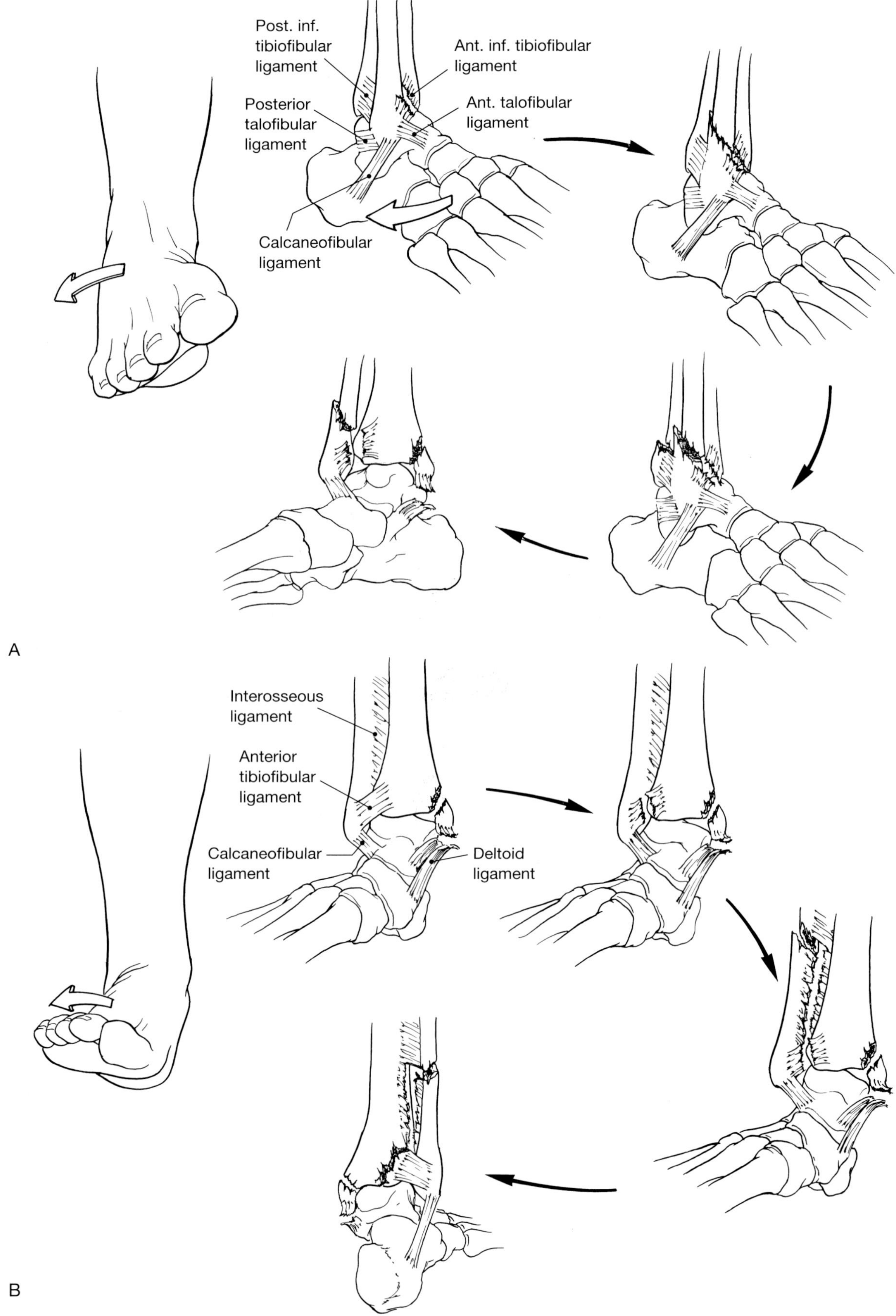

Figure 5. A: The supination external injury. **B:** The pronation external rotation injury (Lauge-Hansen).

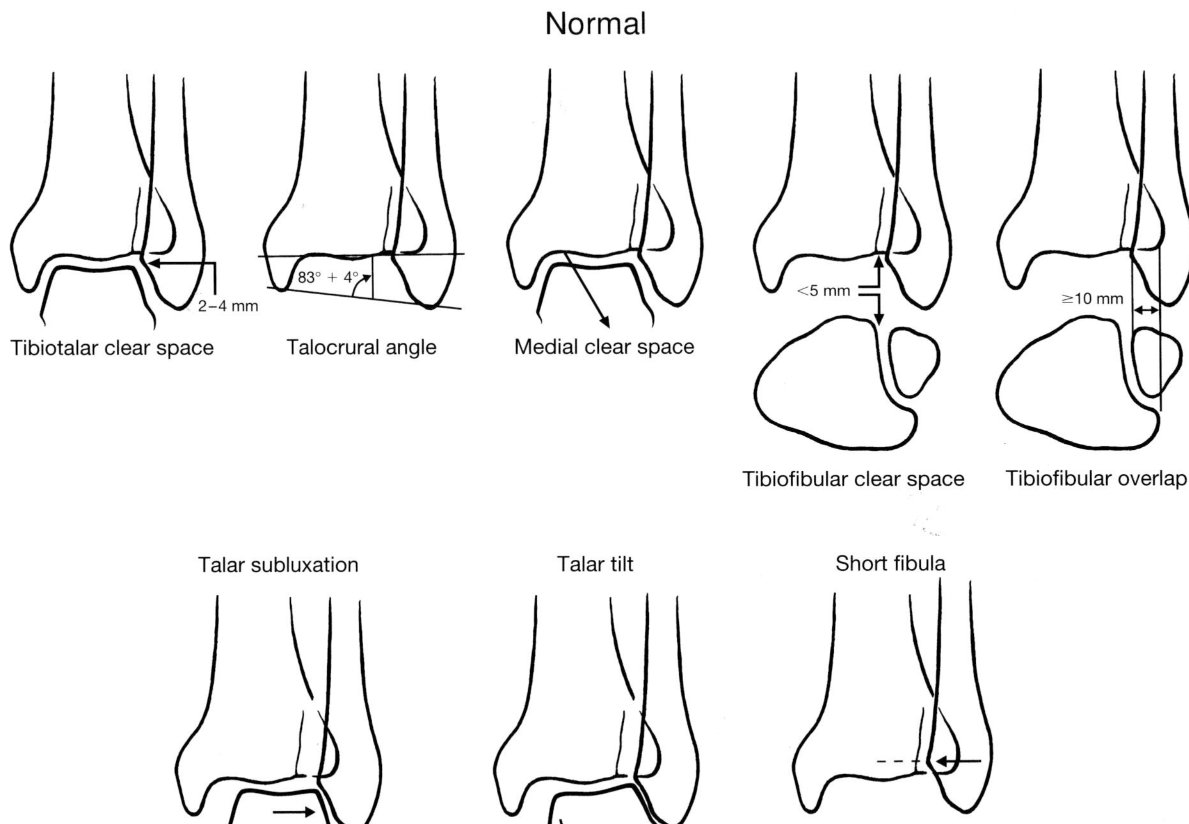

Figure 6. X-ray criteria consist of the clear space at a point 1 cm proximal to the ankle consisting of the distance between the lateral posterior tibia and the medial posterior fibula.

lateral malleolus was sectioned. Harper (13) evaluated the deltoid ligament and concluded that the lateral malleolus and supporting ligaments are primary restraints of both anterior and lateral talar shift and that the deltoid ligament was the primary restraint against valgus tilting of the talus. The deep and not the superficial deltoid was a secondary restraint against the lateral talar shift. Harper (13) noted that the deltoid ligament would allow up to 3 mm of lateral talar shift in the absence of the lateral malleolus. Close (4) resected all the lateral ligaments and noted that only a 2-mm widening of the mortise until the deep deltoid ligament was sectioned; then the diastasis almost doubled. In our cadaver evaluations without injuring the deltoid ligament and doing a complete syndesmotic ligament resectioning, 2.4 mm was the average widening; with additional sectioning of the deltoid, this space doubled (8). Rasmussen et al. (14) felt that complete sectioning of the tibiofibular ligaments resulted in only minor abnormalities of motion; however, this was greatly increased by cutting the entire deltoid ligament.

The significance of a lateral talar shift has been felt to increase the peak pressures and decrease the contact areas. In the classical work by Ramsey and Hamilton (15), the tibiotalar contact area was reduced by 42% with 1 mm of lateral talar displacement, even though they rigidly fixed the fibula. Michelson's group (2) showed that normal cadavers with axial load had lateral displacement of up to 2 mm.

In our biomechanical laboratory, we used a transducer to measure the spread or diastasis of the syndesmosis and found that with complete rupture of the syndesmotic ligament there was an average distal tibiofibular diastasis of 0.24 mm. No statistical change was seen in the tibiotalar contact area or peak pressure with the deltoid intact. With sectioning of the deltoid in addition to complete syndesmotic disruption, the distal tibiofibular interval widened to an average of 0.73 mm, which was associated with a 39% decrease in the tibiotalar contact area and an average

42% increase in peak pressures (8). Our study also showed that with complete syndesmotic rupture, the normal deltoid ligament strain increased by 10% from baseline, suggesting that the stable articular configuration is held in place by the deltoid ligament (8). This may indicate that the deltoid should be protected from increased stress until the syndesmosis and interosseous membrane heal. Our study also demonstrated that with minimal radiographic changes there can be significant alterations in tibiotalar joint dynamics (8).

In our opinion, the clinical implications of the literature data and our cadaver studies are that the syndesmotic complex does not need to be stabilized if there are good lateral and medial fixations of fractures. However, if the deltoid ligament is torn or there is very poor medial fixation stability, then appropriate stabilization of the syndesmosis is warranted. It is also noted that with a completely torn syndesmosis there is increased stress on the deltoid and one would not want to have deltoid stretching during the healing phase with an unstable syndesmosis. Therefore, early mobilization without protection or syndesmotic stabilization is not indicated.

Our indication for syndesmotic fixation is somewhat different from that of Boden (16), who felt that syndesmotic stabilization would not be indicated unless the proximal extent of the type C Danis–Weber fracture was greater than 4.5 cm. We feel that this is rather arbitrary and will not allow protection of the intact deltoid ligament from abnormal stresses. A stress test should be done under fluoroscopy after initial fixation to determine syndesmotic stability in Danis–Weber B and C injuries. Unfortunately, it takes a long time for degenerative changes to occur with inappropriate syndesmotic fixation. Most of the outcome studies available to us are short term in nature.

From our further laboratory work, we felt that the utilization of a single 4.5-mm fully threaded screw with no lag technique and three-cortex fixation were appropriate. The fixation was secure if it was anywhere between 2 and 4 cm from the ankle joint. Stabilization should be done with the ankle in dorsiflexion to allow the widened part of the talus to be in the mortise. It is our opinion that the syndesmotic screw should be removed between 3 and 4 months after its insertion. Needleman's group (11) felt that syndesmotic fixation prevented the normal external rotation of the fibula, which is required for its dynamic participation in ankle mechanics. We also feel that one single screw does not completely immobilize the syndesmosis and still allows some forces to be passed through the ligamentous structures, which aid in strengthening the collagen bonding.

REFERENCES

1. Zwipp H. Severe foot trauma in combination with talar injuries. In: Techerne H, Schatzker J Jr, eds. *Major fractures of the pilon, the talus and the calcaneus.* New York: Springer-Verlag, 1994:123–135.
2. Clarke HJ, Michelson JD, Cox QGK, Jinnah RH. Tibiotalar stability in bimalleolar ankle fractures: a dynamic in vitro contact area study. *Foot Ankle* 1991;11:222–227.
3. Ogilvie-Harris DJ, Reed SC. Disruption of ankle syndesmosis: diagnosis and treatment by arthroscopic surgery. *Arthroscopy* 1994;10:561–568.
4. Close JR. Some application of the functional anatomy of the ankle joint. *J Bone Joint Surg [Am]* 1956;38:761–781.
5. Vukicevic S, Stern-Padovan R, Vukicevic D, Ileros P. Holographic investigations of the human tibiofibular interosseous membrane. *Clin Orthop* 1980;151:210–214.
6. Adelaar RS. Fractures of talus. *AAOS Instructional Course Lectures* 1990;34:147–156.
7. Earll M, Wayne J, Adelaar RS, et al. Contribution of the deltoid ligament to the joint contact characteristics in the ankle. *Foot Ankle Int* 1996;17:317–324.
8. Burns WC II, Prakash K, Adelaar R, Beaudoin A, Kraus W. Tibiotalar joint dynamics: indication for the syndesmotic screw—a cadaver study. *Foot Ankle* 1993;14:153–158.
9. Joy G, Patzakis MJ, Harvey JP Jr. Precise evaluation of the reduction of severe ankle fractures. Technique and correlation with end results. *J Bone Joint Surg [Am]* 1974;56:979–993.
10. Harper MC, Keller TS. A radiographic evaluation of the tibiofibular syndesmosis. *Foot Ankle* 1989;10:156–160.
11. Stiehl JB, Needleman RR, Skrade DA. The biomechanical effect of the syndesmotic screw on ankle motion. *AO/ASIF Dialogue* 1989;2:1–3.
12. Yablon IG, Heller FG, Shouse L. The key role of the lateral malleolus in displaced fractures of the ankle. *J Bone Joint Surg [Am]* 1977;59:169–173.

13. Harper MD. The deltoid ligament. An evaluation of need for surgical repair. *Clin Orthop* 1988;226: 156–168.
14. Rasmussen O, et al. Distal tibio-fibular ligament analysis of function. *ACTA Orthop Scand* 1982;53: 681–686.
15. Ramsey PL, Hamilton W. Changes in tibiotalar area of contact caused by lateral shift. *J Bone Joint Surg [Am]* 1976;58:356–357.
16. Boden SD, Pabropaulos PA, McCowin P, Lestini WF, Hurwitz S. Mechanical considerations for the syndesmotic screw. *J Bone Joint Surg [Am]* 1989;71:1548–1555.

Complex Foot and Ankle Trauma,
edited by Robert S. Adelaar,
Lippincott–Raven Publishers, Philadelphia © 1999.

2

Complex Ankle Fracture Dislocations with Syndesmotic Diastasis

James B. Stiehl

Complex fracture dislocations of the ankle joint with diastasis have been recognized since the early nineteenth century (1a–c). Many authors have recognized injuries with syndesmotic disruption as the most severe type of ankle fracture not involving the articular surface of the distal tibia or talus (1d,2). Treatment results have improved in recent years with the application of internal fixation, as advocated by the Swiss AO Group (3–6).

The term *diastasis* comes from the Greek word meaning ''to separate,'' implying gross separation of the tibia from the fibula. From the classification of Ashhurst and Bromer and later Lauge-Hansen, this group would include pronation–external rotation type IV, pronation–abduction, mainsonneuve, and certain supination–external rotation type IV fractures (7,8). More recently, Weber of the AO group described any fracture of the fibula above the distal joint line as type C, which would include all diastasis injuries (Fig. 1) (9).

Although several authors have described the ''mixed oblique'' distal fibula fracture as occurring only at the level of the joint line, Colton (3) and Pankovich (10) have suggested that the supination–external rotation type IV injury may occur significantly above the joint line and involve all structures of the syndesmosis.

J. B. Stiehl: Department of Orthopaedics, Medical College of Wisconsin, Milwaukee, Wisconsin 53226; Department of Orthopaedics, Columbia Hospital, Milwaukee, Wisconsin 53211.

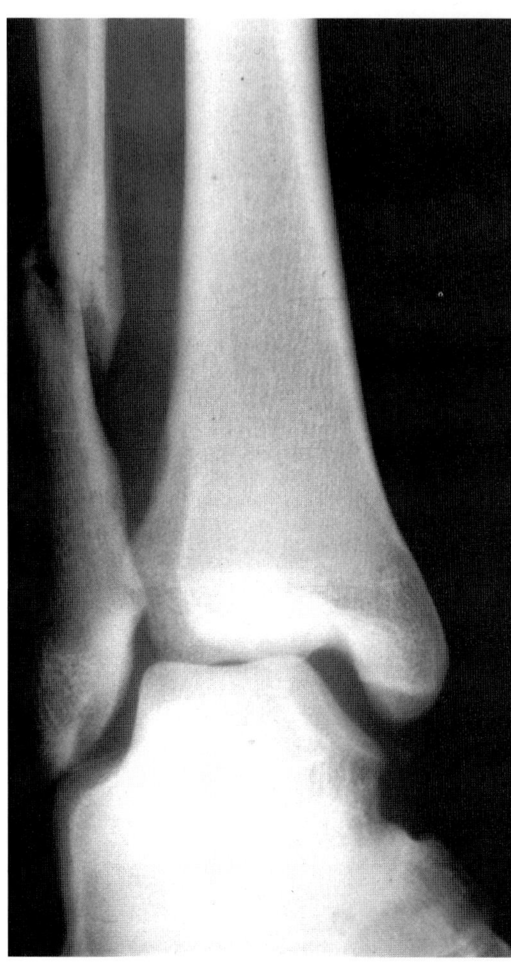

Figure 1. Radiograph of typical diastasis injury with high fibula fracture, syndesmotic disruption, and medial deltoid ligament disruption with significant talar shift.

ANATOMY OF THE SYNDESMOSIS

The ligaments of the syndesmosis form a complex articulation that maintains the fibula closely approximated in the fibular notch. From the coronal plane, this articulation is posterior and lateral, such that the axis of the tibia and fibular notch are directed anteriorly about 30 degrees (11). The anterior tubercle is more prominent than the posterior tubercle and provides an easier landmark for reduction.

The fibula is held in the joint by four ligaments (Fig. 1), as follows. The tibiofibular interosseous ligament is a massive ligament that spans the tibia to the fibula by oblique fibers that run steeply in a distal lateral direction. In the distal segment, the fibers are nearly transverse, and a few fibers run in the proximal lateral direction toward the tibia (Fig. 2A). The anterior–inferior tibiafibular ligament arises from the anterior tubercle and passes obliquely distally and laterally to the anterior lateral malleolus (Fig. 2B). The posterior–inferior tibiofibular ligament arises from a broad origin on the posterior tubercle of the tibia and passes obliquely distally and laterally to the posterior–lateral malleolus (Fig. 2C). The transverse tibiofibular ligament is separate from the posterior–inferior ligament and passes from the posterior tibial margin to the osteochondral junction on the posterior and medial margins of the distal fibula (Fig. 2D) (12).

The function of the syndesmosis is to allow for normal articulation of the ankle joint by determining the precise relationship of the distal tibia and fibula. From the work of Inman (13) and Close (14), we know that the talus normally articulates within the ankle mortise throughout the range of motion. Intermalleolar distance increases approxi-

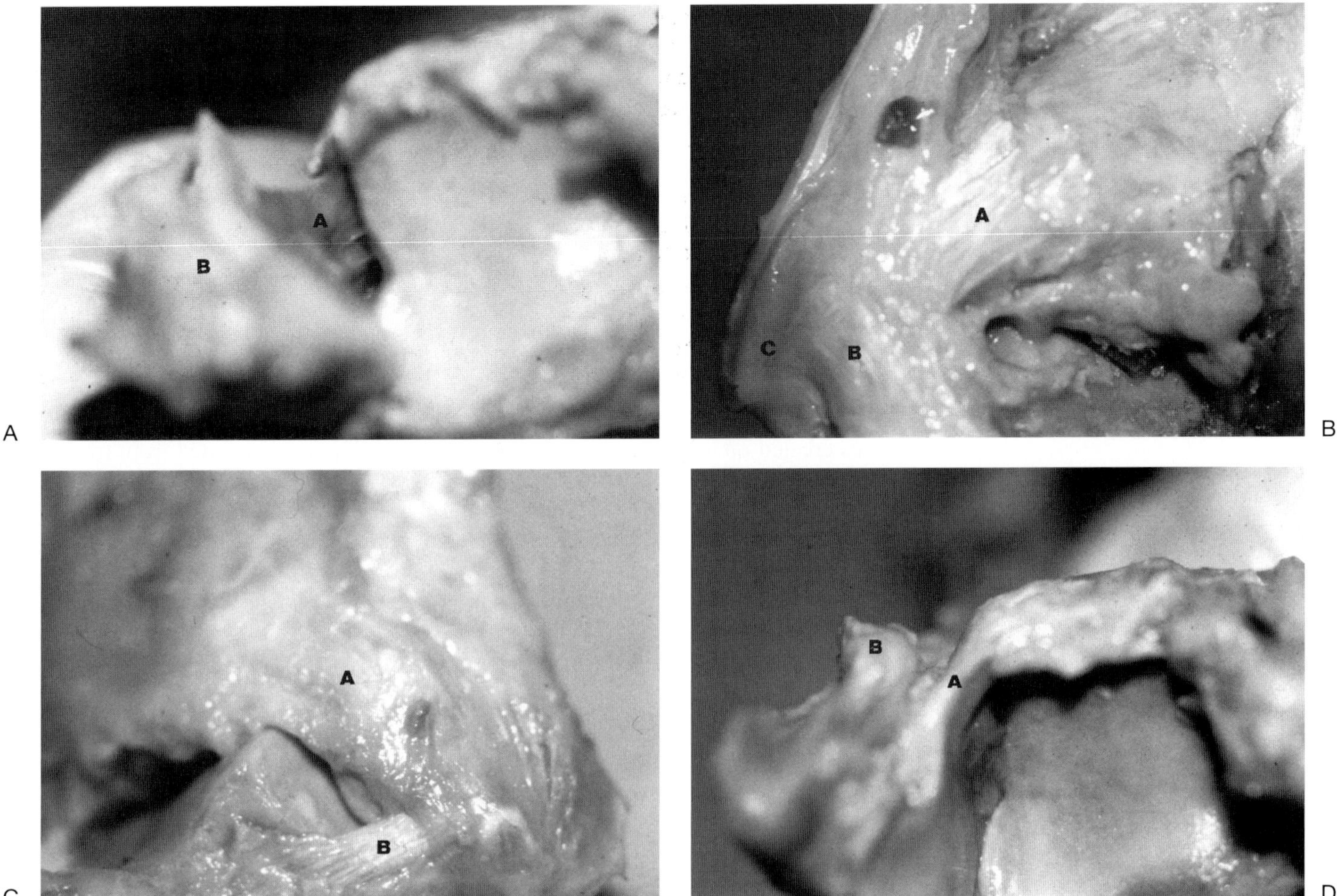

Figure 2. **A:** Tibiofibular interosseous ligament and membrane (*A,* interosseous ligament; *B,* distal fibula); **B:** Anterior–inferior tibiofibular ligament (*A,* anterior–inferior tibiofibular ligament; *B,* anterior talofibular ligament); **C:** Posterior–inferior tibiofibular ligament (*A,* posterior–inferior tibiofibular ligament; *B,* posterior talofibular ligament; *C,* fibular peroneal tendon groove); **D:** Transverse tibiofibular ligament (*A,* transverse; *B,* cut posterior–inferior).

mately 1.5 mm from plantar flexion to dorsiflexion. Also, the fibula demonstrates motion in virtually all planes [including mediolateral, anteroposterior (AP), and proximal–distal] and in rotation. Close estimated this rotation to be 5 to 6 degrees.

With use of cineradiography, Weinert and colleagues (15) demonstrated that the fibula moves distally on heel strike from the pull of the peroneals. This would seem logical, as the mortise then deepens to provide the greatest stability at a moment of greatest loading or impact.

Studies have been made regarding the individual function of ligaments of the syndesmosis. Close sectioned all the ligaments of the syndesmosis and found minimal widening (2 mm) of the mortise. However, when the deep horizontal section of the deltoid ligament was cut, this diastasis increased dramatically to 3.7 mm. Close found that the deltoid ligament stretches only about 2 mm at its greatest dimension. Thus, for gross diastasis of the ankle to occur, the deltoid ligament or medial malleolus must be disrupted (14,16).

The effect of the syndesmosis screw on the normal ankle function has been investigated. Olerud (17) found that dorsiflexion was limited by 0.1 for every degree of plantar flexion when the syndesmosis screw was inserted and suggested that these screws be set with the ankle in maximal dorsiflexion. This potential anatomic constraint was felt to be negligible as an explanation for potential ankle stiffness. We investigated the effect of the syndesmosis screw on other parameters, including talar tilt, AP drawer, and rotation, and found that external rotation was significantly limited in the loaded specimen (18). Theoretically, the screw should be removed prior to resumption of normal weight bearing to allow for physiologic movement of the fibula. Clinical opinions differ widely on this subject.

The author's clinical experience with the use of syndesmosis screw is comparable to that reported in the literature, which suggests that up to 50% of patients can have problems of discomfort, synostosis, and screw breakage with syndesmosis screws that are left in place (19,20). The AO group has recommended *elastic fixation,* inserting the screw through only three cortexes of the fibula and lateral tibia. For the reasons outlined above and from clinical experience, this technique would seem nonphysiologic and destined to create clinical problems in a certain number of patients (12).

With regard to specific mechanisms of injury, we studied in the laboratory various fractures created on anatomic specimens with appropriate loads created from trial and error. Interestingly, a minimum of three times body weight was needed to create a fracture as opposed to a ligament avulsion. Osteoporosis definitely plays a role: older female specimens have a typical distal fibular fracture, and younger males have diastasis with greater ligamentous injury. The only consistent position noted was ankle flexion as opposed to supination, pronation, or version, as suggested by earlier classifications (21).

CLINICAL MANAGEMENT

In addition to pain, swelling, and the inability to bear weight, certain objective findings are apparent on clinical evaluation. Tenderness may be present along the anterolateral lower leg to the level of a high fibular fracture. Clinical instability can be assessed using the Cotton test. This test, described by Cotton in 1910 (22), is done by stabilizing the distal lower leg with one hand while grasping each side of the foot at the talus with the thumb and forefinger of the other hand (Fig. 3). By applying mediolateral force, one can assess crepitus and instability.

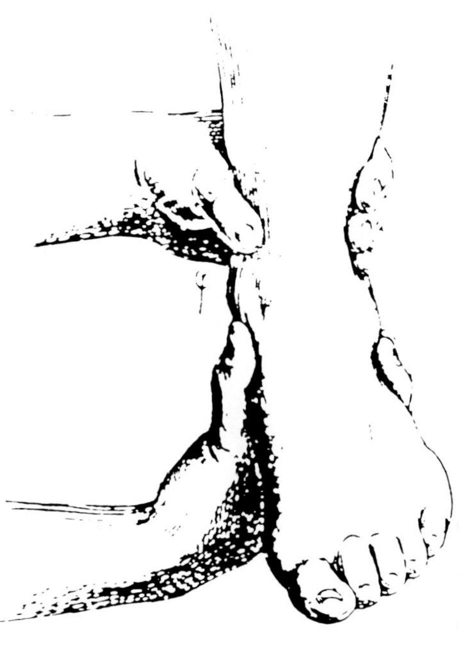

Figure 3. Cotton test for clinical ankle instability assesses mediolateral motion in the sagittal plane (positive greater than 3 to 5 mm).

At surgery, and postoperatively, the Cotton test is quite helpful in determining the function of the syndesmosis. The ankle in neutral flexion should be stable, and any degree of motion in the mediolateral plane is considered to represent possible diastasis. Instability of less than 3 to 4 mm can be treated nonoperatively, but greater amounts imply damage to both the fibula and syndesmosis and the medial structures. Unstable ankle fractures are best treated with internal fixation.

RADIOGRAPHIC CONSIDERATIONS

For preoperative planning and postoperative assessment, normal radiologic criteria are essential (23,24). The following are derived from a review of the literature:

1. Talocrural angle. This angle is the superior medial angle of a line perpendicular to the distal tibial articular surface and a line joining the tips of both malleoli on the mortise view (Figs. 4 and 5). The adult talocrural angle is 83 ± 4 degrees and normally is less than 2 degrees different from the opposite side. Any difference over 5 degrees is abnormal (25).

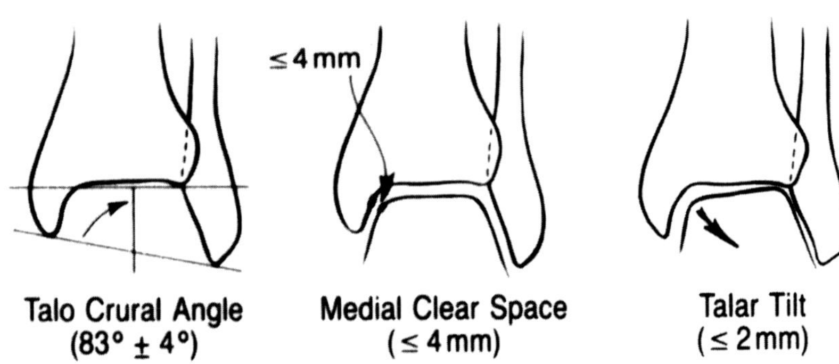

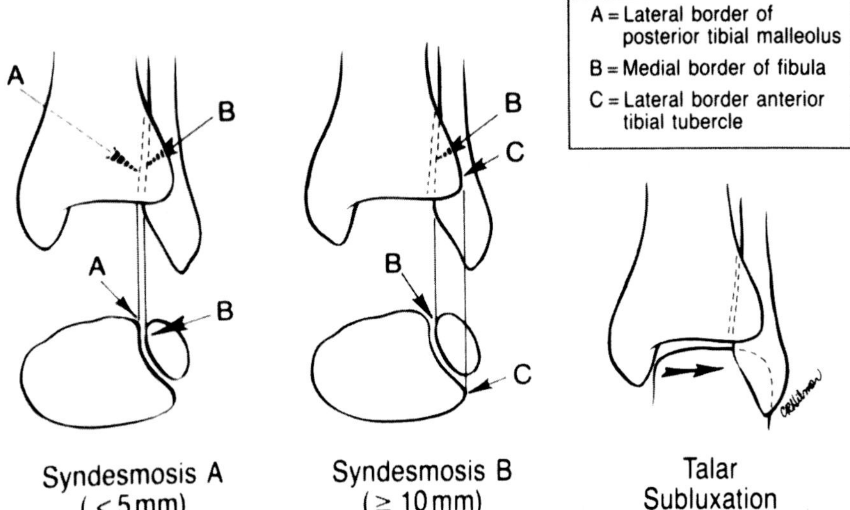

Figure 4. Syndesmotic radiographic criteria. See text for details.

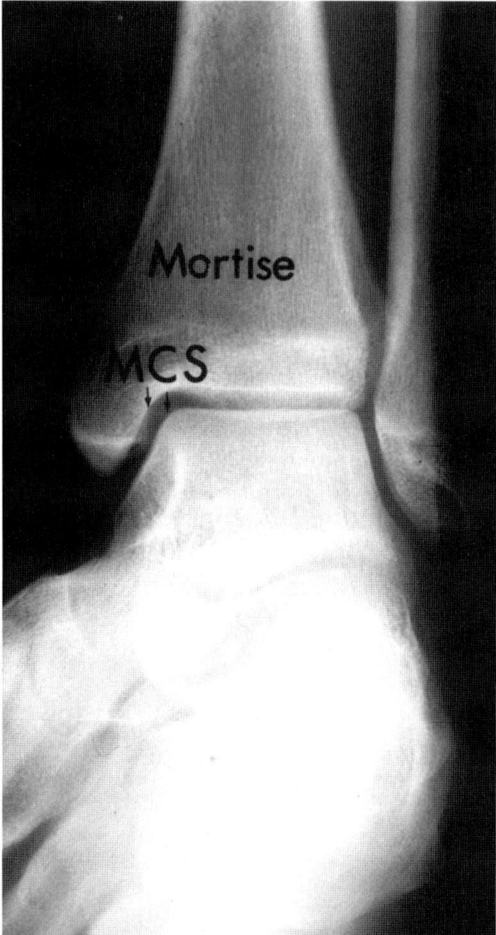

Figure 5. Mortise view assesses medial clear space (*MCS*) and talar tilt.

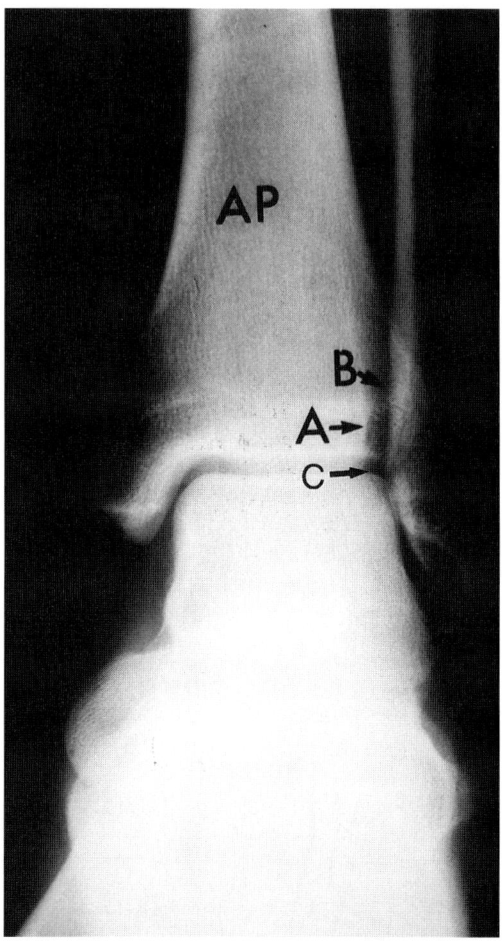

Figure 6. Anterior–posterior (*AP*) view assesses syndesmosis A (*A* to *B,* less than 5 mm), syndesmosis B (*B* to *C,* more than 10 mm), and talar subluxation.

2. Medial clear space. This is the distance from the lateral border of the medial malleolus to the medial border of the talus at the level of the talar dome on the mortise radiograph (Figs. 4 and 5). A space greater than 4 mm is abnormal (26).
3. Talar tilt. This represents any differences in the width of the joint spaces proximal to the medial and lateral talar ridges on the mortise radiograph (Figs. 4 and 5). A difference of 2 mm is considered the upper limit of normal.
4. Syndesmosis A. This measures the tibiofibular clear space from the lateral border of the posterior tibial malleolus (point A) to the medial border of the fibula (point B) on the AP radiograph (Figs. 4 and 6). This is normally less than 5 mm and represents syndesmosis disruption if abnormal (5).
5. Syndesmosis B. This measures the tibiofibular overlap from the medial border of the fibula (point B) to the lateral border of the anterior tibial prominence (point C) on the AP radiograph (Figs. 4 and 6). This is abnormal if it is less than 10 mm.
6. Talar subluxation. This is a subjective asssessment of congruity of the tibial articular surface and talar dome on the anterior radiograph (Figs. 4 and 6). This is abnormal if any incongruity exists. Boden (27) has created criteria for treatment of the diastasis and recommends a syndesmosis screw if the proximal fibula fracture is 3 to 4.5 cm above the joint line. Fractures below 3 cm above the joint line and fractures in which the medial malleolus with attached deep deltoid can be rigidly fixed do not need

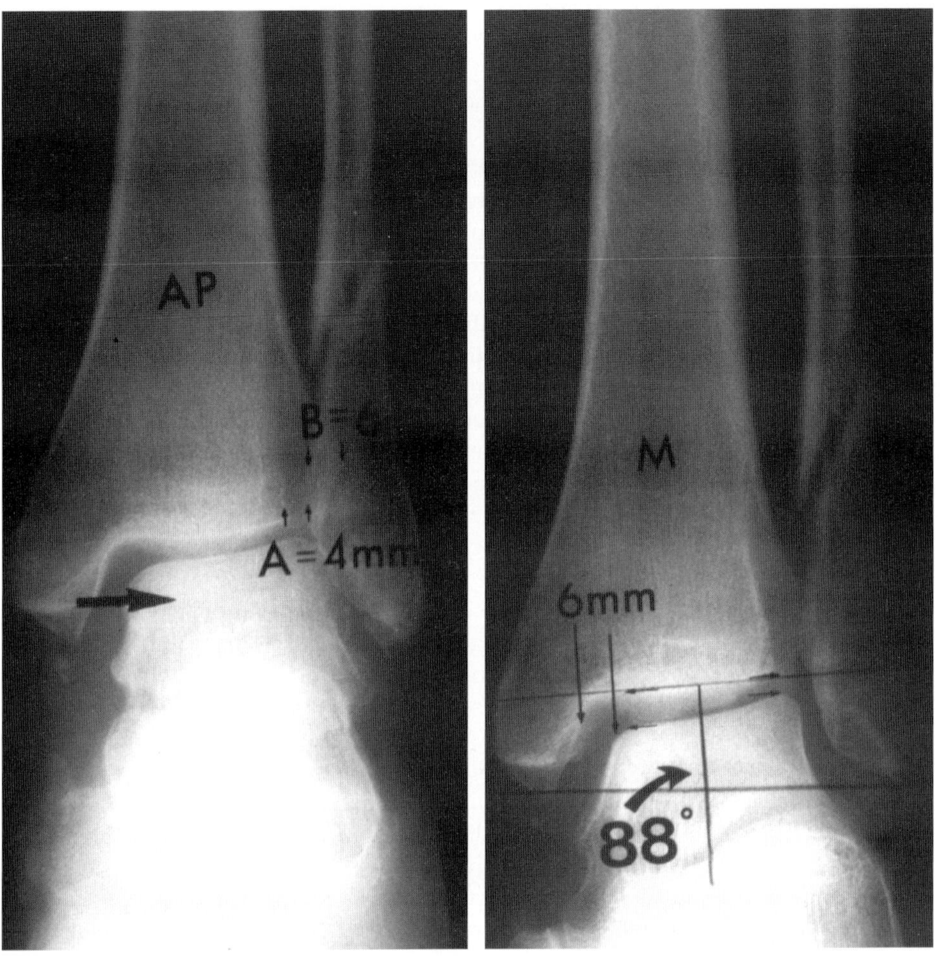

Figure 7. A: Mortise view 1 year after a displaced pronation external rotation IV fracture demonstrates abnormal medial clear space, talocrural angle, and talar tilt. This patient had severe symptoms. **B:** Anterior–posterior view at 1 year demonstrates abnormal syndesmosis B and talar subluxation.

screws. Some caution should be applied if a posterior malleolar fracture is present because of the strong ligaments that may be functionally lost, hence the need for snydesmosis screw (Fig. 7).

OPERATIVE TREATMENT

Because of the severity and instability of these injuries, swelling is marked. Early operative reduction within 12 hours is mandatory to avoid wound healing problems from compromised soft tissues. The most dangerous time is after 3 or 4 days, when fracture blisters and contused skin increase the risk of infection. In these instances, it is best to perform an adequate closed reduction and to wait 2 to 3 weeks. One must keep in mind that infection of the ankle joint can result in fusion or ultimately amputation.

For satisfactory stability of the ankle joint, open reduction and internal fixation require repair of all structures needed to stabilize the ankle joint in the anatomical condition. The medial malleolus, if fractured, is usually initially reached through a separate medial incision. If it is intact and the deep deltoid has been completely disrupted, no medial repair is needed or for that matter possible (28). The posterior malleolus may not need repair if less than 25% to 30% of the articular surface is involved (29).

However, posterior malleolar repair may be needed to stabilize certain cases; the fibula tends to sublux posteriorly if the posterior malleolus is not fixed. In cases with significant diastasis and a high fibula fracture, posterior malleolar fixation is usually needed (11).

To restore the normal mortise, the fibula must be held out to its length and fixed with a one-third lateral semitubular plate (Fig. 8). A typical fracture can be stabilized with a five- or six-hole plate; it is very important to contour the plate accurately to the normal bend of the distal fibula. This should be done with a lateral bend and with internal rotation distally to match the lateral malleolus. If no bend is placed, a painful ankle can result from the straightened distal fibula. The posterior antiglide plate may be useful in certain spiral oblique fractures (30). Lag screws can be used to reduce oblique fractures anatomically prior to plate application. Comminution can be spanned by a plate, and the appropriate length can usually be determined by assembling major fragments (31). Nonunion is uncommon in the distal fibula, and bone graft can fill small defects. Fractures of the fibula located in a more proximal location should be plated if any shortening or displacement exists. Attempts to pull the distal fibula out to proper length are unrealistic given the degree of tension of soft tissues in the lower leg.

If total syndesmosis disruption has occurred and the posterior tubercle of the distal tibia is fractured, the fibula drifts posteriorly and is nearly impossible to hold reduced by closed methods. A transverse position or ''syndesmotic'' screw is needed to hold the fibula reduced; before the screw is inserted, all other bony structures must be stabilized and the joint reduced. The posterior tubercle and malleolar fragment should be fixed if it is large enough to have articular cartilage present (11). Important weight-bearing surfaces may be gained, and stability is enhanced as the posterior and transverse tibiofibular ligaments are attached to this fragment. The posterior malleolus is best fixed directly through a posterolateral approach.

Before the syndesmosis screw is inserted, the Cotton sign is assessed; usually it will be 5 mm or more. This measure must revert to zero after screw placement. Another sign is widening of the anterior tibiofibular gap of at least 5 mm, if a bone hook is

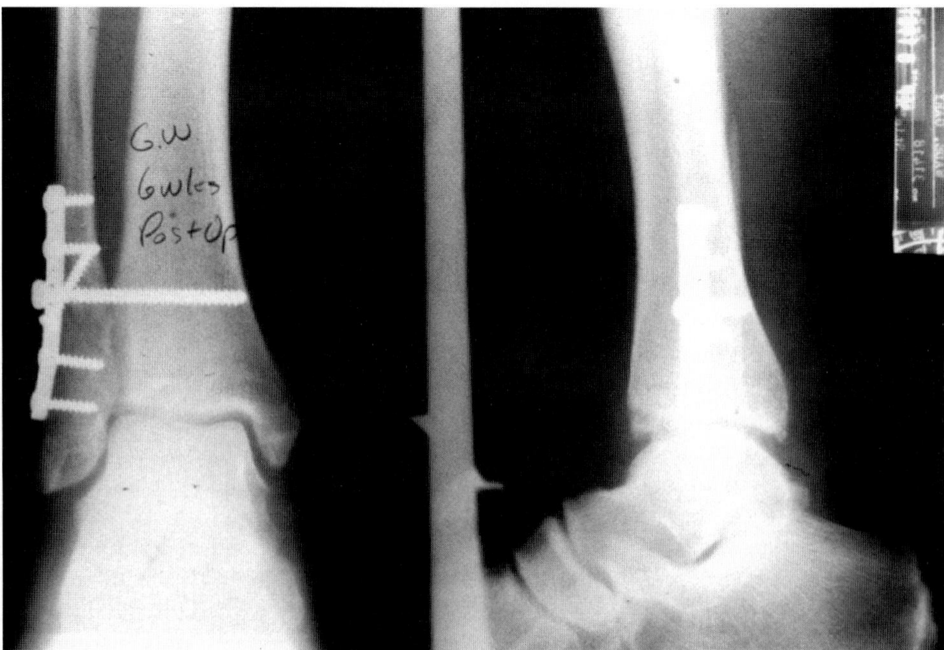

Figure 8. Clinical example at 6 weeks after operation demonstrates fibular plate fixation and anatomic restoration of the mortise.

used to apply external rotation force to the distal fibula (32). The screw is usually inserted 2 cm above the joint and may be placed through the plate. It must be directed anteriorly about 30 degrees from the coronal plane of the lower leg to center the screw (11). Otherwise, the screw may deflect the posterior surface of the tibia. Reduction of the tibiofibular joint is done by reversing the mechanism of injury with internal rotation and firm thumb pressure, holding the fibula firmly in a slight anterior direction against the anterior tubercle of the distal tibia. The cortexes of the fibula and tibia are drilled carefully and taped while reduction is held. A 4.5-mm AO screw or 3.5-mm cortical screw through four cortexes is recommended. Ordinarily, one syndesmosis screw is adequate and can be placed through a hole in the semitubular plate. If there is a proximal undisplaced fibular fracture, then two syndesmosis screws may be desirable. The three-cortex elastic fixation described by the AO group is suspect and can lead to screw failure and painful screw micromotion when screws are left in place indefinitely (20).

POSTOPERATIVE MANAGEMENT

There is no clear literature consensus on postoperative management for ankle fractures. To allow early syndesmosis and fracture healing, the patient should not bear weight for 6 weeks unless external cast immobilization is applied (33,34). Several studies have shown that osteopenia is present in the ankle joint regardless of initial early full weight bearing. The author prefers early active range of motion, which is started at 5 to 7 days after wound healing is ensured (35). The patient may be safely protected in a short leg orthosis and usually remains non-weight bearing. For the reasons outlined above, all syndesmosis screws should be removed at 6 to 8 weeks to allow for return of normal fibular motion. Following screw removal, full weight bearing can be initiated in the short leg orthosis and should be protected for at least another 4 to 6 weeks. At final release to normal activity, there should be no tenderness about the ankle, and the Cotton sign or stress x-ray film should be physiologic. Stretching, strengthening exercises, and physical therapy are then recommended until normal function is achieved. Plate removal may be considered in younger patients at 12 to 18 months after injury. The above regimen is the author's personal preference, but recent controlled studies have shown no difference in late results after early protected weight bearing, non-weight bearing, or active range of motion (20).

LATE RESULTS

Several clinical studies have found the best results in younger male patients under the age of 40; women and older patients tended to have poorer results (2,3). In terms of specific treatment, anatomic reduction retained throughout treatment has been shown to provide the best results regardless of the severity of fracture type according to earlier classifications. The author studied a group of pronation–external rotation injuries with late follow-up of 70 months, finding the best results in cases in which anatomic final result was obtained. Compared with a historical control (only medial malleolar fixation with cast immobilization used for diastasis injuries), a statistically superior result was obtained with anatomic repair (20).

Clinical evaluation using the Cotton test and radiographic review is important in the late evaluation of these injuries. Normally, there is absolute stability with the Cotton test in the normal ankle. Significant slop or looseness can indicate a wide mortise, which usually results from a shortened fibula with a poorly reduced distal tibiofibular joint. The hallmark clinical presentation is a painful joint with tenderness and swelling. Salvage may done in these cases by correcting the malunion, but results are less predictable. Early osteoarthritis and the need for fusion is seen when an anatomic result has not been obtained.

REFERENCES

1a. Dupuytren G. *Lecons orales de clinique chirurgicale,* Ed. 2, Vol. 1. Paris: Germer–Bailliere, 1839:378.
1b. Cooper AP. *A treatise on dislocations and on fractures of the joints.* London: AP Cooper, 1823.
1c. Maissonneuve MJG. Pecherches sur la fracture du perone. *Arch Gen Med* 1840;52: 165–187, 433–473.
1d. Brodie IAOD, Denham RA. The treatment of unstable ankle fractures. *J Bone Joint Surg [Br]* 1974;56:256–263.
2. Burwell HN, Charnley AD. The treatment of displaced fractures at the ankle by rigid internal fixation and early joint movement. *J Bone Joint Surg* 1965;47:634–660.
3. Colton CL. Fracture-diastasis of the inferior tibiofibular joint. *J Bone Joint Surg [Br]* 1968;50:830–835.
4. DeSouza J, Gustilo RB, Meyer TJ. Results of operative treatment of displaced external rotation-abduction fractures of the ankle. *J Bone Joint Surg [Am]* 1985;67:1066–1073.
5. Hughes JL, Weber H, Willenegger H, Kuner EH. Evaluation of ankle fractures; nonoperative and operative treatment. *Clin Orthop* 1979;138:111–119.
6. Mast JW, Teipner WA. A reproducible approach to internal faxation of adult ankle fractures: rationale, technique, and early results. *Orthop Clin North Am* 1980;11:661–679.
7. Ashhurst A, Bromer RS. Classification and mechanism of fractures of the leg bones involving the ankle. *Arch Surg* 1922;4:51–129.
8. Lauge-Hansen N. Fractures of the ankle: II. Combined experimental surgical and experimental-roentgenologic investigations. *Arch Surg* 1950;60:957.
9. Heim U, Pfeiffer KM. *Small fragment set manual technique recommended by the A.S.I.F. Group.* New York: Springer-Verlag, 1982.
10. Pankovich A. Fractures of the fibula proximal to the distal tibiofibular syndesmosis. *J Bone Joint Surg [Am]* 1978;60:221–229.
11. Heim U. Malleolar fracturen. *Unfallheilkunde* 1983;86:248–258.
12. Stiehl JB. Complex ankle fracture dislocations with syndesmotic diastasis. *Orthop Rev* 1990;19:499–507.
13. Inman VT. *The joints of the ankle.* Baltimore: Williams & Wilkins, 1976.
14. Stiehl JB. *Inman's joints of the ankle,* 2nd ed. Baltimore: Williams & Wilkins, 1991.
15. Weinert CR, McMaster JH, Ferguson RJ. Dynamic function of the human fibula. *Am J Anat* 1973;138:145–150.
16. Stiehl JB. Ankle fractures with diastasis. *AAOS Instructional Course Lecture* 1990;39:98–112.
17. Olerud C. The effect of syndesmotic screw on the extension capacity of the ankle joint. *Arch Orthop Trauma Surg* 1985;104:299.
18. Needleman RL, Skrade DA, Stiehl JB. The effect of the syndesmotic screw on ankle motion. *Foot Ankle* 1989;10:17–24.
19. Grath GB. Widening of the ankle mortise. *Acta Chir. Scand* 1960;263[Suppl]:7–10.
20. Stiehl JB, Schwartz H. Long term results of pronation-external rotation ankle fracture dislocation treated with anatomical open reduction. *J Orthop Trauma* 1990;4:339–345.
21. Stiehl JB, Skrade DA, Johnson RP. Experimentally produced ankle fractures in autopsy specimens. *Clin Orthop* 1993;285:244–250.
22. Cotton FJ. *Fractures and joint-dislocations.* Philadelphia: WB Saunders, 1910:549.
23. Pettrone FA, Gail M, Pee D, et al. Quantitative criteria for prediction of the results after displaced fractures of the ankle. *J Bone Joint Surg [Am]* 1983;65:667–677.
24. Phillips WA, Schwartz HS, Keller CS, et al. A prospective, randomized study of management of severe ankle fractures. *J Bone Joint Surg [Am]* 1985;67:67–78.
25. Sarkisian JS, Cody SW. Closed treatment of ankle fractures: a new criterion for investigation; a review of 250 cases. *J Trauma* 1976;16:323–326.
26. Joy G, Patzakis MJ, Harvey JP. Precise evaluation of severe ankle fractures, technique and correlation with end results. *J Bone Joint Surg [Am]* 1974;56:979–993.
27. Boden SD, Pabropaulos PA, McCowin P, Lestini WF, Hurwitz S. Mechanical considerations for the syndesmotic screw. *J Bone Joint Surg [Am]* 1989;71:1548–1555.
28. Harper MC. The deltoid ligament. An evaluation for surgical repair. *Clin Orthop* 1988;226:156–168.
29. Harper MC, Hardin G. Posterior malleolar fractures of the ankle associated with external rotation-abduction injuries. *J Bone Joint Surg [Am]* 1988;70:1348–1364.
30. Winkler B, Weber BG, Simpson L. The dorsal antiblide plate in the treatment of Danis-Weber Type-B fractures of the distal fibula. *Clin Orthop* 1990;259:204–209.
31. Limbird RS, Aaron RK. Laterally comminuted fracture-dislocation of the ankle. *J Bone Joint Surg [Am]* 1987;69:881–885.
32. Solari J, Benjamin J, Wilson J, Lee R, Pitt M. Ankle mortise stability in Weber C fractures: indications for syndesmotic fixation. *J Orthop Trauma* 1991;5:190–195.
33. Ahl T, Dalen N, Selvik G. Ankle fractures: a clinical and roentgengraphic stereophotogrammetric study. *Clin Orthop* 1989;245:246–255.
34. Finsen V, Benum P. Osteopenia after ankle fractures. *Clin Orthop* 1989;245:261–268.
35. Finsen V, Saetermo R, Kibsgaard L, Farran K, Engebretsen L, Bolz K, et al. Early postoperative weight-bearing and muscle activity in patients who have a fracture of the ankle. *J Bone Joint Surg [Am]* 1989;71:23–27.

EDITORIAL COMMENTS

Complex on Ankle Fracture Dislocations with Syndesmotic Diastasis

James B. Stiehl

In this chapter Dr. James Stiehl emphasizes that anatomic reduction is critical and has given you several helpful suggestions to obtain it. The maintenance of anatomic reduction of the fibula is critical in contouring the semitubular plate with a lateral bend and slight internal rotation. If the fracture is oblique and greater than 45 degrees or a spiral without much comminution, then a lag screw anatomic reduction should precede plate fixation. The medial complex is usually fixed second and a stable reduction is done to the medial complex; usually a syndesmotic screw is not necessary, except when the proximal fracture of the fibula is more than 4.5 cm or if the stress or Cotton test is positive after fixation. We cannot overemphasize the stress test at the conclusion of the case with the use of image intensifier to determine whether a syndesmotic screw would be necessary. The question of timing of removal of the screw is somewhat controversial, but there is no question that the screw needs to be removed because it prevents external rotation of the fibula and will leave a non-physiologic situation. I would not recommend leaving the screw in to allow it to break. We usually remove a screw at approximately the third or fourth month. The syndesmosis with the interosseous membrane has been damaged, and the collagen tissue takes a long time to reach adequate strength; we know that syndesmotic fixation is not rigid, so tension is allowed through the syndesmosis as long as movement or weight bearing is allowed.

When there is no fracture of the medial side and there is a deltoid injury, then a syndesmotic screw in our laboratory situation has been helpful to protect the deltoid from increased stress. Even when the medial side has been rigidly fixed, we found that there is increased stress in the intact deltoid in our cadaver models. Therefore, I believe that protection of the deltoid is appropriate during the healing period. The use of the syndesmotic screw when the deltoid is ruptured in an unstable fracture will prevent abnormal laxity in the deltoid, which in turn will decrease lateral shift of the center of motion of the ankle and an increase in the contact pressure. The most important part of the deltoid ligament, as far as our studies have shown, has been the superficial tibial calcaneal component, which is primarily from the anterior colliculus. The deep deltoid was not found to be as important, and its main function is to keep the talus from rotating externally.

Dr. Stiehl also mentioned that timing for ankle fractures is important; one should make sure that blisters are not forming and that the skin will wrinkle prior to fixation. We have found that a foot pump with intermittent pressure on the plantar plexus is helpful in addition to a Jones dressing and elevation to decrease swelling. There are many risk factors to be aware of, particularly in the elderly population. The risk factors include age, osteopenia, obesity, diabetes mellitus, vascular disease, neuropathy, and spastic disorders. One's goal should also be to restore the gastroc soleus length by casting or immobilizing the foot in neutral to prevent contractures of this muscle group. Postoperative care is up to the individual, with early motion, non-weight bearing, or weight bearing in a cast giving equal results. Physical therapy is usually not needed except when there are severe soft tissue problems. Even with an anatomic reduction, long-term swelling and arthralgias tend to be the routine rather than the exception.

Robert S. Adelaar, M.D.

Complex Foot and Ankle Trauma,
edited by Robert S. Adelaar,
Lippincott–Raven Publishers, Philadelphia © 1999.

3

Fractures of the Posterior Malleolus

James B. Carr

In 1911, Destot (1) employed the term *posterior malleolus* to describe a fracture involving the posterior tibial margin. Fifteen years later, Trethowan (2) used the term *third malleolus.* These two terms have found common usage in current practice. A fracture of the posterior malleolus frequently accompanies injuries to the lateral and medial malleoli. This relatively common injury was aptly termed *trimalleolar fracture of the ankle* by Henderson and Stuok (3) in 1933. Rarely, a posterior malleolar fracture can occur in isolation. This chapter reviews the relevant anatomy, physiology, and treatment of this common fracture.

GROSS ANATOMY

The posterior tibial margin completes the curvilinear shape of the distal tibial articular surface (Fig. 1). It extends most distally on the fibular side. The transverse tibiofibular ligament inserts on the distal aspect of the posterior malleolus. This ligament, in combination with the transverse talofibular ligament, serves to deepen the ankle mortise posteriorly. Proximally, the posterior tibiofibular ligament inserts on the posterior tubercle of the tibia. This portion of the tibia has been termed *Volkman's triangle* and is analogous to the anterior tubercle of Chaput. Segmental vessels from the posterior tibial artery enter the posterior malleolus via the transverse tibiofibular ligament. The ankle capsule completes the soft tissue attachments on the most distal aspect of the posterior margin.

J. B. Carr: Department of Orthopaedic Surgery, Medical College of Virginia, Richmond, Virginia 23298; Department of Orthopaedic Surgery, MCV Hospitals, Richmond, Virginia 23298.

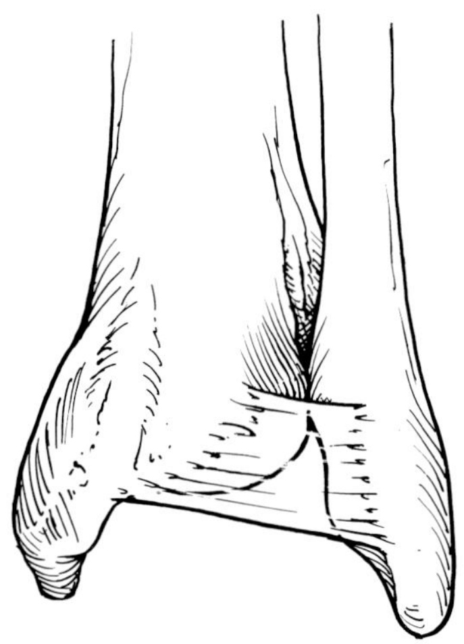

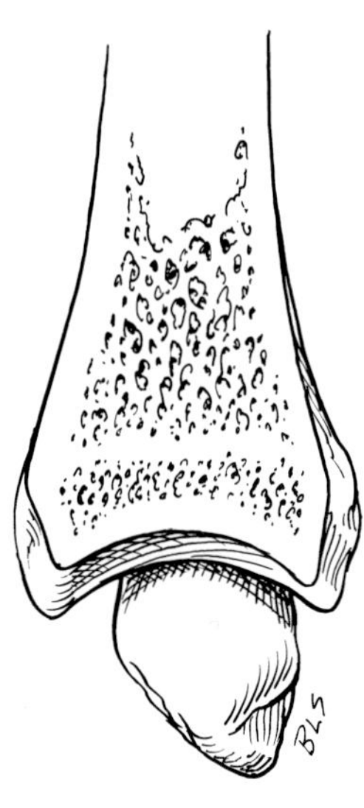

Figure 1. Lateral and posterior views of the distal tibia. Note the posterior ligaments, which deepen the mortise posteriorly.

FUNCTIONAL ANATOMY

The posterior malleolus serves two major functions. The first is transmission of weight-bearing loads through its articular surface. A recent contact pressure film study noted alteration in articular pressures with fractures involving 25% of the posterior malleolus (4). These authors noted a loss of 35% ankle contact area for posterior fragments involving 50% of the distal tibial surface. The second, and more controversial, function is the role of the posterior malleolus in conferring posterior stability to the ankle. Given the shape of the distal tibia, this function makes intuitive sense. This concept is reinforced by the clinical observations of McLaughlin and Ryder (5) and later McDaniel and Wilson (6). These authors noted a high percentage of ankles with residual posterior tibiotalar subluxation in conservatively treated trimalleolar fractures, if a large (greater than 25%) posterior malleolar fragment was present. It is likely that a fibular malunion contributed to the residual talar subluxation in these series.

The role of the osseous posterior malleolar structure in conferring posterior stability to the ankle has recently been challenged by Harper in two studies (7,8). In the first, a clinical study, he demonstrated no advantage for fixation of a large posterior malleolus fragment, as long as the other components of the ankle were reduced and stabilized, and a near anatomic reduction of the posterior malleolus was obtained (7). In a laboratory study, he demonstrated no posterior instability with posterior malleolar fragments comprising up to 40% of the posterior tibial margin (8). He emphasized the importance of the intact collateral malleoli, the syndesmosis, and the posterior talofibular ligament. This latter concept is analogous to anterior ankle stability, in which the anterior talofibular ligament is a well-recognized restraining factor. Somewhat different results have been obtained by Scheidt et al. (9) in a recent cadaver study. Using an experimental model to simulate weight bearing, increased posterior and internal rotation instability were noted with large posterior malleolar fragments.

In summary, it is obvious that large displaced posterior malleolar fragments interfere with the weight-bearing function of the distal tibial articular surface. The issue of posterior stability is not as clear. It is vital to restore the fibular buttress anatomically with its associated ligamentous structures when considering the treatment of large posterior malleolar fractures.

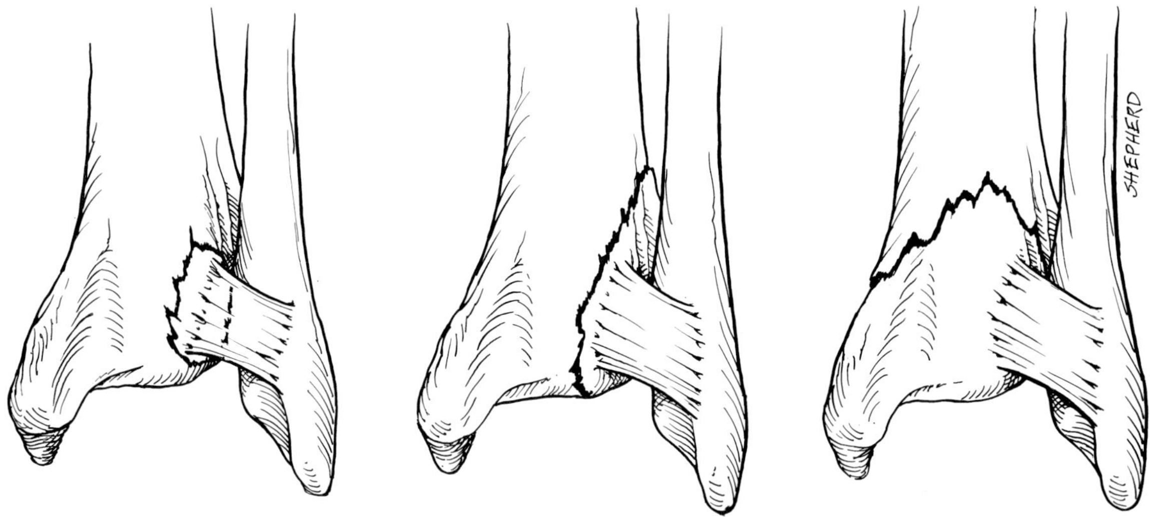

Figure 2. The three types of posterior malleolar fractures. **A:** Extraarticular **B:** Posterolateral **C:** Large fragment extending posteromedially.

PATHOLOGIC ANATOMY AND MECHANISM

The incidence of an isolated posterior malleolar fragment in reported series ranges from 0.8% to 2.5% (10). The mechanism appears to be a direct posterior force, or perhaps a vertical load applied in plantar flexion. Brostrom et al. (11) felt that occult syndesmotic damage accompanied most ''isolated'' posterior malleolar fractures. They emphasized the necessity for a careful search for other injuries in the setting of an apparently isolated posterior malleolar fracture.

Most commonly, a posterior malleolar fracture occurs in conjunction with other malleoli and ligamentous lesions. The typical forces involve abduction, external rotation, and axial loading (7). Thus, the posterior malleolar fracture occurs in the later stages of the Lauge-Hansen classifications, e.g., SE3, PE3.

Regarding the pathology of the posterior malleolus fracture, three major types are encountered (10) (Fig. 2). The first is extraarticular and is analogous to the avulsion of the Chaput tubercle in the anterior distal tibia. The second type is intraarticular and involves the posterolateral corner of the tibia. The third involves the posteromedial tibial margin. This latter fracture may involve a large portion of the tibial plafond. In certain instances, it is nearly a shear fracture of the entire posterior one-half of the distal tibia. Recognition of these latter two types is important if one is considering surgical treatment of this lesion.

RADIOLOGY

The posterior malleolus is visualized on the lateral radiograph of the ankle (12). A double cortical shadow above the plafond can sometimes be visualized on the anterior–posterior view and may give a clue as to the location of the fracture, i.e., lateral or medial. The size of the posterior malleolus is classically described as a percentage of the total curvature of the distal tibia (Fig. 3). This is a clinically useful guideline, but in certain instances, based on the rotation of the x-ray beam, it may underestimate the size of some injuries (13). Computed tomography may be obtained to determine definitively both the size and location of the posterior malleolar fracture (Fig. 4). This is rarely necessary, except in certain complex situations.

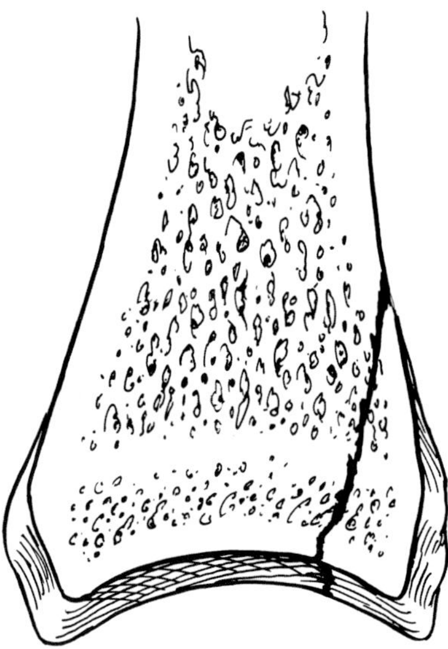

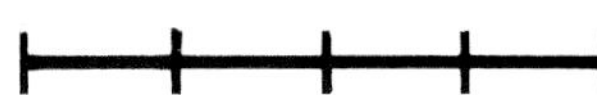

Figure 3. The method of estimating posterior malleolar fracture size on the lateral radiograph. In this case, 25% of the surface is involved.

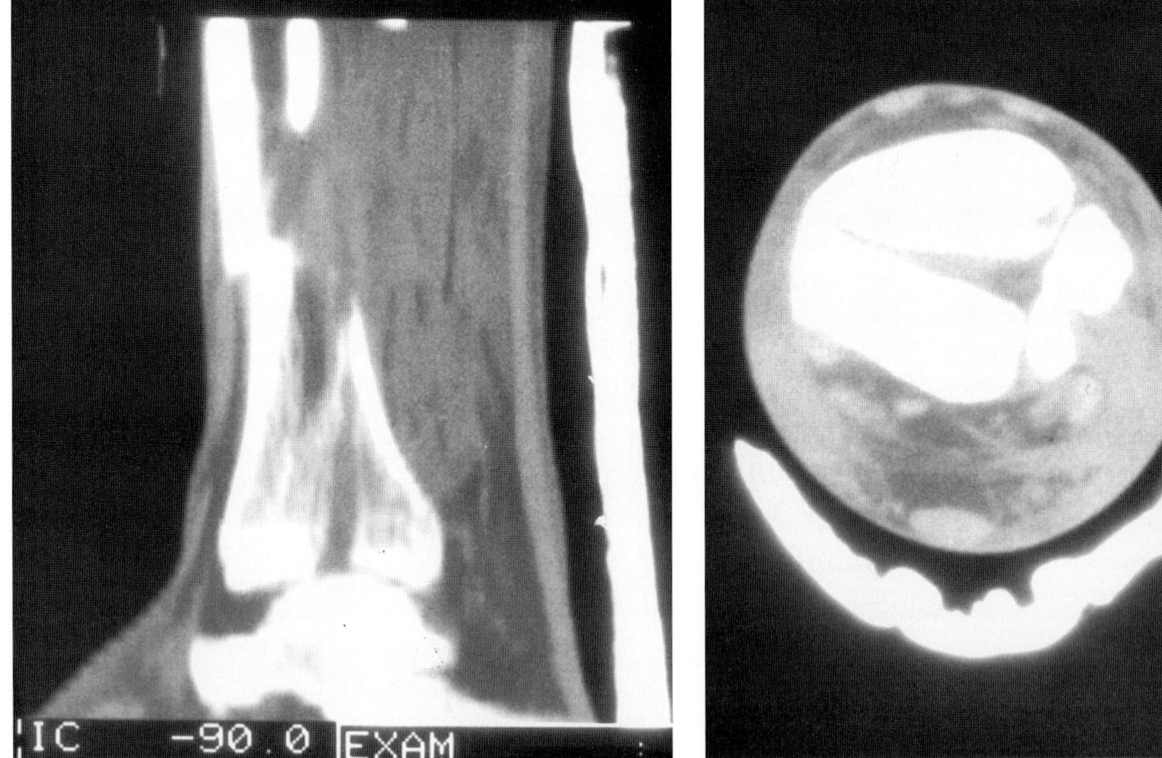

Figure 4. A,B: Computed tomography is the best method of estimating the size of a posterior malleolar fracture.

TREATMENT

Since the posterior malleolus is rarely fractured in an isolated fashion, its treatment must be considered in the context of the overall ankle pathology, as well as the characteristics of the injury at hand. Nonoperative treatment of ankle fractures with a large posterior malleolar fragment (greater than 25%) is not recommended, since many heal with residual posterolateral subluxation (6). The remainder of this section assumes that operative treatment has been selected for the particular injury at hand and focuses specifically on treatment decisions regarding the posterior malleolus.

The size of the posterior malleolar fragment is a useful guideline for treatment. A second guideline involves the reduction obtained by anatomic fixation of the other ankle components. Most authors agree that posterior malleolar fractures comprising less than 15% of the joint surface, or extraarticular fractures, may be ignored. Fractures comprising 20% to 25% represent a gray zone regarding fixation. For fragments comprising 25% or greater of the distal tibial joint surface, accurate reduction is advisable. As previously discussed, the issue of fixation is somewhat controversial. Traditionally, fixation has been recommended.

In my practice, I tend to fix the large posterior malleolar fragments in as anatomic an alignment as possible. If one does not choose to fixate a large fragment, anatomic and stable reduction of the malleoli are required, and the syndesmosis is stabilized as necessary. The posterior drawer must be negative to omit fixation of a large, well-reduced posterior malleolar fracture.

Occasionally one encounters an ankle fracture with a posterior malleolar fragment comprising up to 50% of the weight-bearing surface. Given the important articular function of this fragment, priority must be given to exact reduction and secure fixation (Fig. 5).

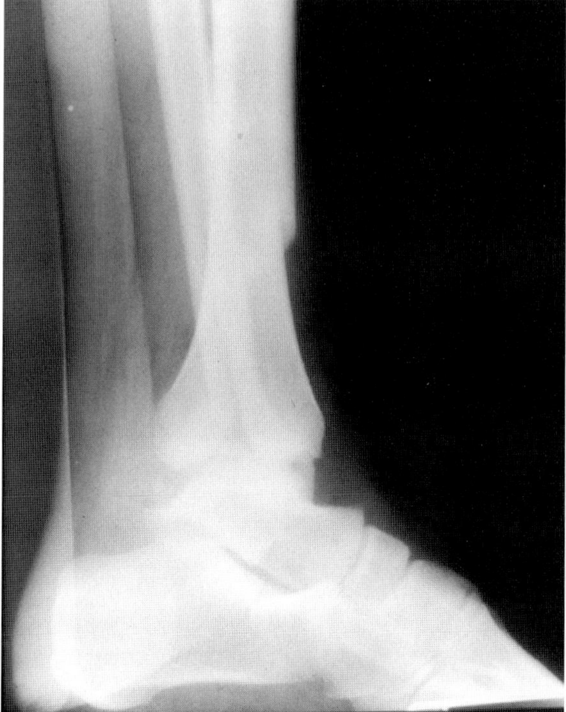
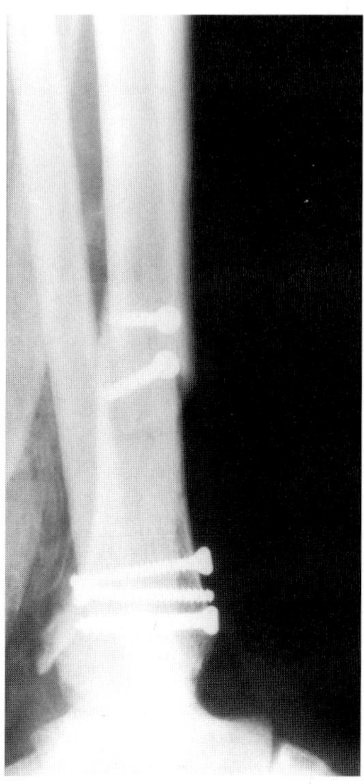
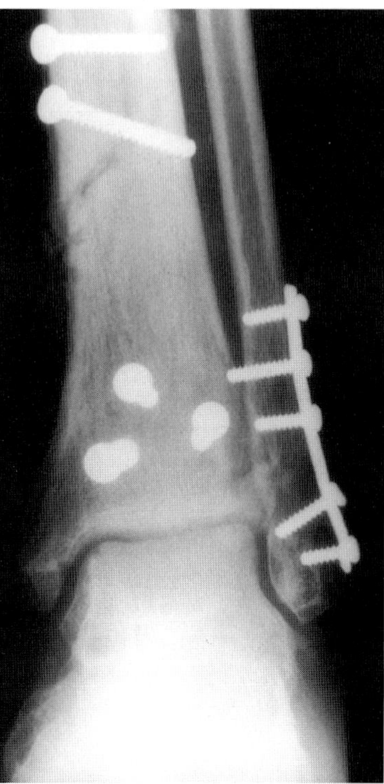

A–C

Figure 5. A large posterior malleolar fracture in association with lateral and medial malleolar fracture. **A:** Preoperative lateral view—the posterior fragment comprises 50% of the joint surface. **B:** Postoperative lateral view. Note the combination of posterior–anterior and anterior–posterior (AP) screws. **C:** Postoperative AP view.

SURGICAL TECHNIQUES

Once fixation of the posterior malleolus is elected, there are numerous choices for surgical approach and fixation. In general, the posterior malleolus is approached after reduction and fixation of the fibula and medial malleolus.

For lesions located in the posterolateral tibia, the posterolateral approach of Henry (14) is recommended. This interval is developed between the peroneal and Achilles tendon, taking care to avoid damage to the sural nerve and to avoid dissection medially in the neurovascular bundle. The flexor hallucis muscle is identified and used as a guide to the fragment (Fig. 6). The patient is positioned in a semilateral decubitus position with a large sandbag under the hip, with flexion of the hip and knee to allow access to the posterolateral corner. Once on the fragment, intraoperative fluoroscopy and extra-articular anatomy alignment is used for assessing the reduction. A ''sloppy lateral'' (i.e., oblique lateral) may be useful for viewing the articular reduction if a fibular plate obscures the straight lateral view (D. Ross, personal communication). One has the choice of an anterior to posteriorly directed screw, or a posterior to anteriorly directed screw. Both are effective, and up to the surgeon's discretion. If an anterior–posterior screw is chosen, the ''glide hole first'' technique with a 3.5-mm cortical screw is recommended (15). With this technique, a 3.5-mm overdrill hole is accurately placed in the tibia from anterior to posterior with the fragment unreduced. This produces a glide hole of proper depth, and one can assess its position within the fracture fragment. The fracture is then reduced and fixated with K-wires. The thread hole is *then drilled* and tapped; the screw is then inserted, usually through the anteromedial wound used for approaching the medial malleolus.

In the posterior to anterior technique, either a cortical lag screw or small-fragment cancellous screw can be used. The screw is inserted following reduction of the fracture

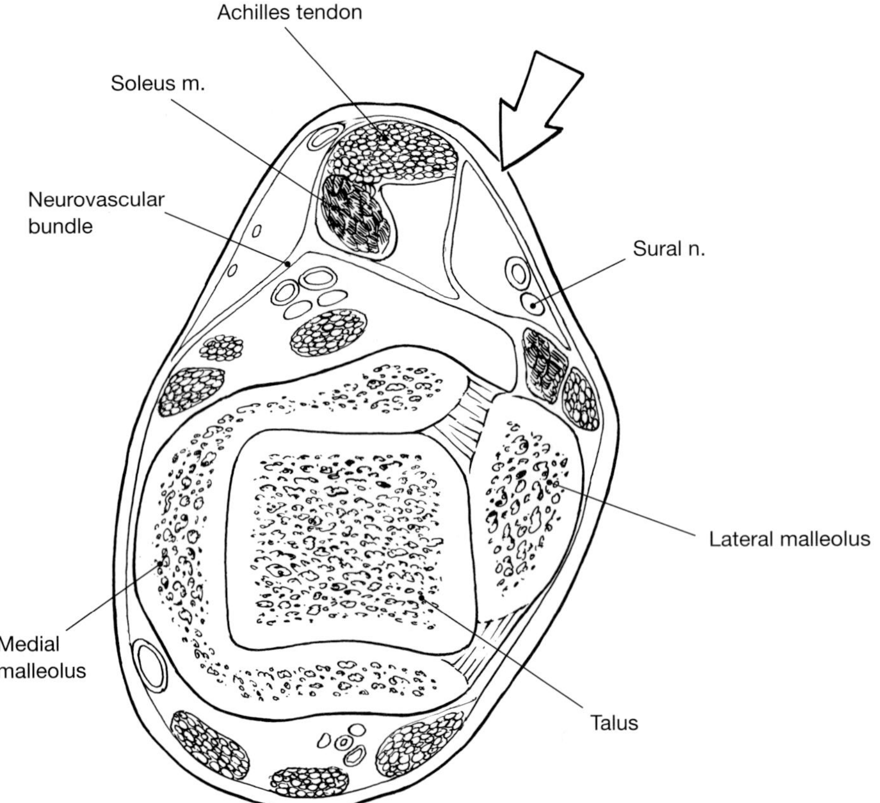

Figure 6. The posterolateral approach of Henry.

and provisional K-wire fixation. A washer may be used to provide a mechanical advantage on the screw head. This screw tends to give excellent fixation since longer length of thread purchase is available (Fig. 7).

A useful intraoperative aid is a large pointed clip reduction forceps (#399.08, Synthes, Paoli, PA). The point of the forceps may be applied through stab incisions, and the clamp is well proportioned for use in the distal tibia (Fig. 8). This can reduce the amount of soft tissue dissection required for manipulation and provide temporary fixation of the posterior malleolus.

The final surgical option for surgical approach and fixation is posteromedial (16). Dr. Shelton (16) reports good experience with this approach. In my practice, it is reserved for the unusual injuries that exit the medial cortex, or are attached to a large portion of the medial malleolus. Although a posterolateral fragment may be visualized with a posteromedial approach, extensive tissue dissection is required. One can then use either screw fixation or, as Dr. Shelton recommends, a small fragment plate.

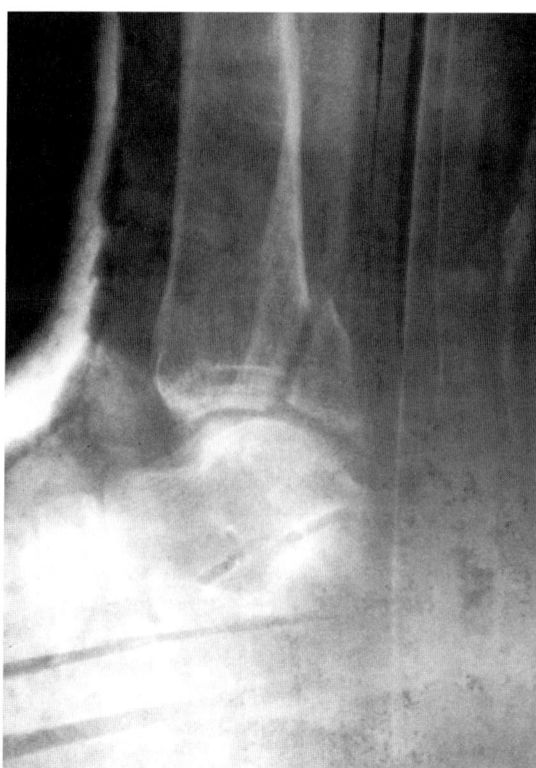
A

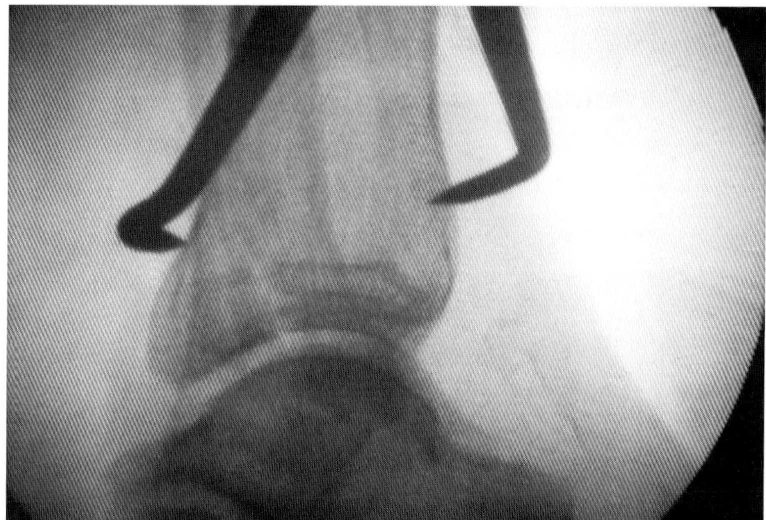
B

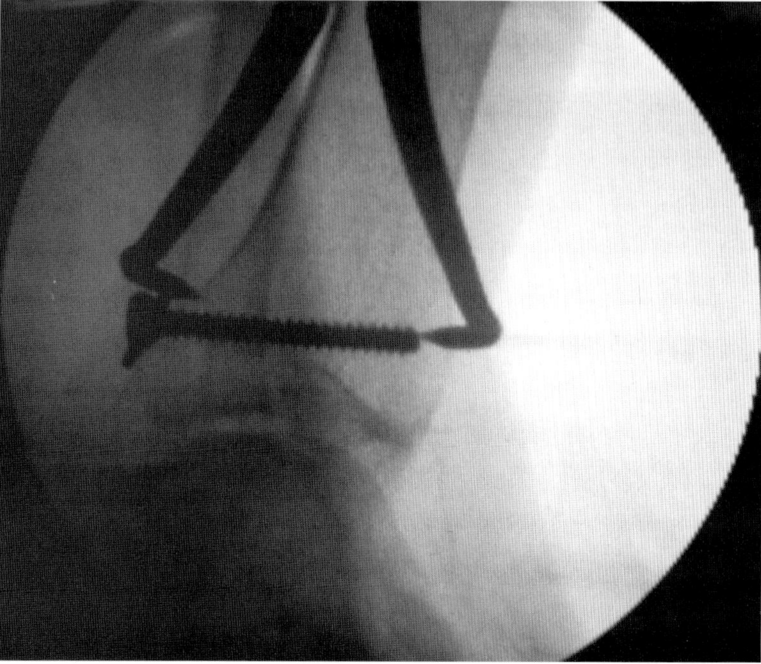
C

Figure 7. The posterior–anterior screw. **A:** Preoperative lateral view demonstrating a posterior malleolar fracture involving 30% of the distal articular surface. **B:** Intraoperative reduction. Note the use of large pointed forceps. A reduction clamp holding the fibula was removed for demonstration purpose. **C:** Postoperative view.

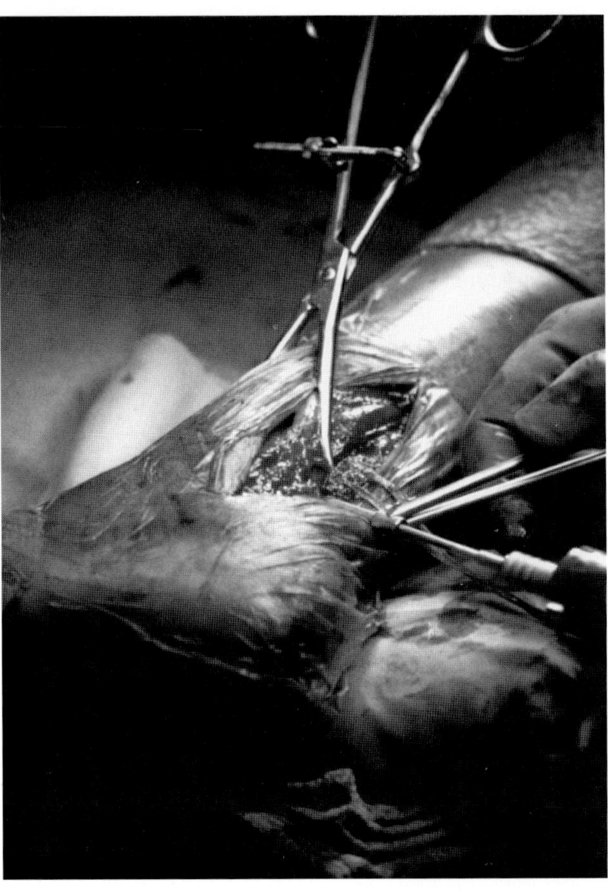

Figure 8. Large Weber reduction forceps (Synthes, Paoli, PA) are well proportioned for use in the distal tibia.

SUMMARY

The posterior malleolus is a frequently fractured structure about the ankle. It functions both in weight bearing and to some degree in conferring posterior stability on the ankle mortise. For large fractures comprising 25% or more of the distal tibial articular surface, a minimum of anatomic reduction and appropriate operative treatment of other malleoli fractures is required. For most situations, I would recommend fixation with these large fragments of screws.

REFERENCES

1. Destot E. Fracture du pilon et de la mortise. In: *Traumatism du pied en rayon X.* Paris: Masson, 1911:109–134.
2. Trethowan WH. The operative treatment of ankle fractures. *Lancet* 1926;1:90–92.
3. Henderson MS, Stuok W. Fractures of the ankle: recent and old. *J Bone Joint Surg* 1933;15:882–888.
4. Macko VW, Matthews LS, Zwirkoski MS, Goldstein SA. The joint—contact area of the ankle. *J Bone Joint Surg* 1991;73:347–351.
5. McLaughlin HL, Ryder CT Jr. Open reduction and internal fixation for fractures of the tibia and ankle. *Surg Clin North Am* 1949;29:1523–1534.
6. McDaniel WJ, Wilson FC. Trimalleolar fractures of the ankle, an end result study. *Clin Orthop* 1977;122:37–45.
7. Harper MC, Hardin G. Posterior malleolar fractures of the ankle associated with external rotation-abduction. *Joint Surg* 1988;70A:1348–1356.
8. Harper MC. Posterior instability of the talus: an anatomic evaluation. *Foot Ankle* 1989;10:36–39.
9. Scheidt KB, Stiehl JB, Skrade DA, Barnhardt T. Posterior malleolar ankle fractures. An in vitro biomechanical analysis of stability in the loaded and unloaded states. *J Orthop Trauma* 1992;6:96–101.
10. Bonin JG. *Injuries to the ankle.* Darien, CT: Hofner, 1970.
11. Brostrom L, Tiljedahl SO, Lindrall N. Isolated fractures of the posterior tibial tubercle. Aetiology and clinical features. *Acta Chir Scand* 1964;128:51–56.
12. Hendeberg T. The roentengenographic examination of the ankle joint in malleolar fractures. *Acta Radiol* 1946;27:23–42.

13. Ferries JS, DeCoster TA, Firoozbaksh KK, Garcia JF, Miller RA. Plain radiographic interpretation in trimalleolar ankle fractures poorly assesses posterior fragment size. *J Orthop Trauma* 1994;8:328.
14. Henry AK. The distal end of the tibia from behind. In: *Extensile exposure applied to limb surgery.* Baltimore: Williams & Wilkins, 1945:148–150.
15. Mast J, Jakob R, Ganz R. *Planning and reduction technique in fracture surgery.* Berlin: Springer–Verlag, 1989:240.
16. Shelton ML, Anderson RL, Jr. Complications of fractures and dislocations in the ankle. In: Epps, CH Jr, eds. *Complications in orthopaedic surgery.* 5th ed., vol 1. Philadelphia: JB Lippincott, 1986: 599–648.

EDITORIAL COMMENTS

Fractures of the Posterior Malleolus

James B. Carr

Fractures of the posterior lateral malleolus are directly related to syndesmotic injury, and it should be noted that this is an avulsion-type injury. The posterior tibiofibular ligament attaches to the posterior lateral tibia, and this portion is usually injured. Treatment for fractures from 20% to 25% of the articular surface in the posterior lateral quadrant depends on a stable reduction of the medial and lateral anterior fracture patterns. After that portion of the fracture is stabilized, anatomic reduction and stress views are critical in making your determination as to whether a separate approach is needed. Biomechanically, the posterior lateral approach gives the best form of fixation with screws, as discussed by Dr. James B. Carr. I would remind all that planning is essential and if one is going to go posterior, then a more posterior lateral approach to the fibular fracture is needed. One then would use the flexor hallucis longus muscle as a guide down to the posterior process of the talus and posterior lateral fragment of the tibia. Fluoroscopy and indirection reduction techniques with clamps are essential.

The more rare posterior medial fragments are usually associated with a posterior colliculus. Sometimes plates are necessary for reduction of this medial fragment. The goal of treatment would be to provide adequate biomechanical fixation to allow motion but not weight bearing within the first 6 to 8 weeks. One should realize that a minimal stripping technique is necessary when going posterior since the blood supply is usually coming directly through the ligament into the fragment.

Robert S. Adelaar, M.D.

Complex Foot and Ankle Trauma,
edited by Robert S. Adelaar,
Lippincott–Raven Publishers, Philadelphia © 1999.

4

Open Fractures of the Ankle Joint

James B. Stiehl

In recent years, the treatment of open joint injuries has focused on the use of internal fixation to restore articular congruity and at the same time allow treatment of soft tissue injury. Improved implants, prophylactic antibiotics, and good surgical techniques have greatly reduced the incidence of infection.

Franklin and associates (1) reported on 38 open ankle fractures treated with initial wound debridement, immediate rigid anatomic internal fixation, and delayed wound closure at 5 days. At follow-up, there were no nonunions and only one possible deep infection in the group, which included 16 grade III open fractures.

Bray and colleagues (2,3), in a similar series, compared surgical debridement and immediate internal fixation with debridement and delayed open reduction. There was one infection in each group, but the immediate fixation group had statistically better motion. Also, hospitalization, which averaged 9 days in the delayed fixation group, was shortened to an average of 6 days. This chapter reviews current thinking on open ankle fractures.

ANTIMICROBIAL MANAGEMENT

Microbiologic investigations have determined that between 60% and 70% of all open fractures are contaminated with bacteria at the time of injury (4). The incidence of wound infection in patients who have open fracture correlates with the extent of soft tissue injury. Robinson et al. (5) determined that *Staphylococcus epidermidis* (32.1%)

J. B. Stiehl: Department of Orthopaedics, Medical College of Wisconsin, Milwaukee, Wisconsin 53226; Department of Orthopaedics, Columbia Hospital, Milwaukee, Wisconsin 53211.

and *Staphylococcus aureus* (25%) are the major organisms associated with open fracture wound infections. In addition, gram-negative rods, one of the most common being *Pseudomomas aeruginosa* (13.1%), may account for 39.3% of open fracture infection. Other skin flora organisms of unknown virulence may include *Propionobacterium acnes, Corynebacterium* species, *Micrococcus* species, or environmental contaminants such as *Bacillus* and *Clostridium* species. Mixed infections due to gram-negative bacteria, such as *Klebsiella,* and gram-positive organisms, such as *S. aureus,* have been reported. Farm-related injuries have substantially different types of contamination, with *Clostridium perfringens* warranting specific consideration. Fresh water injuries are similarly associated with *P. aeruginosa* and *Aeromonas hydrophila* (5).

It is important to recognize that skin flora often seen in the initial culture report seldom result in clinically manifest wound infection. On the other hand, *P. aeruginosa* and *S. aureus* are infrequently identified from the initial cultures, although they are frequently associated with infection. The obvious conclusion is that these virulent bacteria find access to the wound at some point after the injury and often may be hospital acquired (6). This phenomenon underlies the principle of primary antibiotic coverage for early wound sterilization and also provides the rationale for limiting initial antibiotic therapy to minimize the emergence of resistant nosocomial bacteria.

The specific selection and use of antibiotic for the treatment of open fractures are suspected on providing wide-spectrum antibiotic coverage against likely pathogens and as an adjunct to the initial surgical treatment, which is surgical debridement and appropriately timed and implemented stabilization of the fracture. Patzakis et al. (7) have determined that a minimum of 3 days of antimicrobial therapy should be given. After 3 days, culture results are available to determine specific continued antimicrobial therapy, if needed. Antimicrobial therapy is usually warranted beyond 3 days if wounds are obviously infected or if an infection is clinically suspected.

Antibiotic treatment should include at minimum a second-generation cephalosporin such as cefazolin or cephamandole from the outset. A single dose of 2.0 g started in the emergency room and 1.0 g every 6 to 8 hours for 48 or 72 hours is recommended for type I open fractures. For type II or III open fractures, combined therapy is indicated to cover both gram-positive and gram-negative bacteria as well as the potential mixed infections. Typically, aminoglycosides such as tobramycin at 1.5 mg per kilogram of body weight are given at admission and 3.0 to 5.0 mg per kilogram of body weight each day in divided doses. The dose of aminoglycosides must be adjusted for renal insufficiency. Ten million units of penicillin is added following a contaminated farm injury. These regimens are continued during the surgical management and cease 3 days after the last major debridement or reconstructive procedure. Finally, tetanus toxoid should be given alone or in combination with hyperimmune globulin, if indicated (8).

EMERGENCY MANAGEMENT

Management of the open fracture starts at the scene of the accident. It is appropriate for the emergency medical team to return the foot to the neutral position by applying gentle axial traction. This enhances stability and improves vascular flow to the foot. The wound should be dressed with sterile, saline-soaked gauze. A splint is applied, but tight circumferential wrapping, which could further compromise the distal circulation, is to be avoided.

When the patient reaches the emergency room, evaluation includes checking neurovascular status, defining fracture stability by examination, and obtaining anteroposterior, mortise, and lateral radiographs. Wounds should remain untouched or at least minimally and sterilely exposed until the patient reaches the operating room. Tscherne and Gotzen (6) found a significantly higher infection rate when the wound was exposed in the emergency room.

Table 1. *Classification of open fractures*

Type	Characteristics
1	Open fracture with a wound less than 1 cm long and clean
2	Open fracture with a laceration more than 1 cm long without extensive soft tissue damage, flaps, or avulsions
3	Open fracture with massive soft tissue damage, compromised vascularity, severe wound contamination, and marked fracture instability
A	Adequate soft tissue coverage of a fractured bone despite extensive soft tissue laceration or flaps, or high-energy trauma irrespective of the size of the wound
B	Extensive soft tissue injury loss with periosteal stripping and bone exposure usually associated with massive contamination
C	Open fracture associated with arterial injury requiring repair

PRESURGICAL PLANNING

For any surgical procedure, a satisfactory outcome depends on careful consideration of all potential problems. Important considerations in open ankle fractures include assessing the soft tissue injury (Table 1), determining subsequent fracture management, and being prepared to handle any other exigencies (9). A surgeon capable of repairing small vessels must be on hand to treat injury to the anterior and posterior tibial artery. Proper instruments, drills, and implant sets should be selected in advance. External fixation devices should be available as indicated.

A detailed plan for fracture reduction and anticipated implants should be made from the injury radiographs on tracing paper along with a step-by-step outline of the procedure. With experience, this approach facilitates technique, avoids errors, and shortens the time required for surgery.

SURGICAL MANAGEMENT

In the operating room, the wound is handled sterilely and the debridement starts while the patient is being prepared for surgery. All dirt, grease, or other particulate matter must be removed. Minimal shaving is needed. The ankle is held carefully while the nurse scrubs it. It may not be appropriate to let the leg hang on a legholder.

Adequate debridement of the wound, accompanied by copious intermittent lavage, is the most important step in management. Small puncture wounds or small lacerations must be extended to allow adequate exposure. A transverse medial wound, caused by laceration of the skin as the foot deplaces laterally, is common (Fig. 1). Debridement is done by incising the skin edges and then systematically debriding to deeper layers. Replacement of any large bone fragment detached in the wound is not recommended,

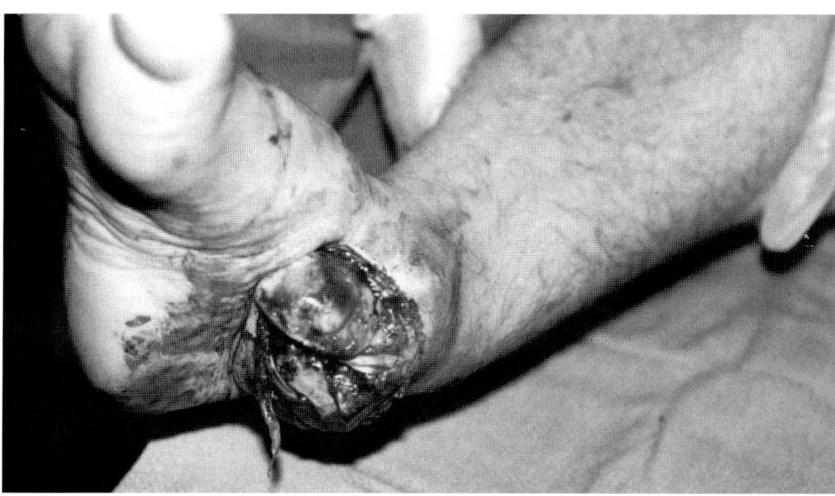

Figure 1. Transverse medial ankle wound following an open dislocation with lateral displacement of the foot.

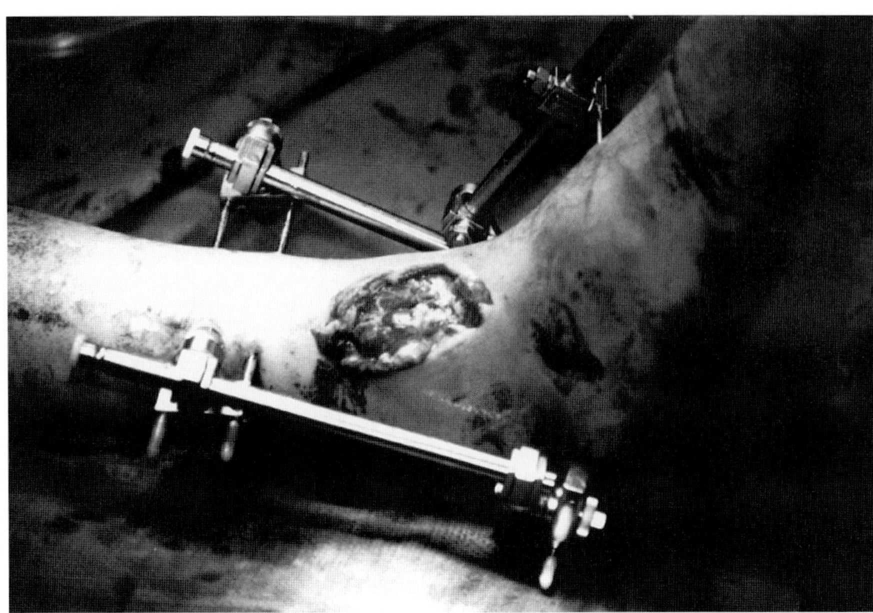

Figure 2. Typical triangular external fixator with pins transfixing the distal fibula, calcaneus, and first metatarsal to immobilize this open pilon fracture.

particularly if gross contamination is present. All questionable tissue must be removed to avoid the possibility of a nidus for future infection. Pulsed mechanical lavage is then done, using 10 L of saline with kanamycin or bacitracin antibiotics. Deep cultures can be made after debridement is complete (8). Cultures in the emergency room or prior to debridement are usually not helpful or cost effective.

The leg is redraped, the surgeons regown and glove, and clean instruments are put on the table. A vascular injury, which does not require bone stability, can be repaired at this point. Concurrent procedures such as deep compartment release of the forefoot and hindfoot should be done at this time. The soft tissue wound determines the type of fracture stabilization to use. For grades I or II fractures and some grade III fractures, a standard internal fixation may be used as recommended by the Swiss AO Group and covered elsewhere. Anatomic restoration and rigid stable internal fixation to allow early active range of motion are the goals. Minimal internal fixation using screws or K-wires can be done in open wounds, but soft tissue coverage should be made of these implants. In ankle fractures, a primary second incision may be needed for the opposite side such as plating a displaced fibular fracture. In this situation, primary wound closure is appropriate (3,10).

For high-energy comminuted fractures such as an exploded pilon distal tibia fracture or severely contaminated wounds (grade IIIA or B), internal fixation may not be indicated. In these situations, external fixation should be used, possibly with minimal Kirschner wire fixation applied through small incisions under fluoroscopic control. A triangular frame or Ilizarov frame may be used in this situation depending on the surgeon's experience or preference. Three-point fixation is obtained by placing pins in the distal tibia, the calcaneus (a safe distance from the neurovascular bundle), the middle talar neck, and the first metatarsal (Fig. 2). These frames are versatile, allowing soft tissue healing and maintaining length when there is bone loss or extensive comminution. They may be removed early after the soft tissues have healed or may be extended for 8 to 10 weeks as primary fracture stabilization. Pin care is important late and includes avoiding any salve or ointment and cleaning the site daily with half-strength hydrogen peroxide. Any skin tension should be relieved. Finally, loose or infected pins should be removed immediately when recognized.

DELAYED WOUND RECONSTRUCTION

Even when the initial debridement of the wound is aggressive, it is very difficult to determine the viability of marginal tissue at that time. An important principle is to redebride at 48 to 72 hours for a second look to establish a viable environment. Factors that increase the risk of infection include poor vascularity, nonviable tissue, and host compromise from various factors (11,12). The surgeon's responsibility is to sterilize the wound by removing nonviable tissue, much like a tumor surgeon. Therefore, at 3 days, if tissue does not bleed, it should be cut out. Recent experience has shown reduced rates of infection if wound closure is delayed (8).

After any delayed wound treatment, the wound should be kept moist and covered with sterile dressings. These dressings should not be changed or disturbed except under sterile conditions and in the operating room. For simple wounds, the delayed closure may be done at the 48- to 72-hour point. There should be no tension on the skin edges at closure. I prefer the use of a horizontal mattress type of stitch with a 3- or 4-0 nylon suture. This allows perfect adjustment of the skin tension. Postoperative immobilization of the wound should be done early to enhance tissue healing. A simple posterior splint can be used in most cases, and only dressings are needed when the entire foot and ankle are immobilized by external fixation.

COMPLEX WOUND RECONSTRUCTION

Soft tissue management is important to prevent deep osteomyelitis. Recent studies have demonstrated markedly reduced rates of infection in type III fractures when wound coverage was employed within 5 to 7 days (12,13). Because vital structures, including bone, tendon, and nerve, can be left exposed for only a limited period, soft tissue flap coverage must be planned within 5 to 7 days. The metabolic demands of these wounds necessitate coverage with tissue that will withstand shear, tolerate mobilization, and bring its own vascular supply. The additional independent blood flow

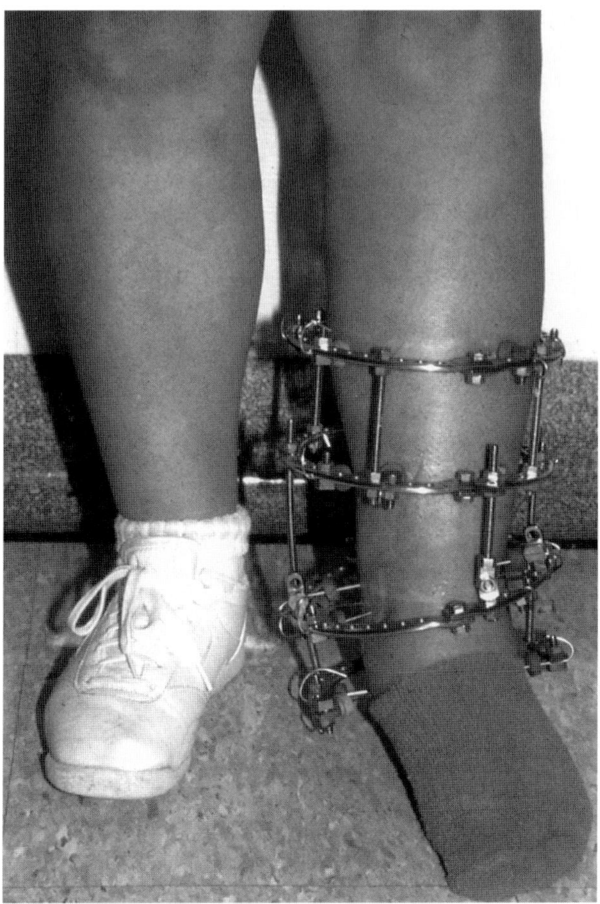

Figure 3. Ilizarov device applied for late external fixation demonstrates potential problems of pin placement, which must be done in concert with the plastic surgeon.

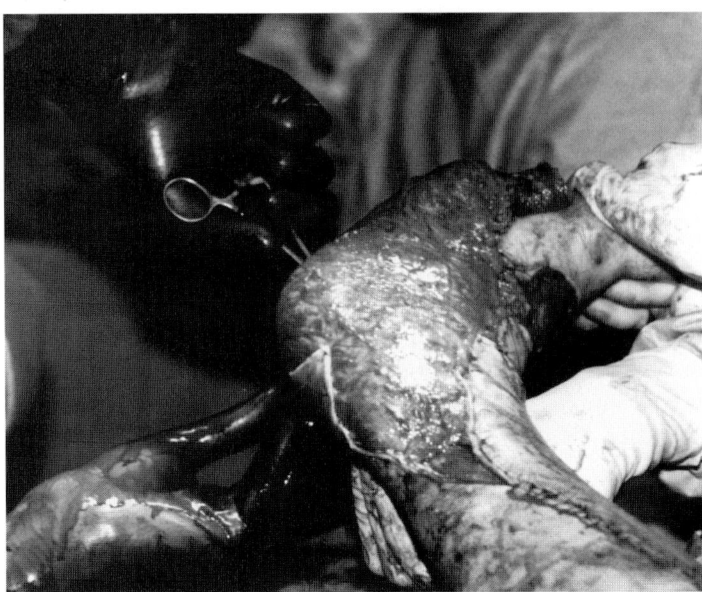

Figure 4. Latissimus dorsi flap provides broad coverage for this severe degloving injury of the foot.

will elevate the oxygen tension within the wound bed and may improve leukocyte function. It is important to anticipate from the outset the need for a flap and to have appropriate personnel on hand to carry out the procedure. Furthermore, certain issues arise from the microvascular surgeon's perspective, such as placement of pins from an external fixation device (Fig. 3). Depending on the wound situation, a microvascular flap may be applied immediately or within the first 72 hours with an excellent chance of survival. With current techniques, flap survival now approaches 96% (14).

Flap coverage over the foot and ankle has certain requirements, and usually free tissue transfer is needed. Local fasciocutaneous flaps have been problematic in providing skin coverage of the malleoli of the ankle and should be avoided. Most problems can be dealt with by muscle transfer with immediate split-thickness skin transfer using one of the following options: lateral arm, latissimus dorsi, rectus abdominis, or gracilis flap. Certain advantages accrue with each graft depending on its size or length. The latissimus dorsi is a large flap and can cover a large portion of the foot (Fig. 4). The gracilis is long and slender and is excellent for smaller isolated dead space defects such as the center of the forefoot. Details of these choices are beyond the scope of this discussion (14) and are covered in Chapter 20.

LATE SKELETAL RECONSTRUCTION

Once initial wound treatment has been successfully applied, i.e., ''clean, closed, and dry,'' late bone defects, delayed union, or reconstruction can be dealt with using bone grafts, etc. An important aspect of current thinking for complex open ankle injuries is to avoid extensive dissection and plating procedures, as advocated in the 1970s by the AO group. The morbidity of chronic osteomyelitis after a high-energy pilon fracture that develops skin problems should dissuade most surgeons from helping create such a disaster.

REFERENCES

1. Franklin JL, Johnson KD, Hansen ST Jr. Immediate internal fixation of open ankle fractures: report of thirty-eight cases treated with a standard protocol. *J Bone Joint Surg [Am]* 1984;66:1349–1356.
2. Bray TJ, Endicott M, Capra SE. Treatment of open ankle fractures: immediate internal fixation versus closed immobilization and delayed fixation. *Clin Orthop* 1989;240:47–52.
3. Bray TJ. Soft-tissue techniques in the management of open ankle fractures. *Techn Orthop* 1987;2:20–28.

4. Dellinger EP, Miller SD, Wertz MJ, Grypma M, Droppert B, Anderson PA. Risk of infection after open fracture of the arm or leg. *Arch Surg* 1988;123:1320–1327.
5. Robinson D, On E, Hadas N, Halperin N, Hofman S, Boldur I. Microbiologic flora contaminating open fractures: its significance in the choice of primary antibiotic agents and the likelihood of deep wound infection. *J Orthop Trauma* 1989;3:283–286.
6. Tscherne H, Gotzen I, eds. *Fractures with soft tissue injuries.* Berlin: Springer–Verlag, 1984:11.
7. Patzakis MM, Wilkins J, Moore TM. Use of antibiotics in open tibial fractures. *Clin Orthop* 1983;178:31–35.
8. Gustilo RB, Merkow RL, Templeman D. Current concepts review. The management of open fractures. *J Bone Joint Surg [Am]* 1990;72:299–304.
9. Gustilo RB, Mendoza RM, Williams DN. Problems in the management of type III (severe) open fractures: a new classification of type III open fractures. *J Trauma* 1984;24:742–746.
10. Hanel DP. Vascularized tissue transfer: an adjunct to the treatment of osteomyelitis. *Orthop Rev* 1989;18:595–608.
11. Lange RH, Bach AW, Hansen ST, Hohansen KH. Open tibial fractures with associated vascular injuries: prognosis for limb solvage. *J Trauma* 1985;25:203–208.
12. Cierny G III, Byrd HS, Jones RE. Primary versus delayed soft tissue coverage for severe open tibial fractures: a comparison of results. *Clin Orthop* 1983;178:54–63.
13. Caudle RJ, Stern PJ. Severe open fractures of the tibia. *J Bone Joint Surg [Am]* 1987;69:801–807.
14. Heim U, Pfeiffer KM. *Internal fixation of small fractures.* Berlin: Springer–Verlag, 1987.

EDITORIAL COMMENTS

Open Fractures of the Ankle Joint

James B. Stiehl

Dr. James B. Stiehl has stressed many important factors in his discussion of open fractures of the ankle joint. The history of the mechanism of the wound is of critical importance to determine how much tissue destruction and contamination have occurred. Early debridement with removal of devitalized tissue is critical, particularly around the ankle joint. It is quite important that wounds about the ankle, particularly the medial anterior aspect, not be left open into the joint and be closed when appropriate. This requires sacrifice of some of the tenets of open wound treatment, but this would be acceptable with the use of redebridement at 48 and 72 hours to avoid leaving any necrotic tissue behind. In the chapters by Dr. Mark Myerson and Dr. Scott Levin, we have a complete discussion of the handling of the devitalized tissue and flap coverage. The fracture should be stabilized. If flap coverage is necessary about the ankle, a free flap would normally be used, done in a timely fashion so as not to compromise ankle joint tissue and desiccate cartilage by continued wound care. The type of antibiotic coverage depends on the wound contamination using the standards established by Dr. R. Guistilo. The antibiotic coverage should be appropriate and should not be used for prolonged periods; resistant forms of bacteria may develop. The most important defense against osteomyelitis is handling of tissue and debridement, not antibiotic coverage. Cultures should be done after debridement and not in an emergency room situation.

It is also important to assess the extent of neurovascular injury at the time of initial debridement. In a type IIIC fracture about the ankle or tibial pilon with nerve and artery involvement, the prognosis is quite poor, particularly with posterior tibial nerve damage. Appropriate deletion should be considered in this situation, but no one will be able to give you a standard approach to making those decisions. Unfortunately, we usually find that our technical skill is greater than our results, particularly when repairing posterior tibial nerves; the fibrotic dysesthetic foot is usually a poor substitute for a functioning below the knee amputation. We do advocate repair of arterial lesions, particularly in compound injuries, to allow for greater tissue survival. Care should also be taken to assess the degree of superficial nerve injury, particularly saphenous and superficial peroneal nerves, with their exposed medial and lateral branches. Injuries to these nerves can usually invoke a significant causalgia.

Robert S. Adelaar, M.D.

Complex Foot and Ankle Trauma,
edited by Robert S. Adelaar,
Lippincott–Raven Publishers, Philadelphia © 1999.

5

Historical Review of the Treatment of Syndesmotic Ankle Injuries

Thomas V. DiStefano, John A. Cardea and Robert S. Adelaar

The syndesmotic ligament complex consists of four structures, the interosseous ligament, the anterior tibiofibular ligament, the posterior tibiofibular ligament, and the inferior transverse ligament. The interosseous ligament consists of numerous short, strong, fibrous bands that connect the tibia and fibula. The anterior tibiofibular ligament sweeps laterally and down between the tibia and fibula on the anterior aspect of the ankle joint. Inferiorly, the fibers are broader and flat. Posteriorly, the ligament lies against the interosseous membrane and talar cartilage. The posterior tibiofibular ligament is positioned like its anterior counterpart on the posterior aspect of the ankle joint. It is smaller and contiguous with the inferior transverse ligament. The inferior transverse ligament is below and anterior to the posterior tibiofibular ligament. It is a thick, tough ligament containing yellow elastic fibers. It also forms part of the articular surface of the talus (1) and is seen easily by arthroscopy.

The deltoid ligament provides stability to the syndesmotic complex. It is composed of a superficial and a deep component. The superficial component consists of tibionavicular, tibiocalcaneal, and posterior tibiotalar parts and originates on the anterior colliculus of the tibia. The tibionavicular part inserts on the navicular and is contiguous

J. A. Cardea and R. S. Adelaar: Department of Orthopaedic Surgery, Medical College of Virginia/Virginia Commonwealth University, Richmond, Virginia 23298.

T. V. DiStefano: Department of Orthopaedics, Tulane School of Medicine, New Orleans, Louisiana 70112.

with the plantar calcaneonavicular ligament. The tibiocalcaneal part inserts on the sustentaculum tali of the calcaneus, and the posterior tibiotalar part inserts medially from the groove for the flexor hallucis on the inner side of the talus. The deep component (anterior tibiotalar) originates on the posterior colliculus of the tibia and inserts on the tip of the medial malleolus and the medial surface of the talus. It has a close relationship with the deltoid artery and its important contribution to the circulation of the body of the talus (1).

BIOMECHANICS

The syndesmotic complex is very important in the normal dynamics of ankle motion and stability. It permits ankle mortise flexibility because of elasticity of the ligaments, which allows intermalleolar distance to change and facilitates tibial and fibular rotation (2). The interosseous membrane is important because it balances the loading of the foot through the fibula. The syndesmosis widens normally with weight bearing as well as when the foot goes from full plantarflexion to dorsiflexion. The interosseous membrane accommodates these changes and up to 120% of its length before failure (3).

The tibial plafond holds 80% to 90% of the body weight. The ankle has peak loads of up to four times body weight. The fibula accounts for 15% of the total load. When loaded, it normally undergoes a few degrees of external rotation and movement in the posterior–lateral direction. The range of motion of the ankle in the loaded position is 32 to 45 degrees and 12 to 56 degrees in the unloaded position. The deep deltoid contributes to internal rotation of the talus from 4 to 8 degrees of plantarflexion. It is the primary restraint against valgus tilting of the talus and a secondary restraint against lateral talar shift (4). The superficial tibiocalcaneal portion is the critical component to providing physiologic contact stresses in the ankle (5).

RADIOGRAPHIC CRITERIA OF SYNDESMOTIC DIASTASIS

Anteroposterior, mortise, and lateral radiographs are routinely taken following ankle injury. Several measurements are commonly assessed to determine syndesmotic diastasis, including the talocrural angle, fibular length, talar shift, medial clear space, tibiofibular overlap, and tibiofibular clear space. The talocrural angle, seen on the mortise view, is measured from the angle of the line parallel to the distal tibia and the intermalleolar line. Normally it is between 8 and 15 degrees. An angle greater than 2 to 3 degrees different from the opposite side indicates fibular shortening. The talar shift, seen on the mortise view, is measured from the angle of the line parallel to the distal tibia and the line parallel to the talar surface. Normally, they are parallel, with a range of 1.5 degrees. Medial clear space, seen on the mortise view, is the distance between the medial talus and the lateral portion of the medial malleolus using like borders (anterior or posterior). Normally it is equal to the distance between the distal tibia and talus. A space greater than 4 mm unloaded is abnormal and signifies lateral shift. With weight bearing secondary to cartilage the gap may be 2 mm. Tibiofibular overlap, seen on the anteroposterior view, is the distance between the medial aspect of the fibula and the lateral border of the anterior tibial prominence. Less than 10 mm signifies division of the tibia and fibula. On the mortise view, the nomal overlap is 1 mm. The tibiofibular clear space, seen on the anteroposterior view, is the distance between the lateral border of the posterior tibial malleolus and the medial border of the fibula. A distance of greater than 5 mm signifies syndesmotic injury. External rotation stress radiographs with mortise and lateral views are used to assess syndesmotic injury (6).

HISTORICAL REVIEW

Two-thirds of complex foot and ankle injuries are ankle and pilon fractures. The proper treatment and indications for stabilization of the syndesmosis remains controversial. In 1726 Petit first reported ankle syndesmotic injuries. Nineteenth century authors included Duputyren, Astley Cooper, and Maisonneuve.

In 1956, the syndesmostic complex was shown to be elastic, with an increase in width from 1 to 2 mm when moving the talus from plantarflexion to dorsiflexion. There is relative external rotation of the fibula in relation to the tibia as the ankle is dorsiflexed (2). In 1960, syndesmotic ossification was observed after injury 10% of the time. However, it was without associated symptoms (7). In 1961, the term *interosseous diastasis* was coined to describe the instability on the lateral side of the ankle that allows talar shift. It was the fractured fibula that was responsible for the poor reduction of the mortise (8). In 1962, it was shown in a large series of supination external rotation fractures treated by open reduction that the anterior tibiofibular ligament was injured in 380 of 405 ankles and that 65.7% of the tears were within the substance of the ligament (9). In 1967, the results of treatment of over 400 abduction/external rotation fractures were reviewed. Late pain, swelling, and degenerative changes were due to persistent laxity of the anterior tibiofibular ligament (10). In 1969, 44% of 36 bimalleolar fractures treated conservatively continued to have pain (11).

In 1970, shortening and lateral displacement of the fibula was observed to be the most common cause of arthritis after fracture (12). In 1971, it was shown that the lateral malleolus carries about 20% of the pressure of the talus (13). One-sixth of the static load is carried through the fibula (little through the interosseous membrane) (14). In 1974, 118 severe bimalleolar and trimalleolar fractures were evaluated after treatment. Three variables were found to affect final clinical results significantly: the amount of displacement prior to reduction, the type of fracture, and the presence of rupture of the deltoid ligament. The length of follow-up, presence of open fracture, age, sex, and body weight did not affect the result (15). In 1976, 1 mm of lateral displacement of the talus was shown to decrease contact area by 42% (16). During stance and pushoff the fibula is pulled distally to deepen the mortise and tighten the interosseous membrane (17). In 1977, a review of cadaveric and clinical studies demonstrated that late degenerative joint disease was related to incomplete reduction of the lateral malleolus and a residual talar tilt. The lateral talus begins to impinge on the proximal fibula, preventing closed reduction. The lateral malleolus is the key to the anatomic reduction of the displaced bimalleolar fracture (18).

In 1983, eight clinical patients treated with fixation of the fibula with the medial malleolus fixed or the deltoid sutured had stable joints and no significant complaints 3 years ago. The interosseous membrane is the main stabilizing force of the ankle mortise (19). In 1984, the interosseous membrane was found to be an important stabilizer of the fibula. It bears little load and when absent, the fibula was not restrained, causing it to translate and rotate rather than carrying load (20). A review of late results of operatively treated bi- and trimalleolar fractures found several significant correlations. This included adequacy of the reduction of the syndesmosis and the development of late arthritis, adequacy of the initial reduction of the syndesmosis and late stability of the syndesmosis, late stability of the syndesmosis and final outcome, and adequacy of the reduction of the lateral malleolus and that of the syndesmosis. An adequate reduction of the syndesmosis is necessary to achieve a stable ankle. The reduction of the syndesmosis will be unsatisfactory if the lateral malleolus is not well reduced. Age, sex, and severity of initial displacement did not show a statistically significant correlation with outcome. Subjective result and development of osteoarthritis did not show a significant correlation (21). In 1989, it was demonstrated that syndesmotic fixation prevents normal external rotation of the fibula, which is required for its dynamic participation in ankle mechanics (22). In a cadaveric study, it was demonstrated that the critical zone for fixing the syndesmosis in ankles with deltoid injury and without medial malleolar fracture was 3 to 4.5 cm above the joint. In ankles with medial malleolar fractures that were fixed, fixation of the syndesmosis was not necessary (23). The lateral malleolus and supporting ligaments are the primary restraints of both anterior and lateral talar shift (4). In a retrospective study of 30 ankles treated with a syndesmotic screw, several observations were made. There was no increase in widening of the mortise or syndesmosis with a syndesmotic screw in place. There was no late syndesmotic widening after screw removal. Seven of the patients developed calcification in the interosseous membrane, and four of them developed synostosis. However, it was more closely related to the site of the fracture than the site of the screw. Two-thirds developed lucency around the screw site but none failed. The transfixion screw provided satisfactory stability of the syndesmosis to promote stable healing of the interosseous membrane and distal ligaments of an ankle fracture (24).

In 1991, it was demonstrated that accurate reduction and internal fixation correlated strongly with final result in Weber B fractures. Degenerative joint disease occurred sooner in Weber C than Weber B fractures (25). Worse results were obtained in ankle fractures that included medial malleolar fractures due to damage to the articular surface of the tibial plafond (26). In 1995, a cadaveric study indicated that diastasis and rotation were related to the amount of injury to the ligament. Measurements on stress mortise radiographs had a weak correlation with diastasis ($r = 0.41$). However, measurements on stress lateral radiographs had a strong correlation with diastasis ($r = 0.81$). Two screws provided better fixation than one screw, which provided better fixation than suture repair (27). In a retrospective study of 43 patients (31 treated with a syndesmotic screw) treated for Weber C fractures, several observations were made. Worse functional results were obtained with dislocated ankles and those with medial malleolar fractures. The best results were seen after accurate reduction of the fibula and syndesmosis. An increase in width of syndesmosis was associated with a worse result (more than 1.5 mm unacceptable). A syndesmotic screw was recommended with a ruptured deltoid ligament and the fibular fracture greater than 3.5 cm above the syndesmosis or with a medial malleolar fracture rigidly repaired and the fibular fracture greater than 15 cm above the syndesmosis (28).

INDICATIONS/TECHNIQUE FOR SYNDESMOSIS SCREW

After initial fixation in Weber B and Weber C fractures, the ankle is stressed under fluoroscopy to determine stability. If it is still unstable, the syndesmosis is stabilized. A single 4.5-mm fully threaded screw, without lag technique, is inserted parallel to and 2.5 to 4 cm above the ankle joint utilizing three cortexes. It should be done in full dorsiflexion to allow the widened part of the talus to be in the mortise. The screw is removed 3 to 4 months from insertion. One screw does not completely immobilize the syndesmosis and still allows forces to be passed through the ligaments to aid in collagen bonding. It is inserted at an angle of 30 degrees from the middle of the fibula toward the tibia. A lateral radiograph is used to ensure location. Some surgeons prefer open fixation methods such as a staple (5).

DATA SUMMARY

We give here preliminary data on 278 ankle fractures treated operatively from January 1992 to December 1994 at the Medical College of Virginia in Richmond.

Open procedures: 21 (7.5%)
Number of patients: 272 (6 bilateral)
- Age range: 12–88 years
- Average age: 36.8 years
- 150 males (55.1%), 122 females (44.9%)
- 141 right (50.7%), 137 left (49.3%)

Number of fractures: 278
- Bimalleolar: 99
- Medial malleolar: 59
- Trimalleolar: 51
- Lateral malleolar with deltoid tear: 30
- Pilon: 16
- Tilleaux: 1
- Other (talus, ankle scopes, etc.): 14

Bimalleolar fractures: 99
  Syndesmosis screws: 14 (14%)
  Staple: 1 (1%)
  Total: 15 (15%)
Trimalleolar fractures: 51
  Syndesmosis screws: 6 (11.7%)
  Staple: 1 (2%)
  Total: 7 (13.7%)
Lateral malleolar fractures with deltoid tear: 30
  Syndesmosis screws: 14 (47%)
  Staples: 2 (6.7%)
  Total: 16 (53.7%)
Overall fractures (bimalleolar, trimalleolar and lateral malleolar with deltoid tear): 180
  Syndesmosis screws or staples: 38 (21.1%)

REFERENCES

1. Gray H. *Anatomy of the human body.* Philadelphia: Lea & Febiger, 1985.
2. Close JR. Some applications of the functional anatomy of the ankle joint. *J Bone Joint Surg [Am]* 1956;38:761–781.
3. Vukicevic S, Stern-Padovan R, Vukicevic D, Keros P. Holographic investigations of the human tibio-fibular interosseous membrane. *Clin Orthop* 1980;151:210–214.
4. Harper MC. Posterior instability of the talus: an anatomic evaluation. *Foot Ankle* 1989;10:36–39.
5. Earll M, Wayne J, Adelaar RS, et al. Contribution of the deltoid ligament to joint contact characteristics in the ankle. *Foot Ankle Int* 1996;17:317–324.
6. Rockwood C, Green D, Bucholz R, Heckman J. *Fractures in adults.* Philadelphia: Lippincott–Raven, 1996.
7. Grath GB. Widening of the ankle mortise. A clinical and experimental study. *Acta Chir Scand* 1960;Suppl 263.
8. Iselin M, De Vellis H. La primauté du perone dans les fractures du cou-de-pied. *Mem Acad Chir* 1961;87:399–408.
9. Cedell CA, Wiberg G. Treatment of eversion-supination fracture of the ankle (2nd degree). *Acta Chir Scand* 1962;124:41–44.
10. Cedell CA. Supination-outward rotation injuries of the ankle. A clinical and roentgenological study with special reference to the operative treatment. *Acta Orthop Scand* 1967;Suppl 110.
11. Phillips WA, Schwartz HS, Keller CS, et al. A prospective, randomized study of the management of severe ankle fractures. *J Bone Joint Surg [Am]* 1985;67:67–78.
12. Muller ME, Allgower M, Willenegger H. *Manual of internal fixation.* New York: Springer, 1970.
13. Sneppen O. Pseudarthrosis of the lateral malleolus. *Acta Orthop Scand* 1971;42:187–200.
14. Lambert KL. The weight-bearing function of the fibula. *J Bone Joint Surg [Am]* 1971;53:507–513.
15. Joy G, Patzakis MJ, Harvey JP. Precise evaluation "of the reduction of severe ankle fractures. *J Bone Joint Surg [Am]* 1974;56:979–993.
16. Ramsey PL, Hamilton W. Changes in tibiotalar area of contact caused by lateral talar shift. *J Bone Joint Surg [Am]* 1976;58:356–357.
17. Scranton PE, McMaster JH, Kelly E. Dynamic fibular function. *Clin Orthop* 1976;118:76–81.
18. Yablon IG, Heller FG, Shouse L. The key role of the lateral malleolus in displaced fractures of the ankle. *J Bone Joint Surg [Am]* 1977;59:169–173.
19. Riegels-Nielsen P, Christensen J, Greiff J. The stability of the tibio-fibular syndesmosis following rigid internal fixation for type C malleolar fractures: an experimental and clinical study. *Injury* 1983;14:357–360.
20. Skraba JS, Greenwald AS. The role of the interosseous membrane on tibiofibular weightbearing. *Foot Ankle* 1984;4:301–304.
21. Leeds HC, Ehrlich MG. Instability of the distal tibiofibular syndesmosis after bimalleolar and trimalleolar ankle fractures. *J Bone Joint Surg [Am]* 1984;66:490–503.
22. Needleman RL, Skrade DA, Stiehl JB. Effect of the syndesmotic screw on ankle motion. *Foot* and *Ankle* 1989;10:17–24.
23. Boden SD, Labropoulos PA, McCowin P, Lestini WF, Hurwitz SR. Mechanical considerations for the syndesmosis screw: a cadaver study. *J Bone Joint Surg [Am]* 1989;71:1548–1555.
24. Kaye RA. Stabilization of ankle syndesmosis injuries with a syndesmosis screw. *Foot Ankle* 1989;9:290–293.
25. Wyss C, Zollinger H. The causes of subsequent arthrodesis of the ankle joint. *Acta Orthop Belg* 1991;Suppl 57:22–27.
26. Broos PL, Bisschop PL. Operative treatment of ankle fractures in adults: correlation between types of fracture and final results. *Injury* 1991;22:403–406.
27. Xenos JS, Hopkinson WJ, Mulligan ME, Olson EJ, Popovic DV. The tibiofibular syndesmosis. *J Bone Joint Surg [Am]* 1995;77:847–856.
28. Chissell HR, Jones J. The influence of a diastasis screw on the outcome of Weber type-C ankle fractures. *J Bone Joint Surg [Br]* 1995;77:435–438.

EDITORIAL COMMENTS

Historical Review of the Treatment of Syndesmotic Ankle Injuries

Thomas V. DiStefano, John A. Cardea, and Robert S. Adelaar

This chapter is included to trace the development of the thinking process for dealing with unstable ankle fractures. It provides the historical sequence of thought in relation to stabilization of ankle injuries over time, combining both the anecdotal and laboratory work to develop the current treatment trend. The text and bibliography will serve as an excellent reference to the rationale behind the treatment we now use in complex syndesmotic ankle injuries.

Robert S. Adelaar, M.D.

Complex Foot and Ankle Trauma,
edited by Robert S. Adelaar,
Lippincott–Raven Publishers, Philadelphia © 1999.

6
The Pilon Fracture

James B. Carr

Pilon is the Latin term for pestle, a term coined by Destot, in 1911 (1), in his treatise on pilon fractures. The term *plafond* is French for ceiling and refers to the relation of the distal tibial articular surface to the talus. In Destot's original work (1), he identified four types of *fracteur du pilon:* (a) anterior margin fracture, (b) posterior margin fracture, (c) explosion fracture, and (d) distal tibia fracture extending into the ankle joint.

When placed in the context of other fractures we treat, the pilon fracture is uniquely prone to iatrogenic complications and poor results (2). This chapter examines the *explosion fracture,* which describes a large group of injuries involving the distal tibial articular surface. An individualized approach is stressed that relies on defining the soft tissue as well as osseous injuries.

ANATOMY OF THE TIBIAL PLAFOND

The distal tibial articular surface, distal fibula, and syndesmotic ligaments provide a stable mortise to support the talus and transmit weight-bearing loads (Fig. 1).

The distal tibial articular surface is concave when viewed from a lateral projection. It is wider anteriorly than posteriorly. A central sagittal ridge is present, which varies in development and size. Anteriorly, the margin of the tibia descends centrally, which can obscure a surgical view of the plafond from a direct anterior approach. Based on pressure film and joint contact studies, the weight-bearing stresses are concentrated in the centromedial aspects.

The distal fibula has a curvilinear articular surface that closely matches the talus. The articular cartilage of the fibula meets the cartilage of the distal tibia to form the analog of *Shenton's line* of the ankle. The fibula is firmly attached to the talus, calcaneus, and tibia via a ligamentous connection. The syndesmosis serves to bind the fibula and tibia together in a firm, yet mobile, articulation. There are four major syndesmotic structures: the posterior and anterior tibiofibular ligaments, the tibiofibular interosseous membrane, and the transverse tibiofibular ligament.

J. B. Carr: Department of Orthopaedic Surgery, Medical College of Virginia, Richmond, Virginia 23298; Department of Orthopaedic Surgery, MCV Hospitals, Richmond, Virginia 23298.

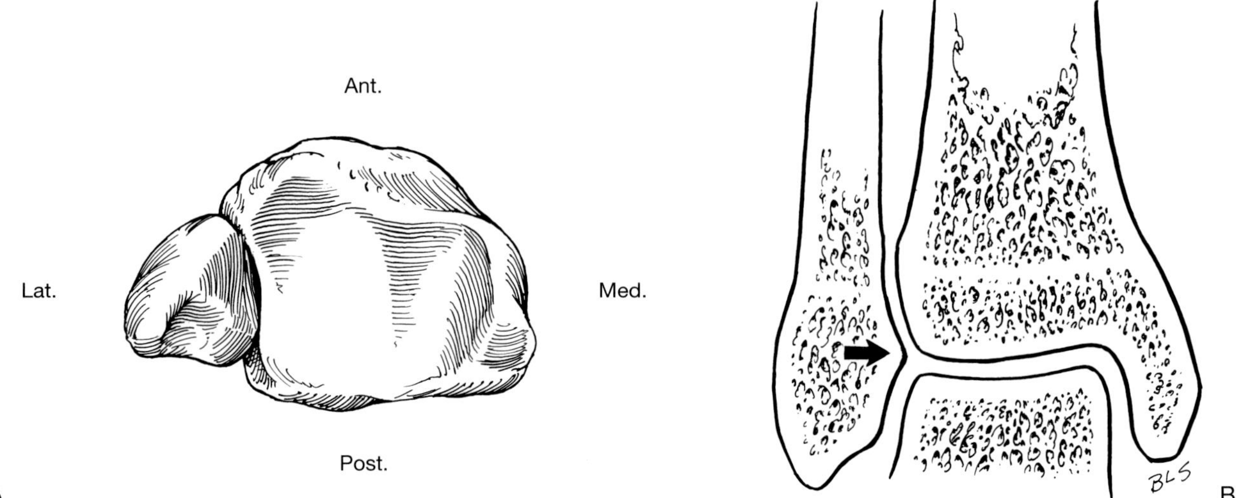

Figure 1. A: End-on view of the tibial plafond. **B:** The tibial and fibular articular cartilage meet laterally and provide a discernable radiographic landmark.

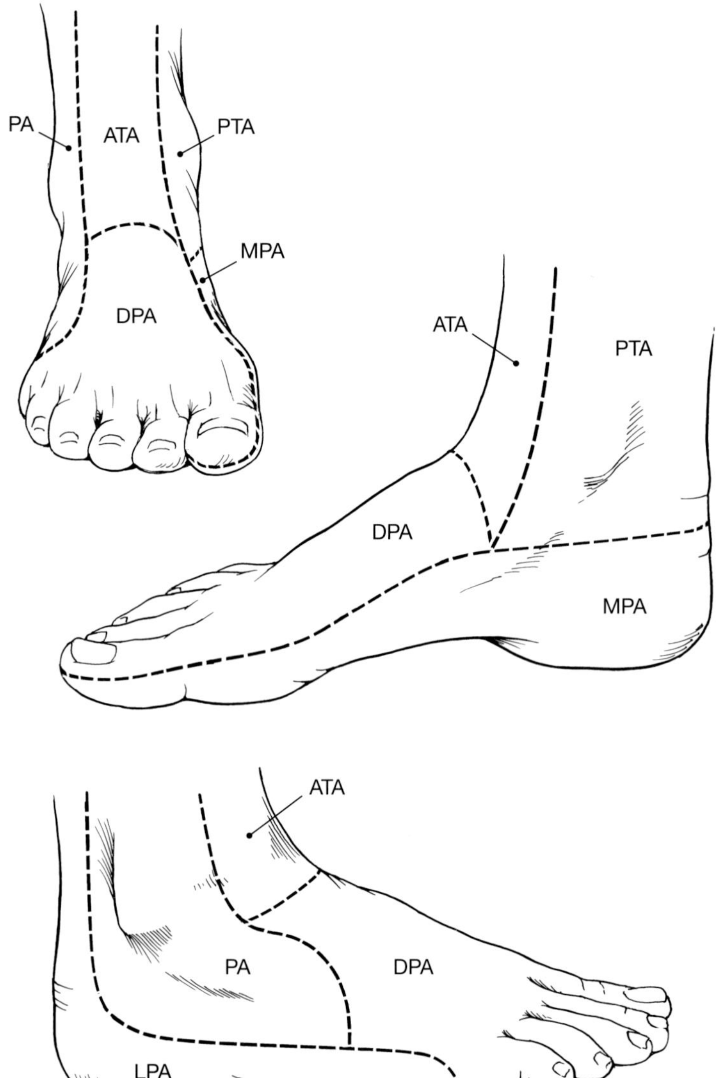

Figure 2. The cutaneous angiosomes about the ankle as described by Salmon (3). *ATA,* anterior tibial artery; *PA,* peroneal artery; *MPA,* medial plantar artery; *PTA,* posterior tibial artery; *LPA,* lateral plantar artery.

CUTANEOUS ARTERIAL DISTRIBUTION

Since pilon fracture treatment commonly suffers from soft tissue complications, it is important to consider some microvascular features of the cutaneous circulation. The cutaneous arterial circulation has been described by Salmon (3) (Fig. 2). The distribution between the posterior tibial artery and anterior tibial/dorsalis pedis meet just medial to the anterior tibial tendon. Laterally, the fibula lies beneath the peroneal artery territory. Incisions are ideally placed in an interarterial location. This is analogous to the concept of intervenous planes of exposure in other skeletal locations. Clinically this ''ideal'' is easiest to accomplish medially. I feel this is important, since the medial incision seems most prone to wound complications.

PATHOLOGIC ANATOMY

Although an infinite variety of pilon fractures are encountered, certain repetitive patterns may be distilled from the confusion of fracture lines (Fig. 3). Six regions are examined for involvement: the fibula, medial malleolus, anterior tibial margin, posterior malleolus, medial tubercle of Chaput, and syndesmosis.

1. Fibular fracture. In 15% of pilon fractures, the fibula is intact. Otherwise, the fibula tends to fracture in the suprasyndesmotic region with a pronation-type pattern. The interosseous membrane is disrupted to at least the level of this fracture, and in some instances higher. Occasionally, a spiral fibular fracture closer to the syndesmosis may be observed.
2. Medial malleolus. The medial malleolus is usually split off at the level of the tibial plafond. In other cases, a larger metaphyseal spike may be present. This metaphyseal spike must be sought out, since it can provide a useful landmark for an anatomic reduction during operative treatment. Marginal articular deformations can occur in this area if the talus abducts during impact.
3. Anterior tibial margin. The anterior margin tends to be comminuted, particularly in dorsiflexion mechanisms. Importantly, the only remaining blood supply may be transmitted by the tenuous anterior capsule. The surgical corollary implies preservation of this thin capsular structure during the operative approach.

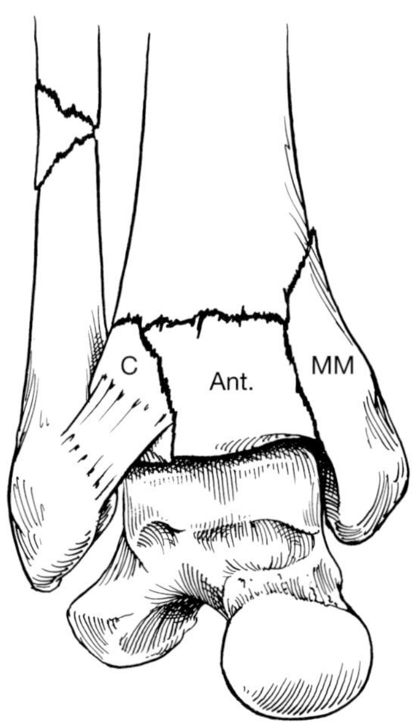

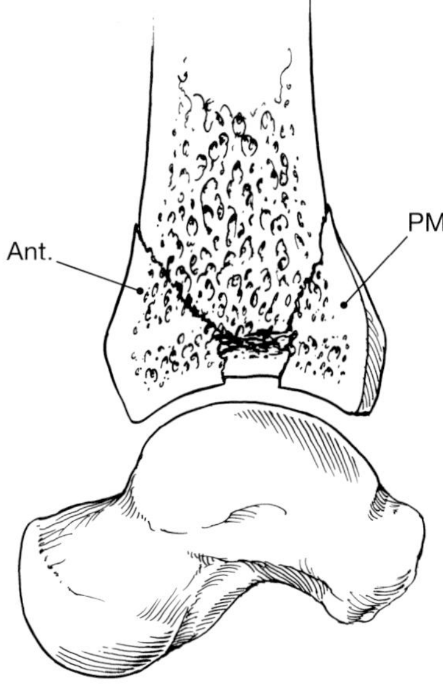

Figure 3. Individual components of the ''typical'' pilon fracture. *Ant.,* anterior joint fragment; *PM,* posterior malleolus; *MM,* medial malleolus; *C,* Chaput tubercle.

4. Posterior malleolus. This tends to fracture a few centimeters above the joint, in the region of the convex curve of the metaphysis.
5. Chaput tubercle. This commonly exists as a fragment attached to the anterior tibiofibular ligament. A variably sized anterolateral fragment of the joint surface may be attached. This important fragment provides a means of stabilizing the syndesmosis and also a landmark for the proper level of the joint line laterally, once fibular length is reestablished.
6. Syndesmosis. As described, this is commonly disrupted to the level of the fibula fracture. In transyndesmotic fibula fracture patterns, a tear of the anterior tibiofibular ligament may be observed.

MECHANISM

Two major forces produce the pilon fracture: rotation and axial compression. The more axial compression plays a role in producing this injury, the more one observes explosion-type comminution (4,5). Conversely, a fracture produced by predominantly rotational forces tends to have lesser comminution and clinically behaves more like a complex trimalleolar fracture (6). If a high fibular fracture is observed, a pronation force was likely involved. A dorsiflexion mechanism produces anterior comminution (1).

CLASSIFICATION/TREATMENT DECISIONS

Numerous classification systems exist (6,7). Common features include indexing the extent and comminution of the articular surface; this is related to prognosis (Fig. 4). Unfortunately, these classifications tend to focus on the obvious bony injury and ignore the soft tissue component. Using these classifications as a reference point, I would like to present a practical algorithm useful in decision making (Fig. 5).

The first step in the algorithm is classifying the fracture as displaced (greater than 2-mm articular stepoff) or undisplaced. The latter are rare, but when encountered may be treated in a cast. Close follow-up is needed to ensure that no displacement occurs in the cast.

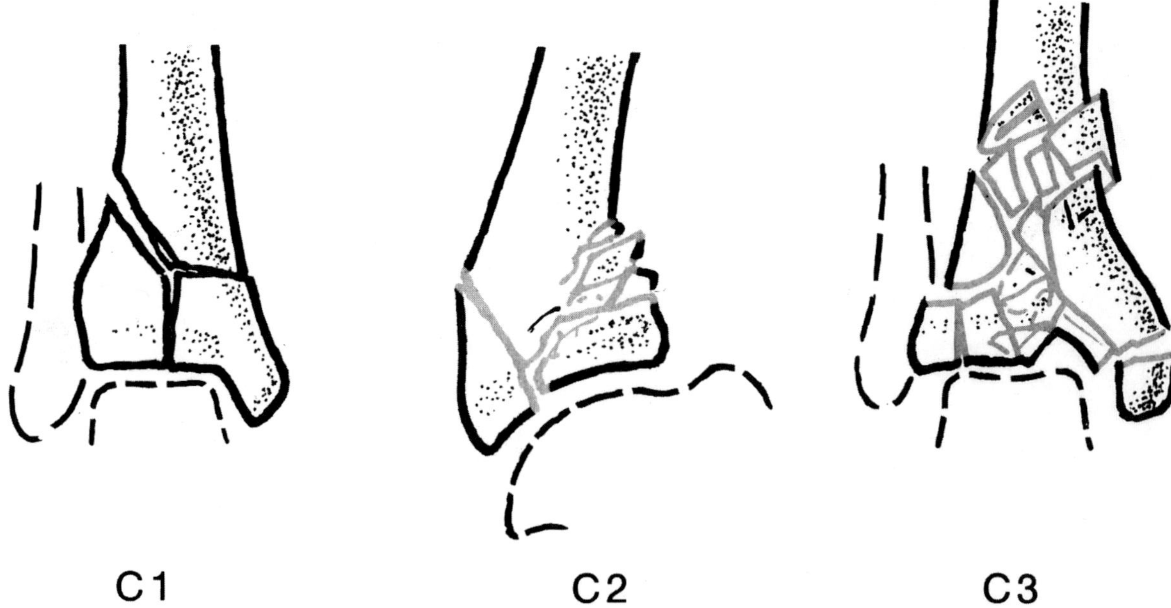

Figure 4. The AO classification of the distal tibia. The pilon fracture is best represented by the C series.

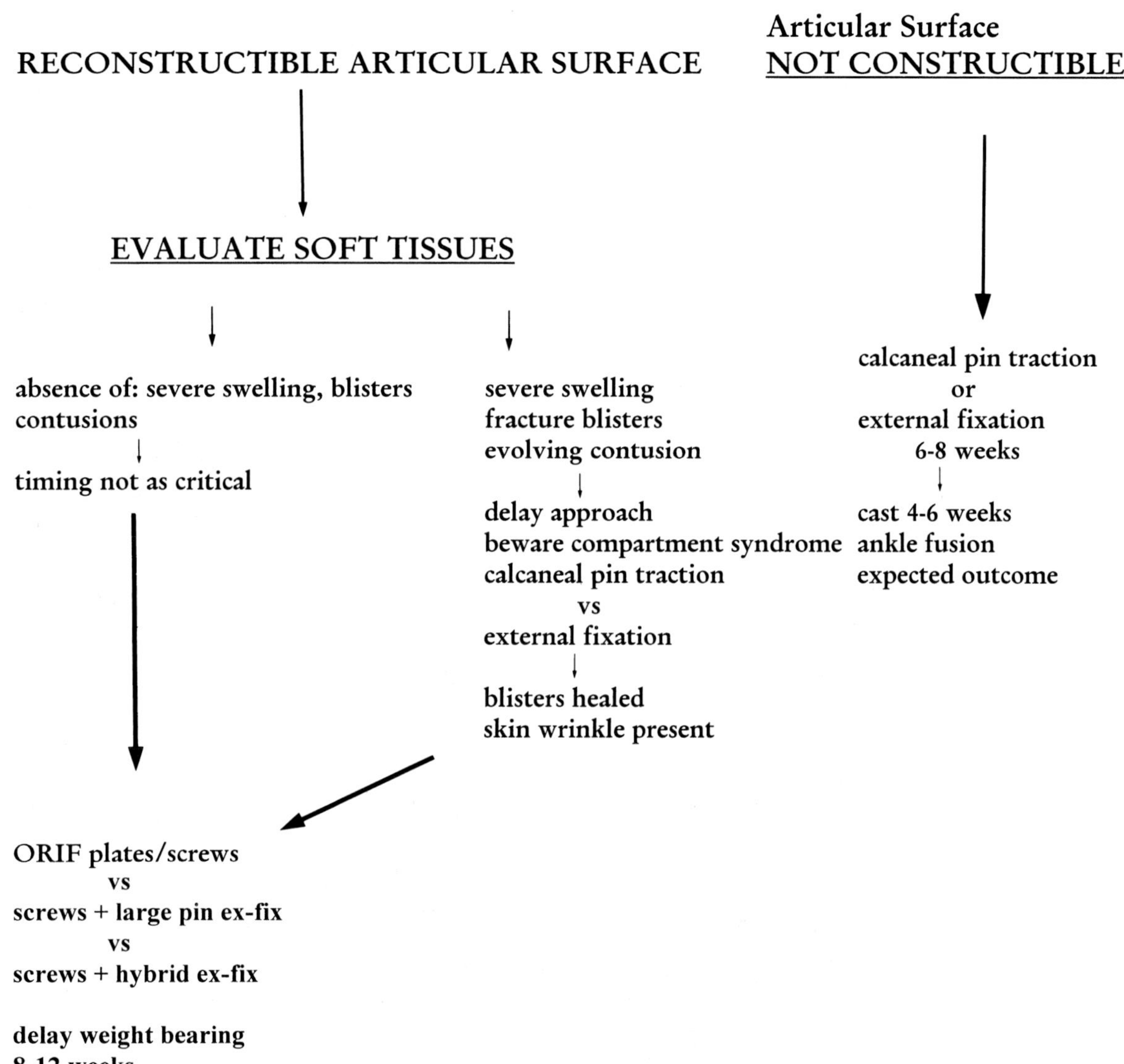

Figure 5. Evaluation of a displaced pilon fracture.

The displaced fractures fall into one of two categories: either the joint surface is amenable to an open reduction internal fixation (i.e., ''fixable''), or it defies surgical reconstruction. This distinction is open to considerable subjective interpretation and will vary according to the individual skills of the surgeon. Although the best surgical results occur with accurate open reduction and internal fixation, the pilon fracture suffers one of the highest rates of iatrogenic surgical complication of any fracture. It makes intuitive sense that it is not worth subjecting the patient to the risks of a large-scale surgery if there is little chance of obtaining any of the benefits. In my practice at a level I trauma center, approximately 10% of the pilon fractures encountered are ''unreconstructible'' (Fig. 6).

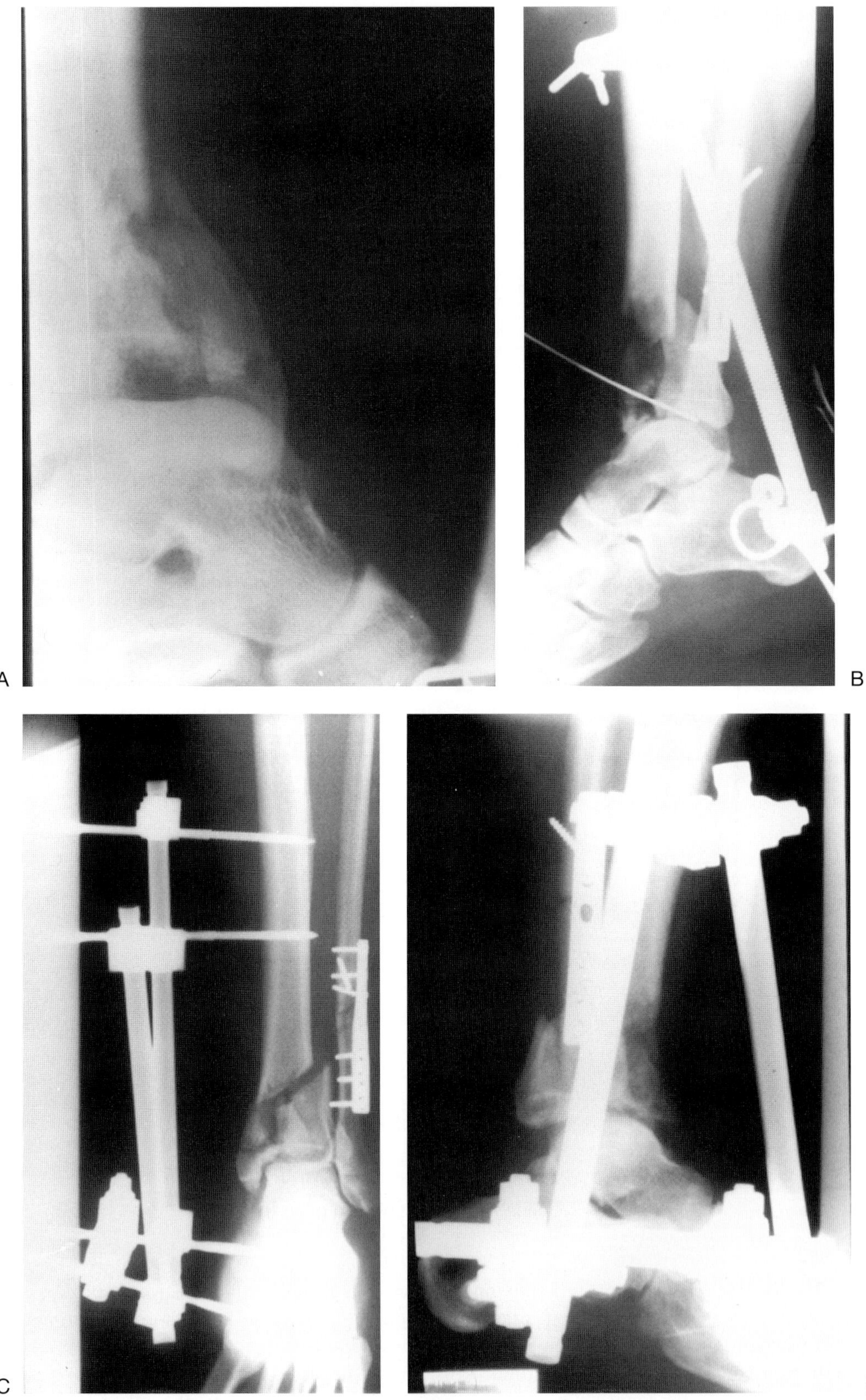

Figure 6. An unreconstructible joint surface. **A:** Preoperative lateral view. Multiple small fragments of the joint are present. **B:** Intraoperative lateral view. An ill-advised open reduction and internal fixation was attempted. **C,D:** Postoperative views in an external fixator. A fusion was eventually required.

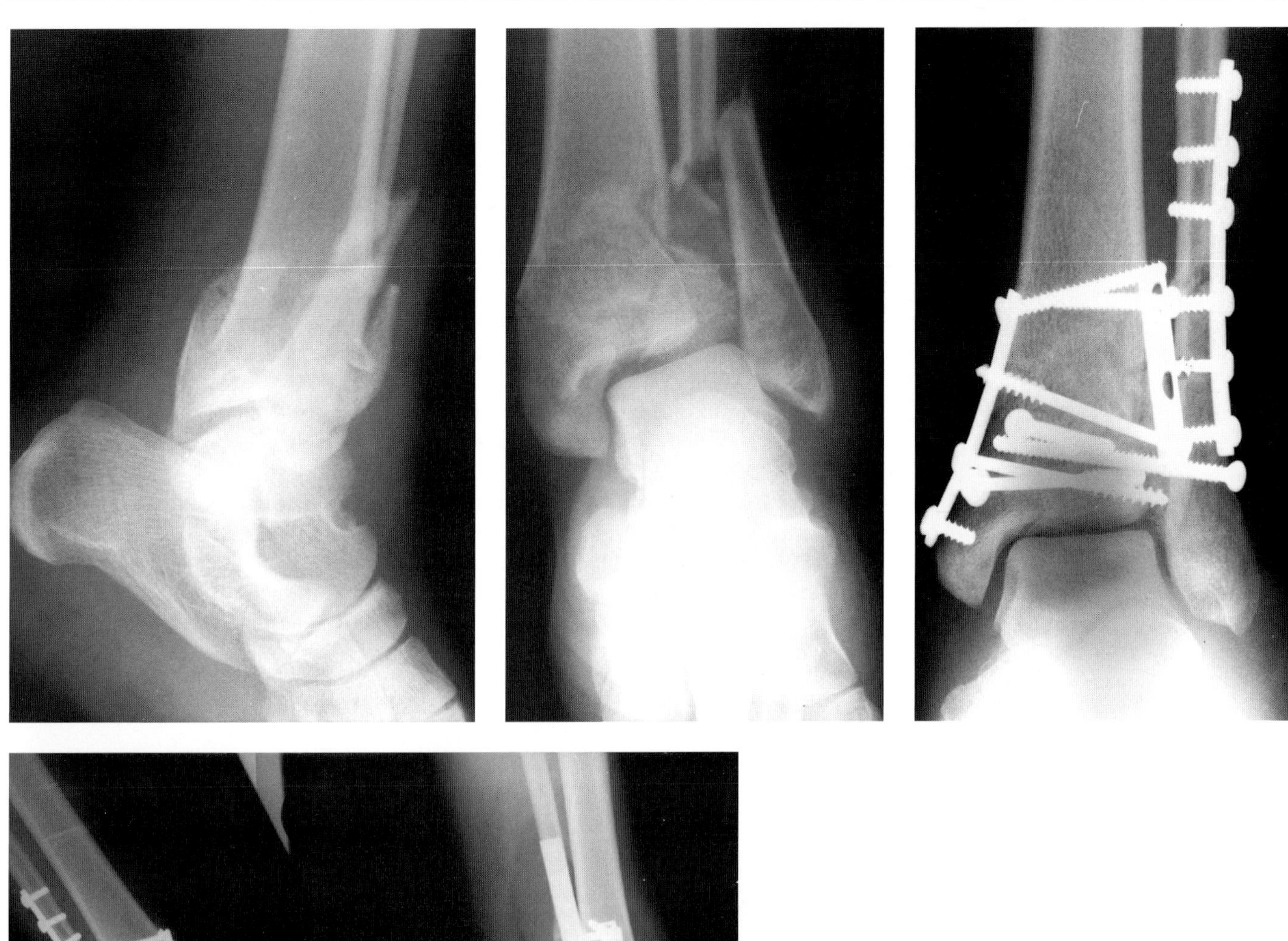

A–C

D

Figure 7. A reconstructible pilon fracture. **A:** Injury film. **B:** Note that the subchondral landmarks are displaced, but identifiable. **C,D:** Postoperative film demonstrating nearly exact reconstruction.

How does one determine if the fracture is ''reconstructible''? The major signs to look for are preserved (albeit displaced) subchondral joint margin landmarks. These are often best assessed by x-ray film obtained with the limb in calcaneal pin traction. If one can identify these joint landmarks, there is an excellent chance they be can restored in an anatomic fashion (Fig. 7). The other major assessment factor is the size of the individual fragments. Again, it is difficult to give an exact size that is ''fixable,'' but ideally one must be able to insert a small fragment screw into or through the fragments to obtain purchase. Finally, one tries to get an idea of the actual size of the joint surface comminution. The one area of the joint that tends to experience extreme comminution is the anterior margin and central lateral portion. This is a sign of a poor prognosis. Unfortunately, avascular necrosis of these fragments, along with late anterior extrusion of the talus, is an all too common occurrence.

The second factor to assess in the decision-making algorithm is the status of the soft tissues, which are tenuous to begin with and are readily damaged by this injury. I try to classify the tissue envelope into one of two categories: good or bad risk for primary healing after surgical approach. Unfortunately, this aspect is even more subjective than the issue of ''reconstructible fractures''; it is extremely important, however, and some judgment must be made. Situations that engender caution regarding open operative treatment include closed degloving, full-thickness contusions, fracture blisters over incision sites, severe swelling, poor circulation (e.g., arteriosclerosis), or diabetes (Fig. 8). If there is any doubt about the soft tissue status, the decision is delayed, the limb is placed in calcaneal pin traction, and serial observations are performed. For example, a full-thickness contusion may originally appear as a deep bruise and may only mature and declare itself after several days of observation.

Calcaneal pin traction is often selected for a number of reasons. First, the limb may be strictly and enforceably elevated. Traction views may be obtained, and the fracture fragments may be assessed further (Fig. 9). The patient may still sit upright in bed, and therefore I use such traction even in the multiply injured patient. A posterior splint is fashioned out of thermal plastic material with Velcro straps to stabilize the limb site temporarily. A pulsatile bladder can then be used to compress the plantar venous plexus. This enables traction to be disconnected while the patient is transported for studies or allowed out of bed. Finally, it avoids large pin tract sites, and the calcaneal pin is easily

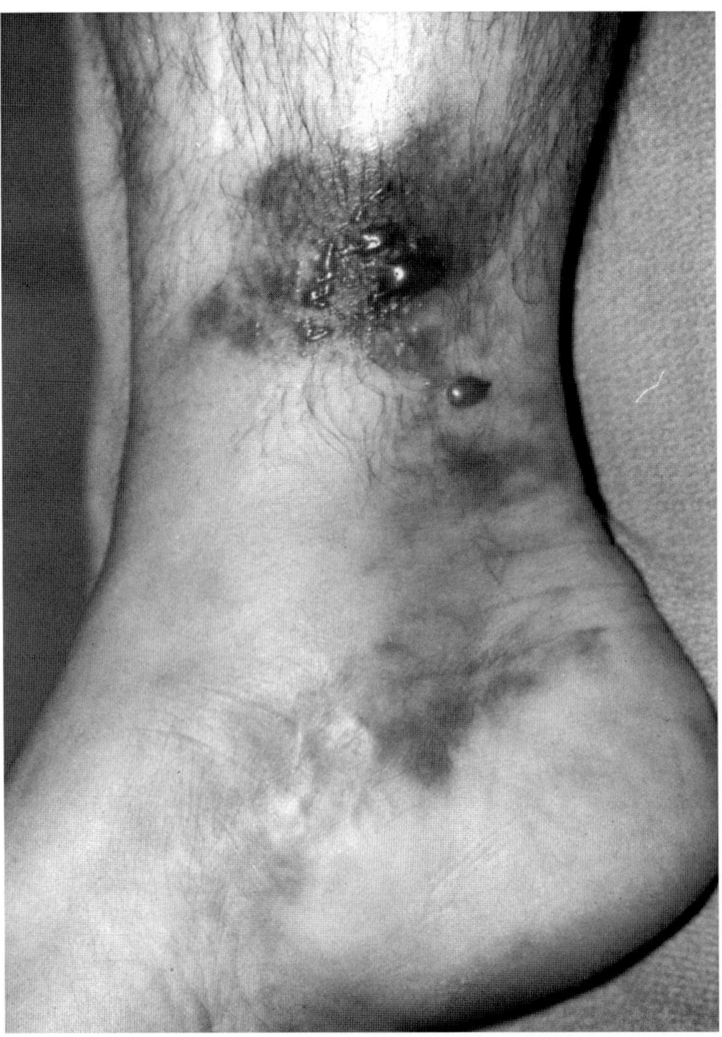

Figure 8. A limb at high risk for operative complications. Blisters are present with significant swelling. The discolored areas represent either pigment changes related to a hematoma or a variable depth contusion. Only time and observation can differentiate the true extent of this type of soft tissue injury.

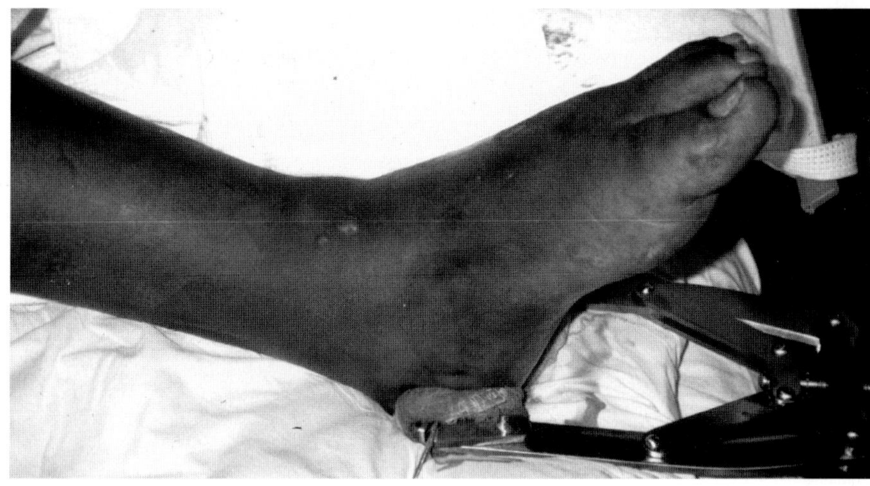

Figure 9. Calcaneal pin traction. The use of a small, smooth K-wire with tensioning bow is recommended.

removed and draped out of the field if further surgery is anticipated. One can use a small, smooth 0.062 K-wire, which is easily inserted in the emergency room. An obvious major deficiency of calcaneal pin traction is the cost of in-hospital treatment. I feel such traction is worth it, if it avoids later complications. If nothing else, calcaneal pin traction is an easy first step that leaves open all possibilities for future treatment. Another alternative is *temporary external fixation,* with pins placed in the proximal tibia and calcaneus or talus (8). A posterior splint is generally required. Pin sites need to be placed well away from intended future incisions. A simpler medial frame may be used if the fibula is plated (9). This latter option can then be combined with a later open reduction, once the soft tissues quiet down.

In summary, for fractures amenable to a formal open reduction and internal fixation, the timing and advisability of surgery is predicated by the soft tissues. A delay of 7 to 14 days may be required which, in my opinion, is best accomplished in calcaneal pin traction. Patience is a virtue, particularly in these times of aggressive fracture care and the ever watchful insurance company. For those injuries deemed ''unreconstructible,'' alternative treatment methods are considered.

TREATMENT MODALITIES

The optimal treatment is based on the following goals (7,10):

1. Exact articular alignment
2. Physiologic metaphyseal alignment
3. Osseous and soft tissue healing
4. Functional restoration
5. Avoidance of iatrogenic complications

These goals are commonly compromised and dictated by the injury itself. Our challenge is to optimize the situation within realistic expectations.

Treatment options may be broadly categorized as follows:

1. Casting—reserved for undisplaced fractures
2. Calcaneal pin traction
3. External fixation—possibly combined with fibular plating and/or *limited internal fixation* of the tibial surfaces (Fig. 10)
4. Open reduction and internal fixation
5. Primary arthrodesis

The remainder of this chapter will center on options 2 to 5.

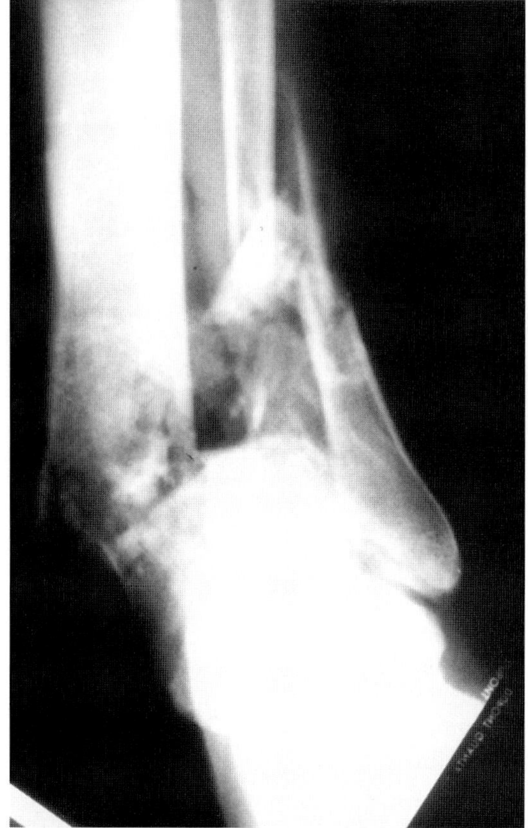

A

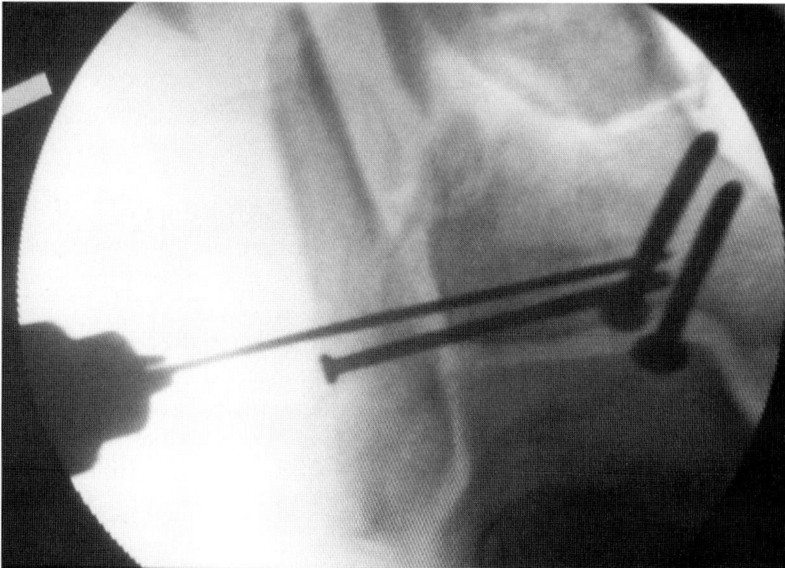

B

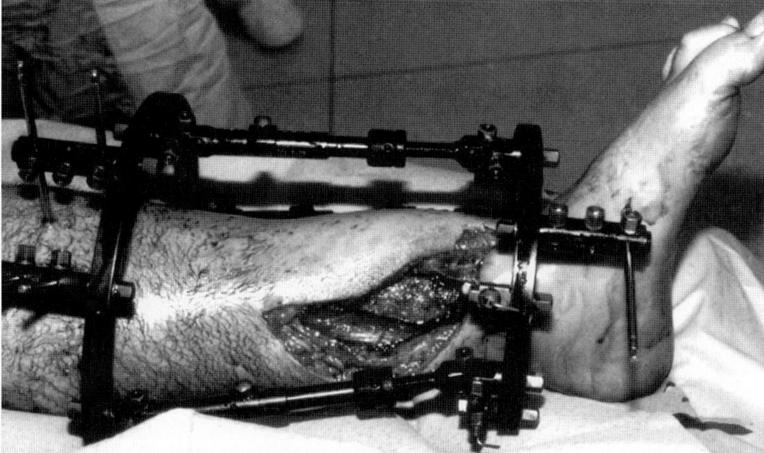

C

Figure 10. Hybrid external fixation. **A:** Injury film. **B:** Intraoperative film demonstrating screw fixation of the joint and the wires in the distal tibia. **C:** Clinical photo of the frame in place. A free flap was required for coverage.

Calcaneal Pin Traction

Calcaneal pin traction depends on ligamentataxis to obtain a reduction. This method has historical precedents and represents one of the earliest attempts to intervene in this difficult injury. The major problem is that although metaphyseal segments may align relatively anatomically, the joint surface often does not. Every so often, one obtains a remarkably close reduction when large pieces of the same joint remain firmly attached to metaphyseal segments. These same fractures are also amenable to internal fixation but are rarely definitively treated in this fashion. Calcaneal pin traction remains useful in two situations:

1. By far the most common use is as a temporizing measure. As previously discussed, the distraction, plus strict elevation, provides an excellent means to assess the soft tissues, define the fracture anatomy, and prepare the limb for an operation.

2. Definitive treatment: This is best reserved for unreconstructible injuries. Ankle motion is instituted in traction to "mold" the surfaces. The goal is to obtain a reasonably aligned distal tibial metaphysis, which is then amenable to a later fusion. It avoids the iatrogenic problems experienced with a failed open reduction and internal fixation. Finally, an occasional patient obtains a satisfactory clinical result despite what one would normally consider an unacceptable alignment of the joint. Although this result cannot be depended on or expected, numerous fracture texts depict long-term follow-up of complex pilon fractures treated in skeletal traction (11–13).

Given the pressures of modern practice, the use of calcaneal pin traction has largely been replaced by external fixation. I still think it is an excellent definitive method for rare, select injuries.

Open Reduction and Internal Fixation

As previously stated, open reduction and exact joint reduction offer the best chance for a functional ankle (6,7,10,14). This statement is made with a healthy respect for the potential complications. The keys to success include a thorough understanding of the fracture anatomy, delicate handling of the soft tissues, and a precise reduction accompanied by a minimum of hardware that offers a maximum of fixation. Even if one chooses to buttress the tibia with an external fixator, the comments in this section will still apply to the fixation of the joint. I have previously discussed fracture anatomy and timing, so the remainder of this chapter is devoted to the specifics of soft tissue handling, obtaining a precise reduction, and the tenets of stable internal fixation.

"Careful handling of the soft tissues" is an oft-made statement in fracture surgery. This remains a difficult subject to teach and convey. I consider it useful to think of the soft tissues in three periods: pre-, intra-, and postoperative. There are practical pointers for each.

In the preoperative period, any gross deformity is reduced with splinting. For high-energy injuries and those with extensive comminution, calcaneal pin traction utilizing a 0.062-force smooth K-wire and tension Steinman pin bow is employed. The limb is observed on an elevated frame, and early motion is encouraged. An external fixation frame may be substituted, as previously discussed. Fracture blisters are allowed to rupture on their own and are painted with an iodophor-based solution. In severe cases, they may take up to 3 weeks to epithelize. The blisters remain colonized until completely healed. Small unpopped blisters that can be widely draped from the operative field do not necessarily preclude operation. The limb is observed until skin wrinkling is present.

Intraoperatively, a number of factors are important in handling the soft tissues. A tourniquet is placed but not routinely inflated. A local anesthetic with epinephrine is injected along incision lines; this often suffices for hemostasis and avoids posttourniquet ischemia and swelling. I routinely employ two incisions, a minimum of 8 cm apart. The first incision lies anteromedial to the anterior tibial tendon, on the border of the anterior tibial and posterior tibial arterial distribution. The anterior tibial tendon sheath is not violated, making later tissue coverage easier, if it is necessary. Additionally, this incision tends to lie over the "medial shoulder" of the plafond and often enters directly into a fracture line of the medial malleolus. This fracture line can then be entered to "book open" the medial malleolus and visualize the joint surface (Fig. 11). The underlying saphenous vein and nerve is an easily handled drawback of this particular incision. Finally, the incision is extensile to the entire tibia which allows later reconstructive options. The lateral incision is based slightly posterolateral and is used even if the fibula is intact, since the Chaput tubercle is frequently involved. It also offers another view of the joint from an anterolateral perspective.

All incisions are made directly to the bone without dissection of subcutaneous tissues, other than identification of sensory nerves and venous structures. Fracture lines are entered and "outlined" with a 15-in. blade, and no periosteal stripping is performed until a specific implant placement is required. One tries to use the soft tissue stripping

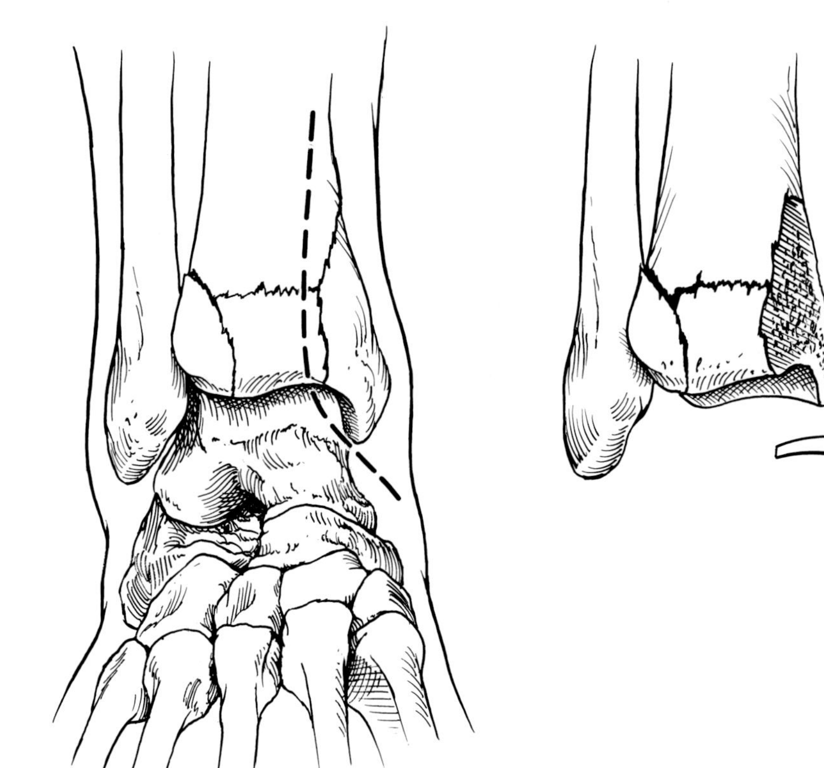

A,B

Figure 11. A: The incision (*dashed line*) lies over the medial "shoulder" of the plafond. **B:** Usually one can then enter directly into a fracture line (*arrow*) and lever the piece open to gain exposure into the joint.

performed by the injury itself as much as possible for exposure. Fracture fragments are manipulated with dental scalers and tissue-sparing pointed reduction forceps.

Once the initial exposure is made, distraction of the zone of injury is performed with a temporary external fixator (Fig. 12) (10). A carbon-fiber Synthes (Paoli, PA) large-fragment external fixator is most useful for this method. A Shanz pin is placed in the proximal tibia, and another half-pin is inserted in the medial talus or calcaneus. The limb is then manually distracted, and the fixator locked into place. C-arm control is used to assess the reduction. Distraction with this method reduces the need for periosteal stripping to expose and manipulate fragments. A nearly anatomic reduction of the metaphysis is usually seen. Overdistraction must be avoided, particularly if appropriate calcaneal pin traction has been performed prior to the surgery.

The use of self-retaining retractors is avoided on the skin. They are useful to lever apart bone fragments to allow exposure to the joint. Large clamps, such as "turkey claws" or Lane forceps, are left on the back table.

As a final soft tissue consideration, the closure consists of 3-0 vicryl on the subcutaneous tissue, followed by Algower–Donati stitches on the skin. If one of the incisions has excessive tension, the medial incision alone is closed. The lateral incision is closed on a delayed basis in 2 to 4 days. A skin graft may be required in extreme cases. These later measures should be uncommon if adequate preoperative traction, elevation, and delay are employed. I also feel that avoiding the use of a tourniquet is useful.

Postoperative soft tissue handling consists of strict elevation, foot pump, and compression wraps. The foot is splinted at a right angle to the leg. Hemovac drains are left in for 24 to 48 hours. Sutures are removed at 2 to 3 weeks postoperatively.

Regarding fixation of the bone itself, the fibula is fixated first. This follows standard principles and small-fragment plating techniques. Although a one-third tubular plate generally suffices, a 3.5-mm D-C plate is occasionally required to hold the fibular reduction. This is particularly true of very high Weber C patterns. Exposure of the anterolateral tibial surface is performed by incising the extensor retinaculum. One must be careful to avoid injuring the communicating peroneal artery, which pierces the interosseous membrane approximately 5 cm above the ankle joint.

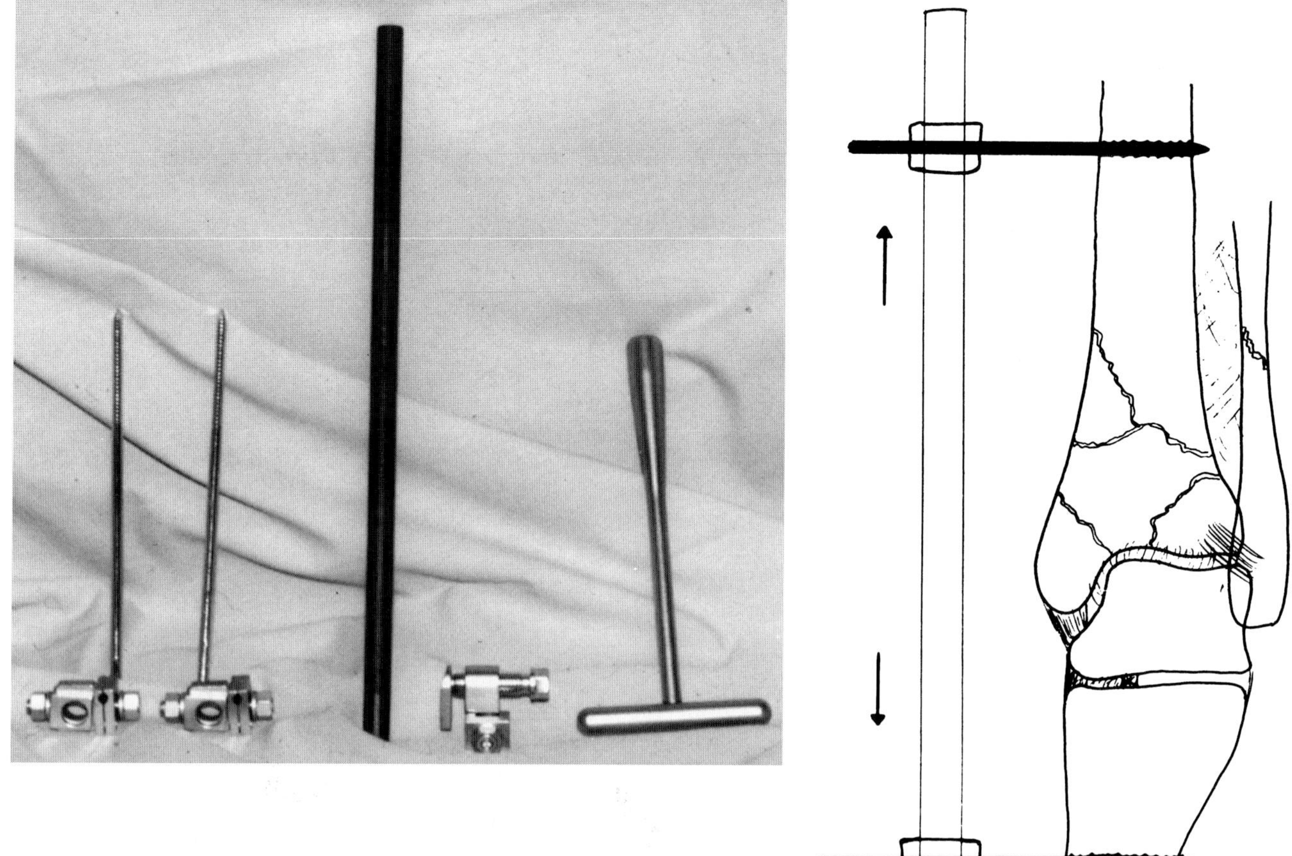

Figure 12. A: The components of the temporary external fixator used for intraoperative distraction. **B:** Ligamentotaxis will usually achieve a nearly anatomic reduction of the metaphysis.

Once the fibula is fixated, attention is turned to the tibia. While the classic tenet of treatment is to plate the fibula first, followed by anatomic reconstruction of the joint, followed by bone grafting and then metaphyseal fixation, I find that metaphyseal and articular reconstruction of the tibia proceed concomitantly. In particular, I look for large metaphyseal fragments that are attached to sizable articular pieces (Fig. 13). These usually occur with the medial malleolus, and also the posterior malleolus. If one can obtain an exact anatomic reduction of these fragments, a useful landmark for the reconstruction of the remainder of the joint is obtained. I find it extremely difficult to reconstruct the joint independently and then attach this segment to the metaphysis. Marginal deformations are corrected by gentle levering with a small osteotome. Bone graft may be packed in above the joint surface to help hold fragments in place (Fig. 14). Laterally, the Chaput tubercle fragment often provides an anatomic reference for the lateral joint line. Fragments may be manipulated with pointed reduction forceps. Posterior malleolar fragments can be a significant challenge and may require a direct posterolateral exposure. This is done through the fibular incision. Small K-wires are introduced through the fragments for provisional fixation, and bone grafting is performed for metaphyseal defects. The K-wires are exchanged for small-fragment lag screws. Cannulated screws can be used. Intraoperative fluoroscopy is routinely used to help assess the joint reduction. Finally, a headlight is essential to see the depths of the joint.

Once the joint is reconstructed, small-fragment plates are used to buttress the metaphysis. Frequently used plates include the one-third tubular, oblique T-plate, and

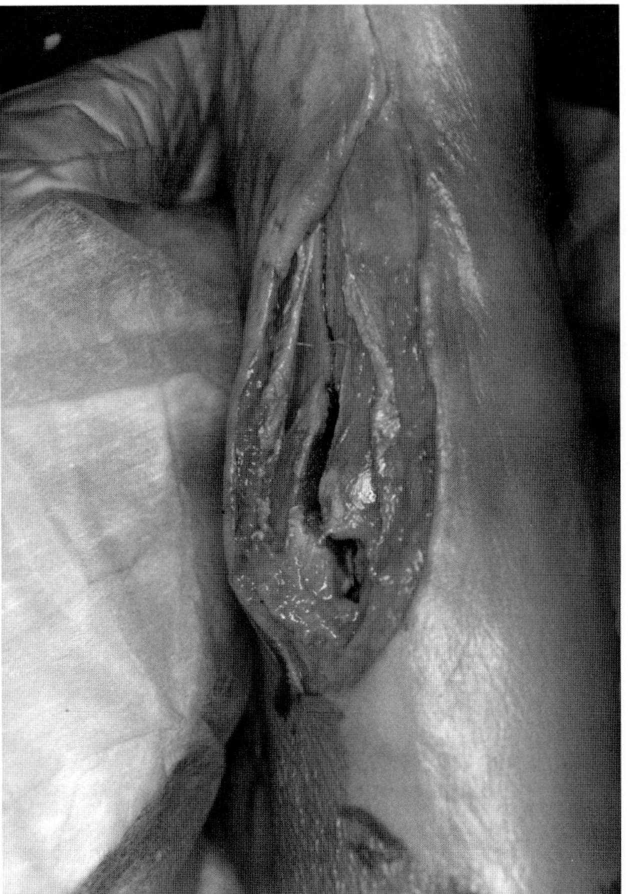
A

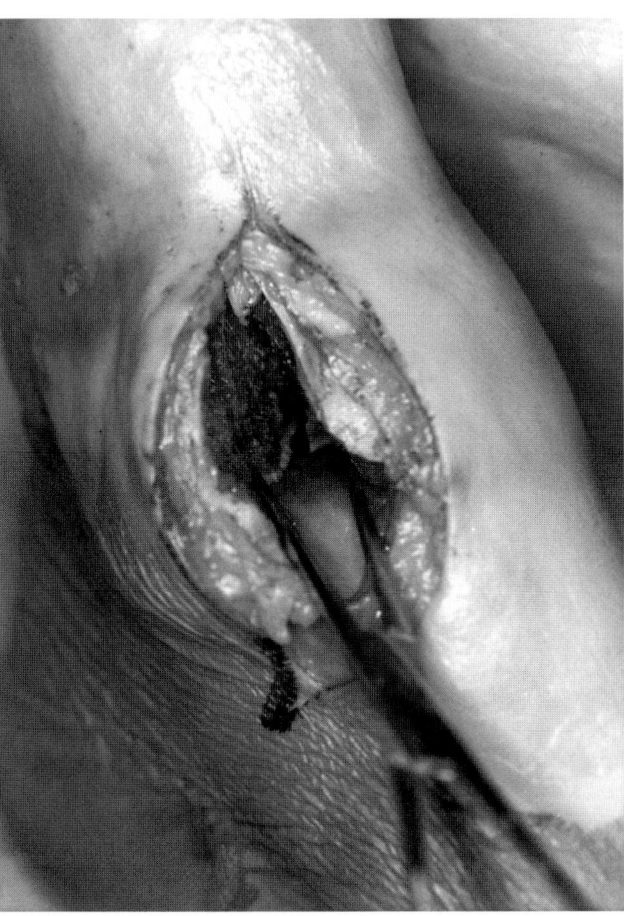
B

Figure 13. The anteromedial incision usually overlies splits in the medial joint. One can then enter the fracture line and hinge the piece back, providing exposure of the joint—the hinged piece remains connected to all its soft tissue connections.

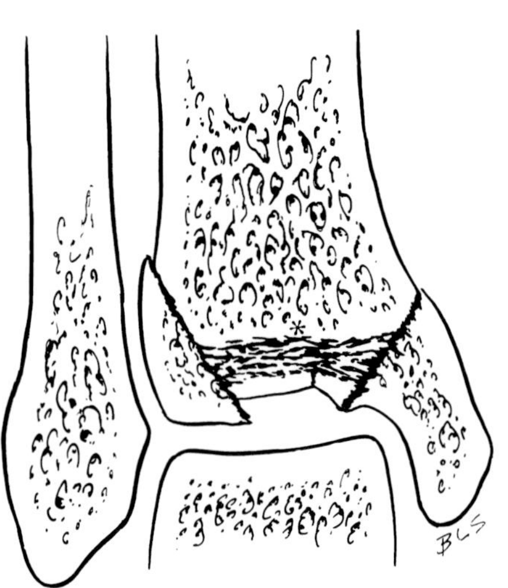

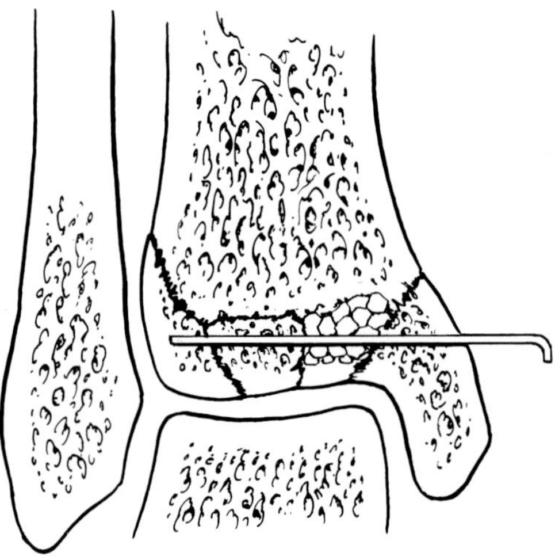

Figure 14. Marginal deformations of the articular surface are reduced and held in place with bone graft. This can now serve as an accurate joint reduction reference. The talus is also a useful template. *, free piece of central articular surface.

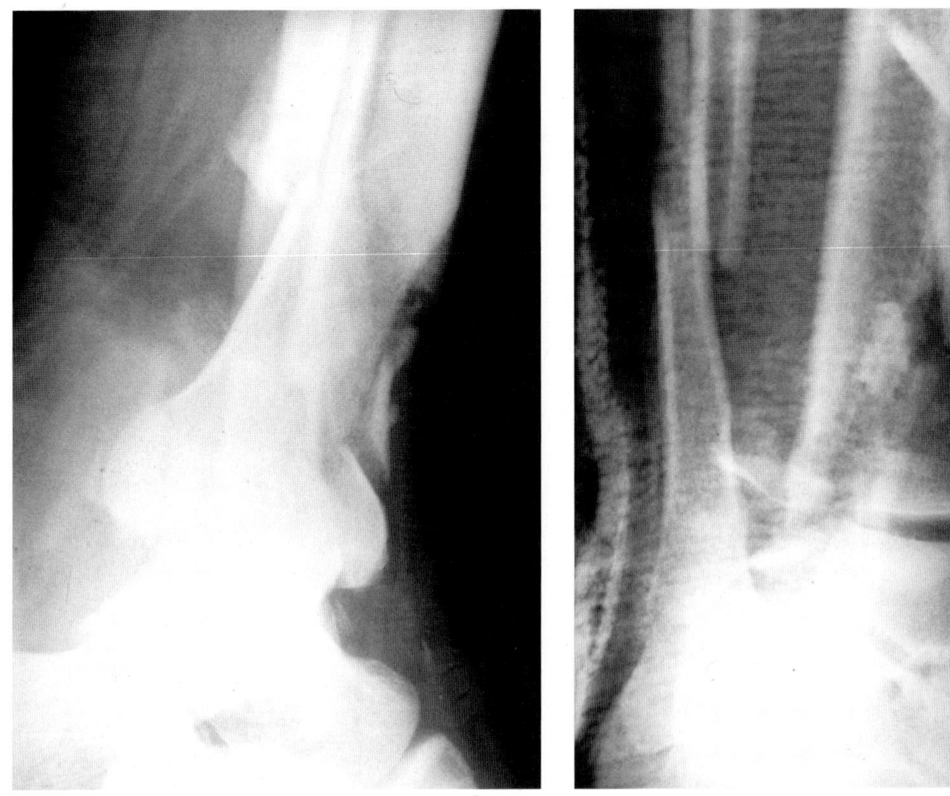

Figure 15. An AO C-3 fracture treated on a delayed basis with open reduction and internal fixation. **A,B:** Injury film.

occasionally the cloverleaf plate. Occasionally, a 3.5-mm D-C plate is used for those fractures with shaft extension. Large-fragment plates are not required for acute fractures. Antiglide plates, compression via plate contouring, and bridge plating are very useful constructs in this area of the skeleton (Fig. 15).

External Fixation

External fixation also has historic precedents and received some interest in the 1960s (15). Because of the complications experienced with ''open surgery,'' this method has recently regained popularity (13,14). If one considers pins and plaster a form of external fixation, this method has a long history. Böhler (11), among others, popularized the *dual pin redresser.* This apparatus applied traction to the leg by tibial and calcaneal pins. Molding of the metaphyseal fragments was performed, followed by a long leg cast incorporating the pins. As with skeletal traction, despite a less than anatomic reduction, some patients retained their ankle joints for many years. Later, in the 1960s, scattered reports of fibular fixation with tibial external fixation appeared. In some instances this was combined with a *limited approach* and a *key fragment fixation* as advocated by Schenk (12). Complications of this method included metaphyseal malunion and pin tract infection. With the modern refinements of external fixation, renewed enthusiasm has arisen for this method. Articulated uniplanar fixators and hybrid fixation utilizing smooth wires have been developed (16,17). The hybrid fixators use small, smooth wires in the distal metaphysis and standard external fixation half-pins in the diaphysis (16). This is often combined with open reduction of the fibula and joint surface. Early results are promising and appear to lessen the incidence of severe complications.

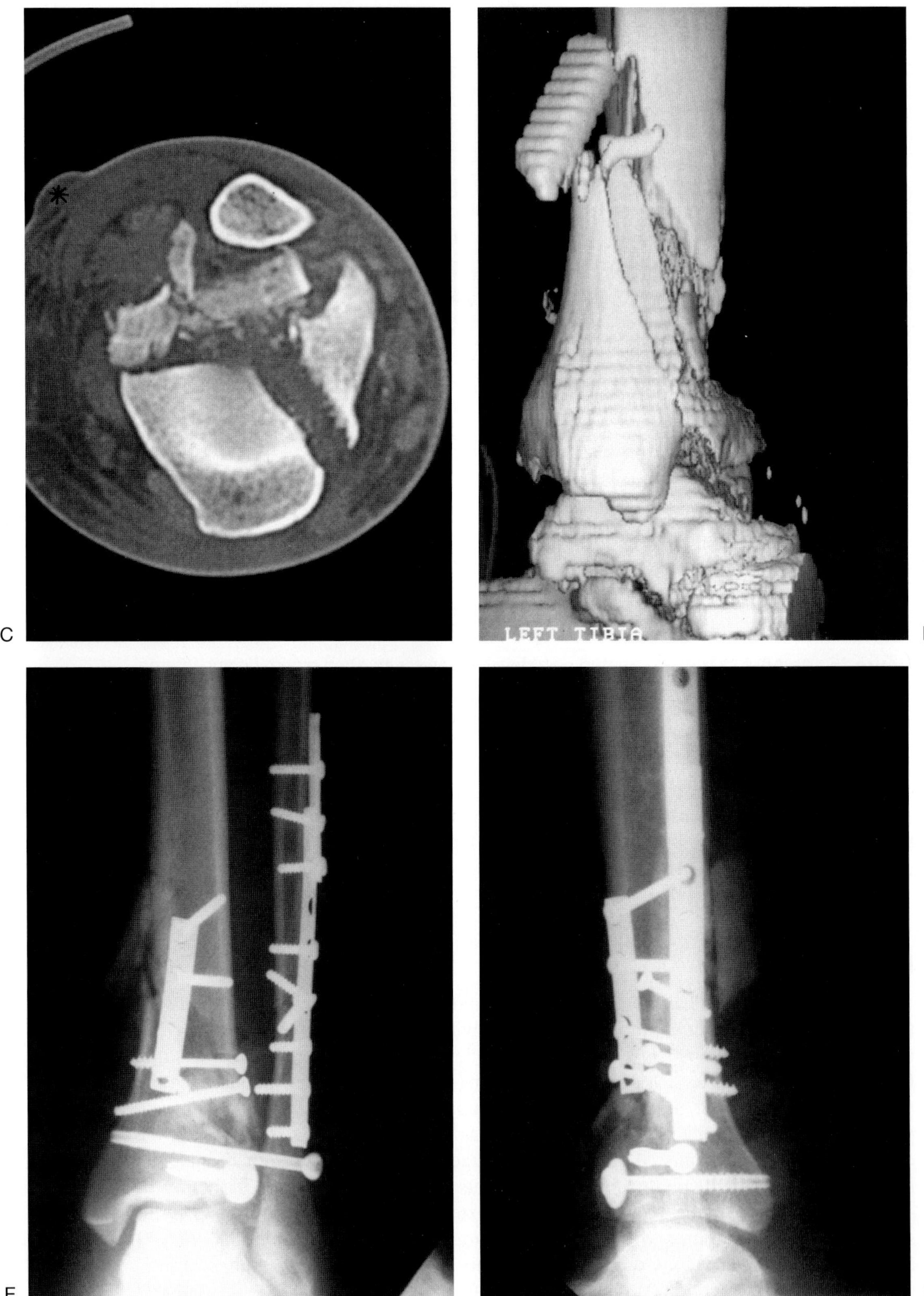

Figure 15. *(continued)* **C,D:** Preoperative computed tomography scan. Note the blister (*) in the area of cortical explosion. **E,F:** Postoperative view. Note medial plate controlling the large medial fragment. Most of the joint reduction was performed using a lateral exposure.

Technique

External fixation may be used in one of two modes:

1. Definitive treatment: external fixation is used instead of calcaneal pin traction. The fracture is pulled out to length via ligamentaxis, and the external fixation is used to maintain the reduction obtained. The frame remains in place for approximately 8 weeks. Overdistraction is avoided. A short leg cast may then be required for full healing. This method is reserved for those injuries deemed ''unreconstructible,'' or for those with such a severe soft tissue injury that primary surgery would entail a significant risk of skin slough or deep infection.

2. The second mode involves the use of an external fixator to neutralize the forces on the tibial side (8,9,16,17). Usually the fibula is approached, plated, and anatomically reduced. One may then perform a limited exposure of the joint surfaces followed by interfragmentary fixation of the key fragments. The goal of an anatomic joint surface must not be compromised. The external fixator is then used to neutralize the remaining forces on the tibial metaphysis until healing occurs. Large half-pins are inserted in the medial tibia, calcaneus, and talus. One must beware of late varus and recurvatum deformities when using this method (Fig. 9).

The technique of hybrid external fixation is very similar, in that fibular fixation and joint reduction are first performed (16). Smooth K-wires are then passed from the fibula through the anteromedial tibia just medial to the anterior tibial tendon. A second wire is passed from just in front of the posterior tibial tendon, out the anterolateral cortex of the distal tibia. The wires are positioned just above the joint surface, but not in the subchondral bone. These wires can then be attached to a circular or semicircular frame and tensioned. The proximal tibia is fixated with half-pins, which are then attached through bars and appropriate rings to the distal frame. Traction may be exerted through the frame and anatomic reduction of the metaphysis obtained. Exposure and stripping of the metaphyseal fragments are avoided, and bone grafting may be used as necessary. This frame remains in place for 8 to 12 weeks depending on the severity of the metaphyseal comminution. Vigilance for pin tract care must be maintained during this time.

Primary Arthrodesis of the Tibiotalar Joint

Primary arthrodesis is a concept that makes intuitive sense for the pilon fracture with extreme comminution (18). It is appealing since it performs the ''inevitable arthrodesis'' early in the course of the injury, rather than waiting for the expected poor result to occur. It has met with limited clinical usage for a number of reasons:

1. Technically, the lack of tibial bone stock makes controlling length and alignment difficult. A long plate or some form of external fixation must be used. Union in this situation is a closely related concern.
2. Although the prognosis is poor for select injuries, it is not uniformly so, and there is morbidity to loss of tibiotalar motion with ankle fusion. As previously stated, the older textbooks on fracture surgery depict long-term follow-up on seemingly destroyed ankle joints that have not required fusion (12).

If a primary fusion is selected, it is best performed when the risk of impaired soft tissue healing is minimized, i.e., on a delayed basis. This may take 4 to 6 weeks in severe injuries. External fixation may be utilized once the bone surfaces are prepared for fusion. Alternatively, a long plate from the talus to the tibia may be utilized. Preservation of the lateral and medial malleolus is recommended.

POSTOPERATIVE CARE

Postoperatively, the foot is splinted in a neutral position. For injuries with rigid fixation, an air brace is used at 2 weeks postoperatively. If fixation strength is in question, a cast is utilized for 6 weeks.

Weight bearing is delayed for 8 to 12 weeks after injury, depending on the comminution present. Therapy is used to regain strength and motion.

For cases treated with external fixation to provide a medial buttress, one must watch carefully for extraarticular malunion. A plating may be required to prevent this complication.

COMPLICATIONS

As previously stated, the pilon fracture has the potential for significant iatrogenic complications. In a recent series, 54% of the operatively treated fractures incurred local complications (2). Most of these were soft tissue-related problems. These complications can be lessened by adhering to the principles outlined in the treatment decision-making section, as well as the recommendations in the open reduction internal fixation section.

Finally, despite the best of treatment, a certain percentage of these injuries will develop posttraumatic arthritis and require ankle fusion. One should always keep this in mind during the treatment. Hopefully, the worst result of nonoperative treatment will be a relatively well-aligned tibia that can then undergo tibiotalar arthrodesis, leaving open the numerous surgical options for this procedure. Clinical results following pilon fractures are related to two factors: the degree of comminution and the exactness of the articular reconstruction. In one review, Ovadia and Beals (7) encountered 70% good and excellent results overall. Importantly, only 60% of patients with class V fractures had good to excellent results. Overall, anatomic fixation gave the most consistent results. Appreciation of these prognostic factors should help one choose the appropriate treatment with realistic goals for the particular fracture at hand.

REFERENCES

1. Destot E. *Traumatismes du pied et rayons malleoles, astragale, calcaneum, avant-pied.* Paris: Masson, 1911:1–10.
2. McFerran M, Smith S, Boulas HJ, Schwartz H. Complications encountered in the treatment of pilon fractures. *J Orthop Trauma* 1992;6:95.
3. Salmon N. *Arteries of the skin.* New York: Churchill Livingstone, 1988:62–67, 151–154.
4. Kellam JF, Wadell JP. Fractures of the distal tibial metaphysis with intra-articular extension: the distal tibial explosion fracture. *J Trauma* 1979;19:593.
5. Bourne RB. Pylon fractures of the distal tibia. *Clin Orthop* 1989;240:42.
6. Ruedi T, Allgower M. Fractures of the lower end of the tibia into the ankle joint: results of nine years after open reduction and internal fixation. *Injury* 1973;5:130.
7. Ovadia DN, Beals RK. Fractures of the tibial plafond. *J Bone Joint Surg [Am]* 1986;68:543.
8. Bone L, Stegeman P, McNamara K, Seibel R. External fixation of severely comminuted and open tibial pilon fractures. *Clin Orthop* 1993;292:101.
9. Ries M, Meinhard B. Medial external fixation with lateral plate internal fixation in metaphyseal tibia fractures. *Clin Orthop* 1990;256:215.
10. Mast J, Spiegel P. Complex ankle fractures. In: Meyers MH, ed. *The multiply injured patient with complex fracture.* Philadelphia: Lea & Febiger, 1984:291–312.
11. Böhler L. *Treatment of fractures,* vol 36. Baltimore: William, Woodard, 1935:446–447.
12. Hamilton WC. Comminuted fractures of the tibial plafond. In: Hamilton WC, et al., eds. *Traumatic disorders of the ankle.* New York: Springer-Verlag, 1984:204–205.
13. Watson-Jones R. Injuries of the ankle. In: Watson-Jones R, eds. *Fractures and other bone and joint injuries.* Baltimore: Williams & Wilkins, 1941:599.
14. Helfet DL, Koval K, Pappas J, Sanders R, DiPasquale T. Intraarticular "pilon" fracture of the tibia. *Clin Orthop* 1994;298:221–228.
15. Scheck M. Treatment of comminuted distal tibial fractures by combined dual-pin fixation and limited open reduction. *J Bone Joint Surg [Am]* 1965;47:537.
16. Tonetta P, Weiner L, Bergman M, et al. Pilon fractures: treatment with combined internal and external fixation. *J Orthop Trauma* 1993;7:489.
17. Bonar SK, Marsh JL. Unilateral external fixation for severe pilon fractures. *Foot Ankle* 1993;14:57.
18. Steihl JB, Dollinger B. Primary ankle arthrodesis in trauma: report of three cases. *J Orthop Trauma* 1988;2:277.

EDITORIAL COMMENTS

The Pilon Fracture

James B. Carr

Dr. James B. Carr has written on his experience with the difficult tibial pilon. The first thing to remember about this fracture is that you can get into trouble; reports in the literature for open reduction and internal fixation average about 35% complication rates. The initial judgment on the reconstructibility of the fracture and soft tissue is of utmost importance. For the reconstructible fractures, timing of surgery is critical; the methods of calcaneal pin traction, elevation, and the recent addition of a foot pump bladder for the plantar plexus intermittent compression all are important in preparation for surgery. The incisions should follow the proper angiosomes, and an 8-cm separation should be maintained. The incision should also be made so that reconstruction is possible if warranted at a later time. The incision should be placed so that if there is skin slough the joint should not be exposed. If necrosis should occur either by injury or by operative intervention, then early coverage, usually by free flap, is mandatory.

When approaching the open reduction, one should not be dogmatic about the stable rigid fixation in this particular fracture. This fracture requires a meticulous soft tissue approach and limited periosteal stripping. Articular restoration of the three or four parts of the fracture is critical; the bone loss gap through the tibia can usually be bridged by later bone grafting and immediate medial fixation. Firm fixation of the fibula will not keep a limited internal medial fixation from going into varus deformity, and these should always be augmented by medial support through external fixation. External fixation should utilize appropriate pin or wire fixators in addition to articular reduction or a medial support. In those cases that are not reconstructible, delay fusion for 6 to 8 weeks at least; surprisingly, some poor articular reductions do fairly well for a certain period. For nonreconstructible cases, the external architecture of the hindfoot and the ankle should be addressed with proper external fixation to avoid varus and difficult late reconstruction or soft tissue and bone contracture. This fracture is always a challenge, and experience has led us to be much more conservative than we have been in the past and to appreciate soft tissue aspects and the zone of injury as well as patient systemic factors.

Robert S. Adelaar, M.D.

Complex Foot and Ankle Trauma,
edited by Robert S. Adelaar,
Lippincott–Raven Publishers, Philadelphia © 1999.

7

Complex Fractures of the Talus

Robert S. Adelaar

Management of talus injuries has always been a challenge because the injury occurs relatively infrequently, the talus is hidden by its anatomic location, making approaches difficult, and the blood supply to the talus is precarious. In this chapter, I give the approach to this injury at the Medical College of Virginia and compare it with current treatment protocols. I emphasize surgical management of the talus and talar neck fractures, which make up over 50% of all talar injuries.

HISTORY OF TALAR INJURIES

The word *talus* has an interesting derivation. Roman soldiers originally made their dice from the heel bones of horses, which became known as the *taxillus* and was eventually shortened to talus. The Greeks made dice from the second vertebrae of sheep and called the bone *astragalus.* Both words, with gambling origins, came to be applied to the same bone in the foot (1). The first account of an accident to the talus was in 1608; Fabricius of Hilden wrote about a man who dislocated his talus (1–3). Many isolated cases have been reported since then; Anderson et al. (4) were the first to collect and classify a series of cases. In 1919, Anderson, a consulting surgeon to the Royal Flying Corps of England, described 18 cases of fractures and dislocations of the talus associated with aircraft accidents (aviator astragalus). Coltart (5), in a review of Royal Air Force studies between 1940 and 1945, reported that of 25,000 fractures and dislocations, 228 were fractures of the talus. Aviator injuries occurred with the foot positioned on the rudder bar in extreme plantar flexion.

Since then many investigators (6–16) have reported series of talar injuries, drawing attention to the problems involved. The modern incidence of talus injuries has been

R. S. Adelaar: Department of Orthopaedics, Medical College of Virginia/Virginia Commonwealth University, Richmond, Virginia 23298.

Reprinted with permission from Adelaar RS. Complex fractures of the talus. In: Springfield DS, ed. *Instructional course lectures.* vol 46. Rosemont, IL: AAOS, 1997:323–338.

Parts of this chapter were reprinted with permission from Adelaar RS. Surgical treatment of fractures of the talus. In: Gould JS, ed. *Operative foot surgery.* Philadelphia: WB Saunders, 1994:377–398.

detailed in a report by the Hanover Medical School (17); 120 talar fractures were seen out of approximately 1,500 complex foot and ankle injuries, as well as over 1,200 ankle injuries and 200 calcaneal injuries. With the advent of mandatory seat belts and more air bags, more of those involved in high-speed crashes survive, which increases the number of injuries to the distal extremities. Almost one-half of talus injuries are secondary to motor vehicle accidents.

ANATOMY

The talus has several anatomic features that predispose it to complex injury (Fig. 1). Because approximately 60% of the talar surface is cartilage, there are often problems with circulation. The talus has seven articular surfaces and is wider anteriorly than it is posteriorly; therefore, dorsiflexion increases stability. However, the talus is weakest at the neck, where the bone is recessed to allow for dorsiflexion. The talar neck deviates medially and is shortened on the medial aspect. The orientation of the talar neck differs from that of the body of the talus in both the horizontal and sagittal planes. In the horizontal plane, the neck shifts medially with a deviation that can range from 10 degrees to 44 degrees, with an average of 24 degrees. In the sagittal plane, the neck deviates downward with range of 5 degrees to 50 degrees and an average of 24 degrees (18). Therefore it is difficult to interpret radiographs with respect to accuracy of reduction. In addition, the alignment of the talus axis affects attempts at screw fixation from the anterior medial approach. Screw fixation is difficult without damaging the navicular, and the short length and the direction of the screw may not give adequate fixation.

When the ankle is plantar flexed, there is increased mobility and anterior instability. In this position, rotational forces may cause subluxation and dislocation. The talar neck is the only extraarticular portion of the talus; it forms a bridge between the posterior and anterior middle facets of the talus. The talocalcaneal ligament is important in stabilizing the talar neck and the distal fragment of talar neck fractures. Dorsal subluxation and varus displacement can occur if this ligament is ruptured. The posterior talocalcaneal ligament is usually the last supporting structure that is ruptured before the body of the talus is completely dislocated from the mortise.

The inferior portion of the talus articulates with the posterior calcaneal articular facet, which keeps the body of the talus in an upright position. The interosseous talocalcaneal ligament plays an important part in reduction of talar neck fractures. The medial and lateral posterior tubercles form a roof over the flexor hallucis longus. The os trigonum is a congenital nonunion of the lateral posterior process and is symptomatic in dancers. The lateral tubercle articulates with the fibula and tibial portion of the mortise; therefore, lateral tubercle injuries can involve articular surfaces. The lateral process also has strong anterior talofibular and posterior talocalcaneal ligamentous attachments (19–21). The lateral process can act as a wedge to disrupt the angle of Gissane or the lateral strut of the calcaneus in calcaneal fractures.

CIRCULATION

Osteonecrosis of the talus is the most harmful complication of talar injuries; to avoid iatrogenic vascular injury, the surgeon must be highly knowledgable of the talus circulation. The blood supply comes mainly from the extraosseous and the intraosseous circulation. The extraosseous circulation, with contributions from the anterior tibial, posterior tibial, and peroneal vasculature, forms a vascular extraosseous ring, described by Wildenaur, around the talar neck and sinus tarsi (22–26). The tarsal sinus artery forms from branches of the anterior tibial artery and peroneal artery. The tarsal canal artery arises from the posterior tibial artery within the deltoid ligament below the medial malleolus (Fig. 2A&B), branching to form the deltoid artery, which is an important source of extraosseous circulation to the body of the talus. Preservation of the deltoid artery is critical during stabilization or reduction of the talar neck and body.

A complete intraosseous anastomosis between all regions of the talus (Fig. 2) has been found in 60% of talar anatomic specimens. The vascular supply varies among the

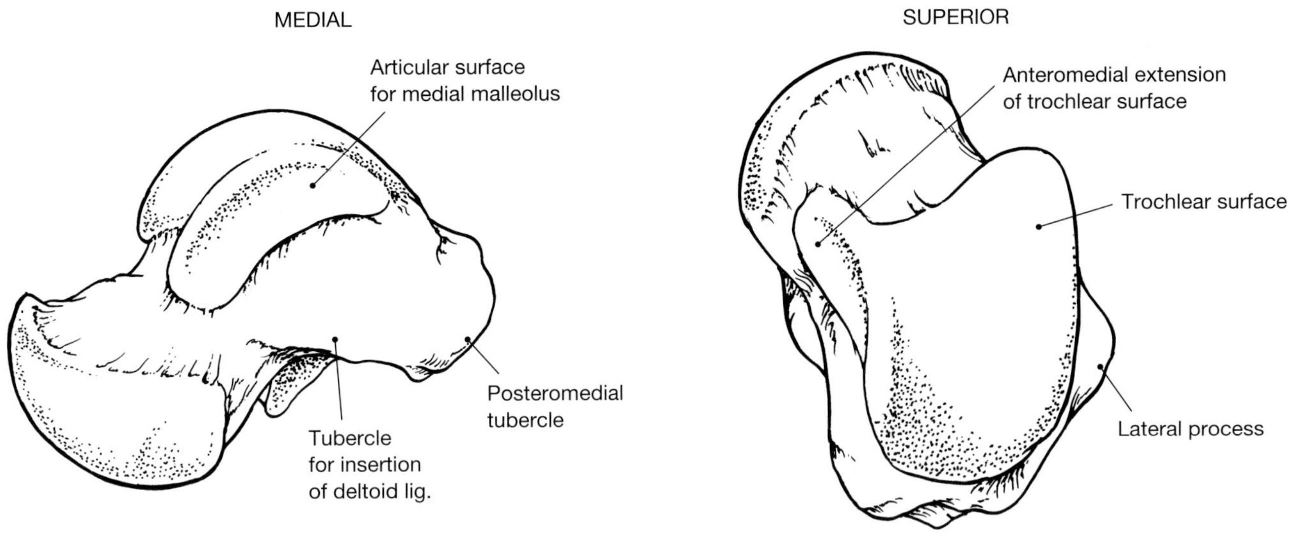

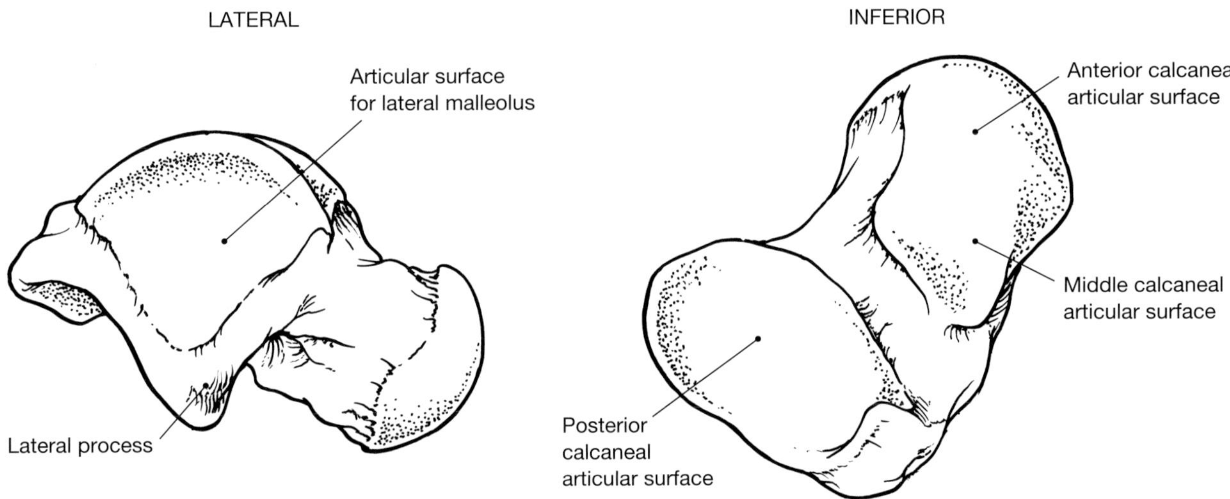

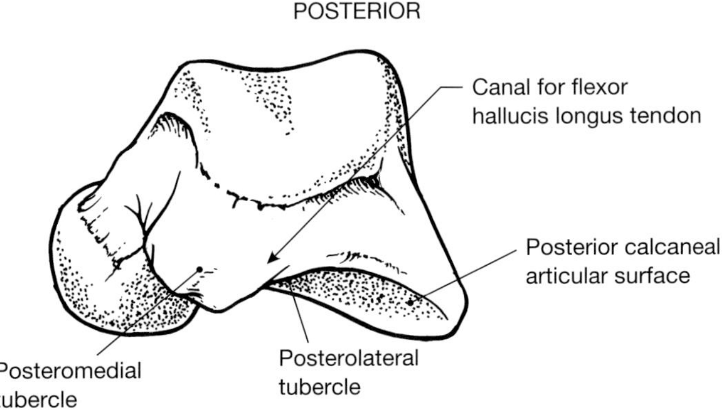

Figure 1. Important anatomic features of the talus.

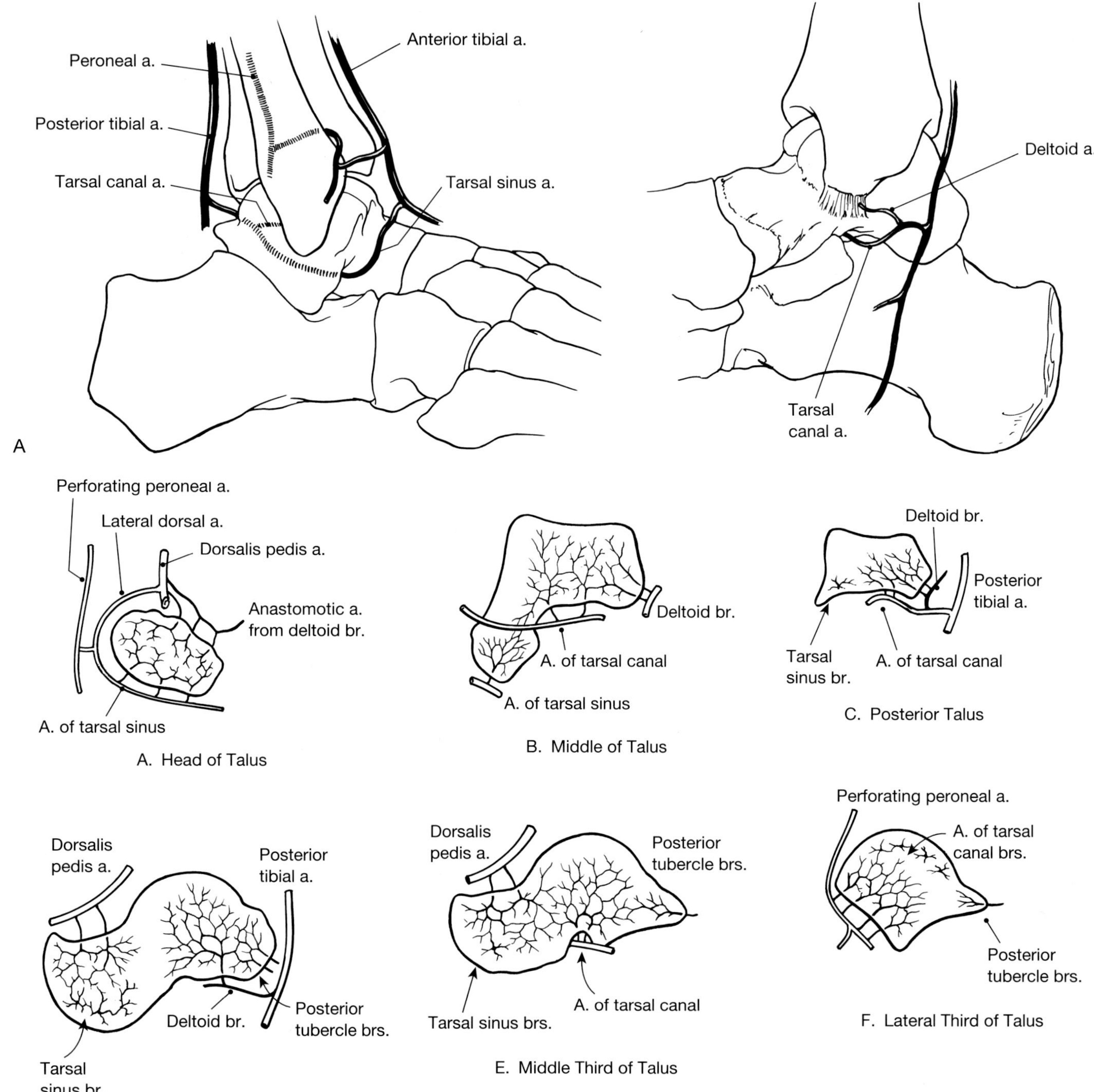

Figure 2. A: The vascular anatomy of the talus from three major vessels. **B:** Deltoid artery branch to body of talus from tarsal canal artery. **C:** Regional blood supply to the talus.

regional sections of the talus. The talar head has an abundant vasculature, which is supplied primarily by the anterior tibial artery. Multiple vascular foramina are seen in the superior and anterior portions of the talar head. The deltoid artery contributes significantly to the interosseous circulation in the medial and proximal portions of the body of the talus. However, the anterolateral surface of the talar body and the posterior tubercles of the talus are relatively avascular.

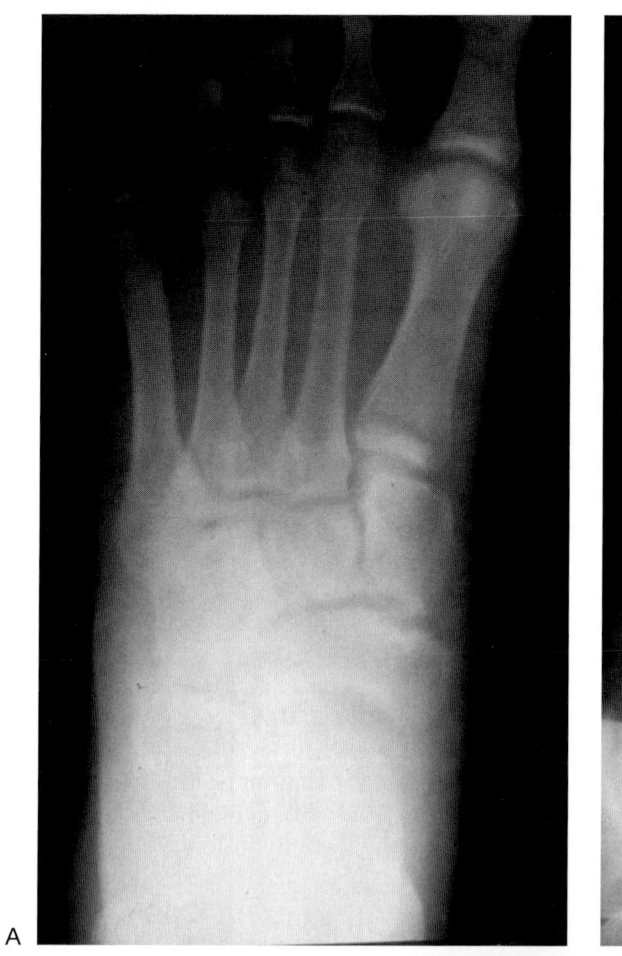

A

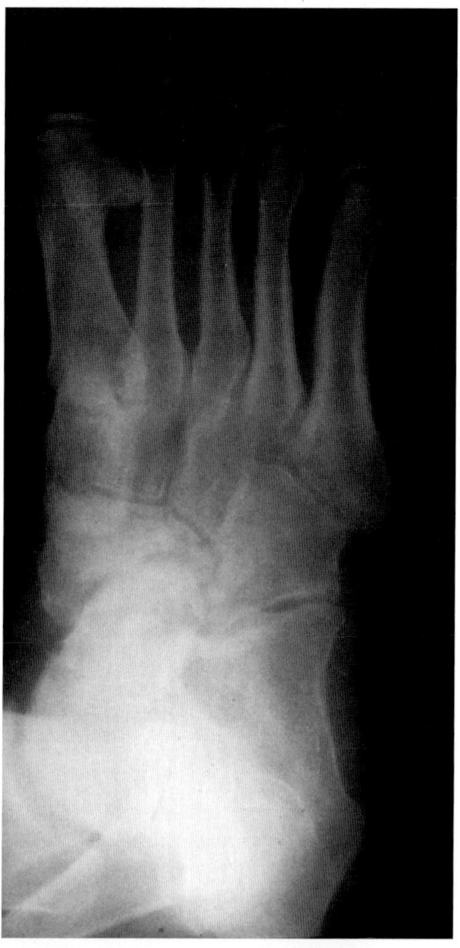

B

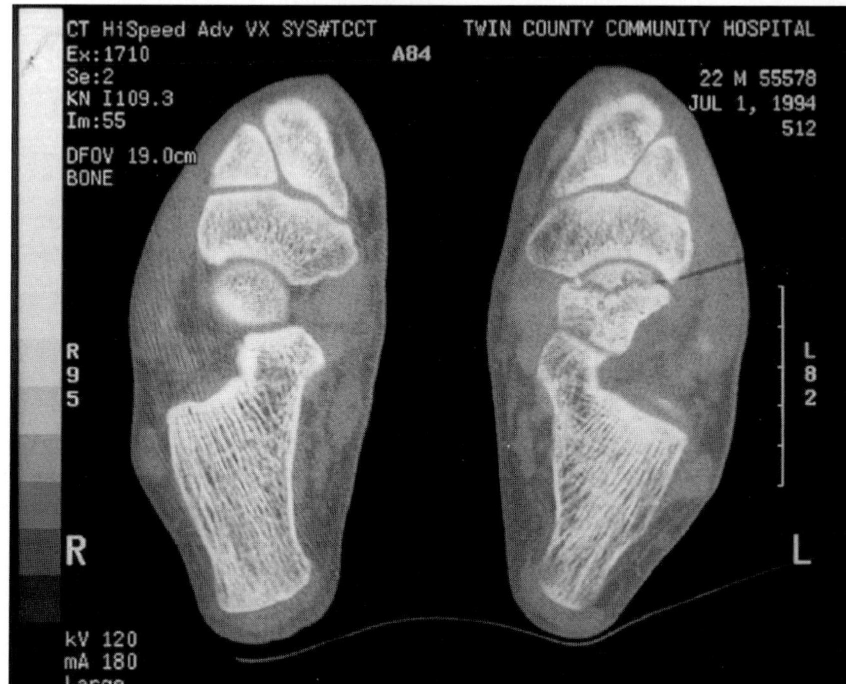

C

Figure 3. A: Radiographic view of the talar head fracture demonstrating an unstable mid-tarsal joint. **B:** A canal view of talar head fracture. **C:** A computed tomography can of talar head fractures.

TALAR HEAD INJURIES

Talar head fractures constitute 5% to 10% of all talar injuries. The mechanism of injury is usually compressive forces secondary to hyperdorsiflexion. Because the talar head is well vascularized, the incidence of osteonecrosis is low. The key problem with this injury is recognition. Instability of the talonavicular joint can be caused by a fracture fragment of greater than 50% (Fig. 3). It is often necessary to obtain special radiographs or Canale views to define the talar neck. Computed tomography (CT) is also used to define the extent and location of injuries. CT is quite helpful in planning for reduction and fixation (Fig. 3).

Unstable talar head fractures, especially those that involve more than 50% of the talar head require rigid fixation (Fig. 4). The surgeon should use a medial approach, taking care not to disturb the posterior tibial tendon attachment to the navicular or spring ligament. A portion of the medial and anterior talonavicular capsule needs to be released. The goal of reduction is rigid fixation to allow early motion after soft tissue healing. Long-term problems with arthrosis are totally dependent on anatomic articular fixation. Subarticular cancellous lag screws are appropriate. Percutaneous K-wires do not provide a stable reduction, and they cause soft tissue problems (Fig. 4B).

Complications that can occur with talar head fractures include instability from nonunion, missed fractures that do not unite, arthrosis of the talonavicular joint as a result of poor articular reduction, and (rarely) osteonecrosis. If complications occur and the fragment cannot be securely fixed, a talonavicular fusion should be considered. The fusion technique that we use at the Medical College of Virginia is screw fixation through the navicular with slotting of a corticocancellous wedge graft from the iliac crest into the talonavicular joint (Fig. 5). In addition, cancellous bone graft is packed into any spaces prior to screw fixation. When attempting a fusion or fracture reduction, it is important not to strip the blood supply entirely from the talar head and to approach the talar head only from the anteromedial aspect. The normal dimensions of the bones should be maintained.

Nondisplaced talar head fractures should be treated nonsurgically. A non-weight-bearing short leg cast is worn for approximately 8 to 12 weeks until healing can be

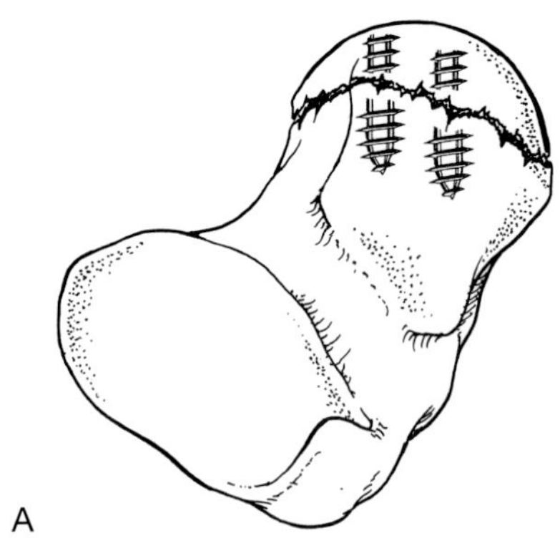

A

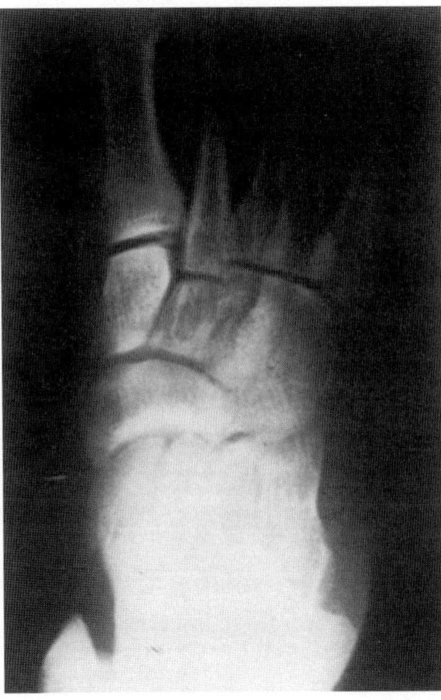

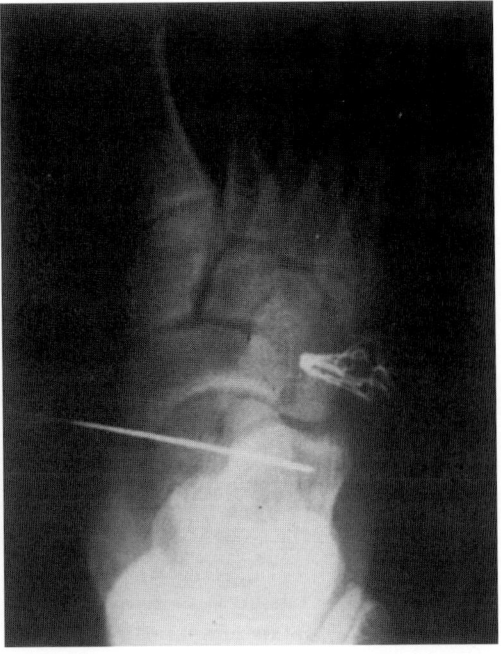

B

Figure 4. A: Talar head fracture can be stabilized with subarticular screws. **B:** Reduction of a talar head fracture with 0.062 K-wires.

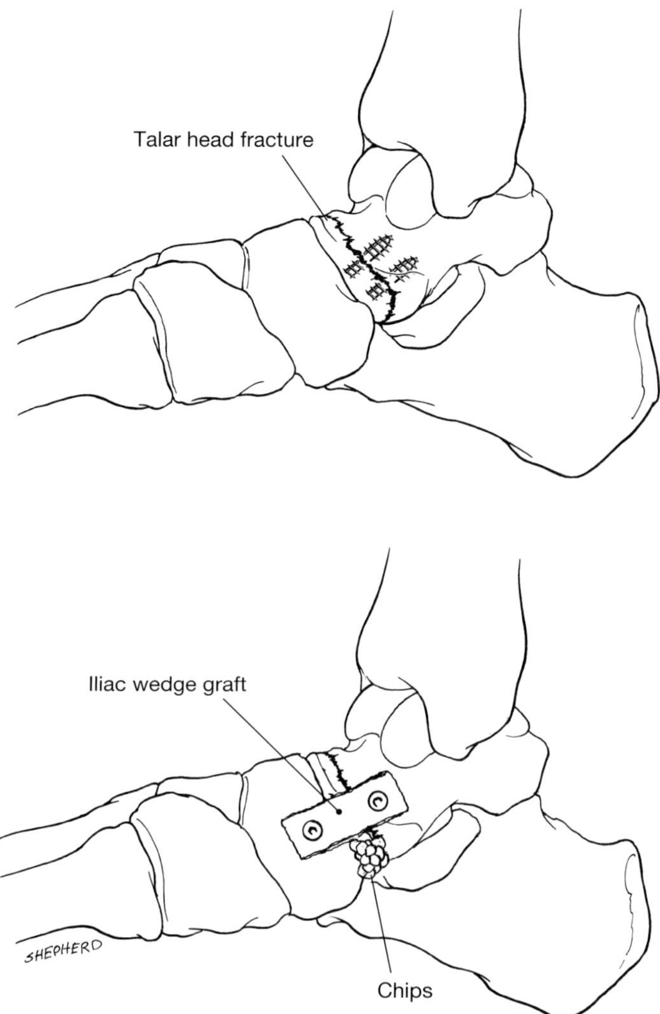

Figure 5. A talonavicular fusion can be performed for articular pain after talar head fracture. A wedge graft is taken from the top of the iliac crest and fixation is with one or two lag screws.

confirmed radiographically. If a displaced fracture involves more than 50% of the talar head, it usually requires internal fixation. If it involves less than 50% with no instability of the talonavicular joint, excision of the displaced fragments can be considered.

TALAR NECK FRACTURES

Talar neck fractures represent approximately 50% of all talar injuries. The principles that apply to the treatment of talar neck injuries also apply to treatment of talar body fractures, with some modifications in exposure. The mechanism of injury has been described as a dorsiflexion of the foot against a stationary tibia (Fig. 6) with impingement of the talar neck, or trochlea, which is the weakest area on the tibial dome (Fig. 7). As this force continues, there is usually medial and dorsal comminution of the talus, disruption of the talocalcaneal ligament, and disruption of the posterior and subtalar capsule. Supination of the ankle with impingement of the talar neck against the medial malleolus will cause subluxation of the subtalar joint and comminution of the medial neck (18). This usually occurs in class II or III injuries (Fig. 8 II and III) (13). When the talar body dislocates, it is usually found at the posteromedial aspect of the Achilles tendon, where it can compress

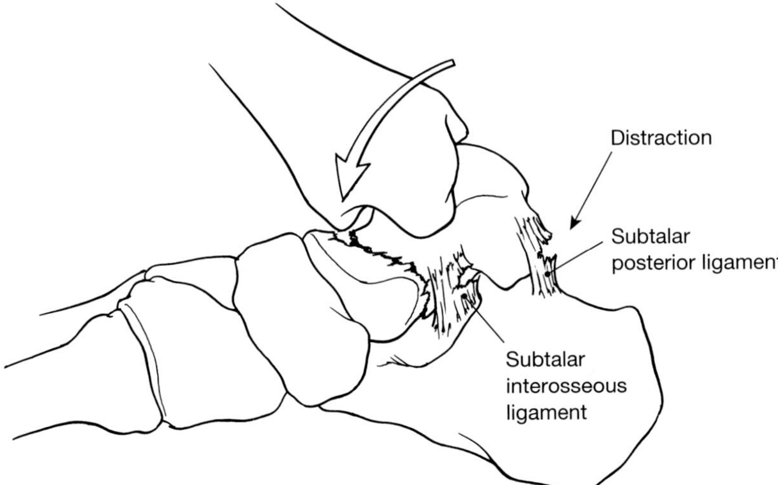

Figure 6. The mechanism of injury for most talar neck fractures is hyperdorsiflexion with an axial load. After impingement of the trochlea (the talar neck) on the tibia, the posterior capsule is put under stretch and supination occurs, thereby stabilizing the subtalar joint.

the adjacent neurovascular structures. Talar neck fractures can also occur from direct blows.

In laboratory experiments, it was difficult to produce talar neck fractures by wedging the talus against the tibial dome in dorsiflexion. These fractures could not be produced unless the ankle was in a neutral position and ankle motion was eliminated by compressing the calcaneus against the overlying talus and tibia (18,27). Peterson and associates (27) felt that these forces could be reproduced in an extended leg if the triceps surae was contracted. Supination forces are more commonly associated with higher classes of Hawkins injuries because they produce fracture dislocation patterns and often cause a direct pushoff injury to the medial malleolus. Fractures of the medial malleolus and lumbar spine injuries have been found in association with talar neck injuries.

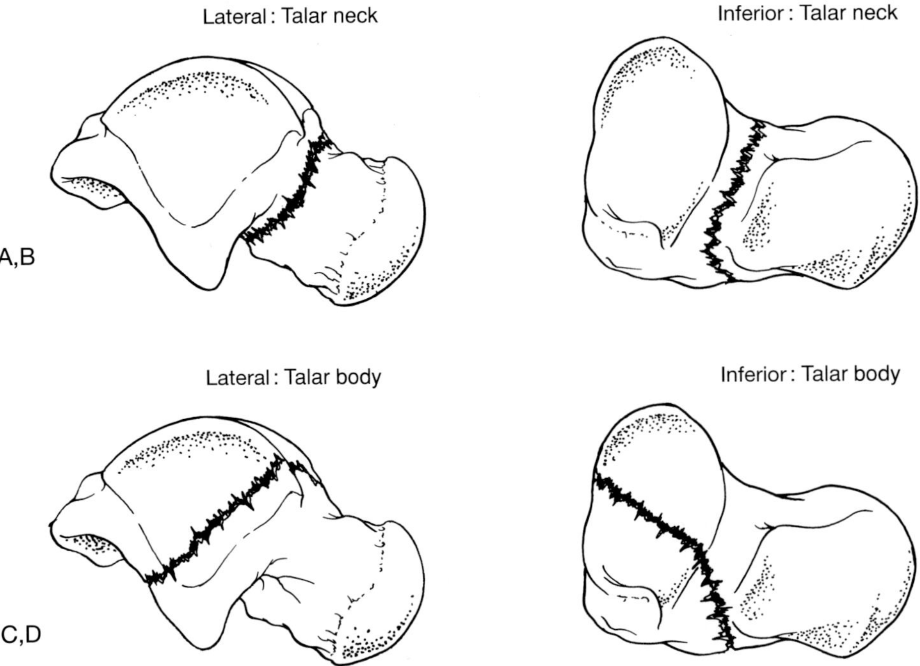

Figure 7. The difference between talar neck (**A** and **B**) and body fractures (**C** and **D**) is dependent on whether the fracture exits in the posterior articular joint.

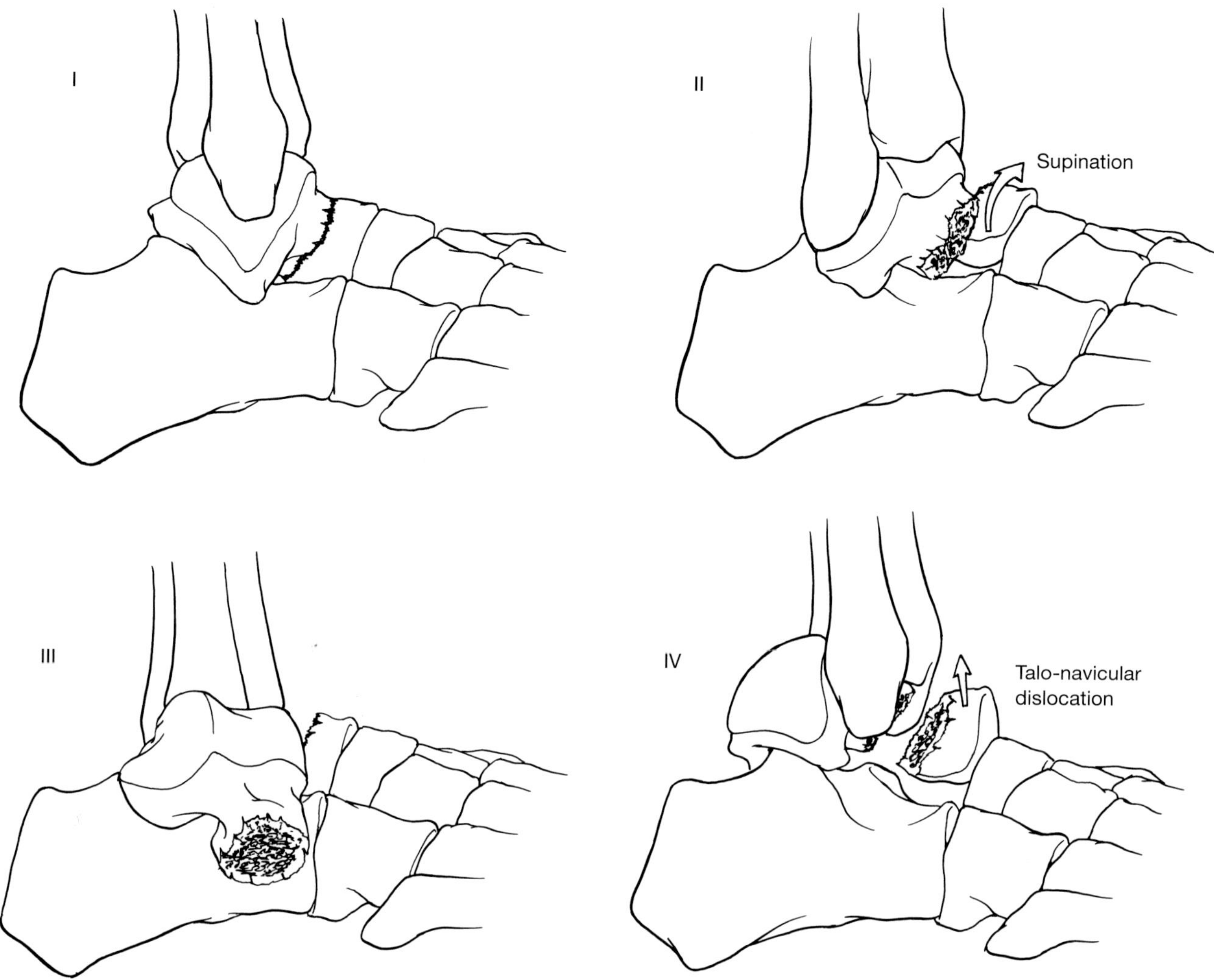

Figure 8. *I,* Nondisplaced; *II,* neck fracture with displacement; *III,* displaced neck with subtalar ± ankle dislocation; *IV,* type II or III with talonavicular subluxation.

Classification

The Medical College of Virginia uses a modified Hawkins classification (Fig. 8) (13). A class I injury is a nondisplaced vertical neck fracture with no subluxation; a class II injury displays mild dorsal displacement of the distal talar neck fragment with subluxation of the subtalar joint (Fig. 9A,B); and a class III injury involves displacement of the talar body with associated subtalar subluxation and talar neck displacement (Fig. 9C). As the displacement of the talar neck increases, the incidence of malunion, osteoarthritis, and osteonecrosis increases (9,11,28,29). The talocalcaneal ligament is ruptured when dorsal displacement of the distal fragment is present. With rupture of this ligament, it is difficult to control the talar neck by closed means because of the supination deformity or varus and comminution that occur. Open techniques are recommended when it is not possible to achieve anatomic reduction and when there is at least 3 mm of dorsal displacement and 5 degrees of varus rotation. Another type of talar neck fracture has been observed by Canale and Kelly (12), who noted that a talonavicular dislocation could accompany a Hawkins class II or III injury. This has been called a Hawkins class IV injury.

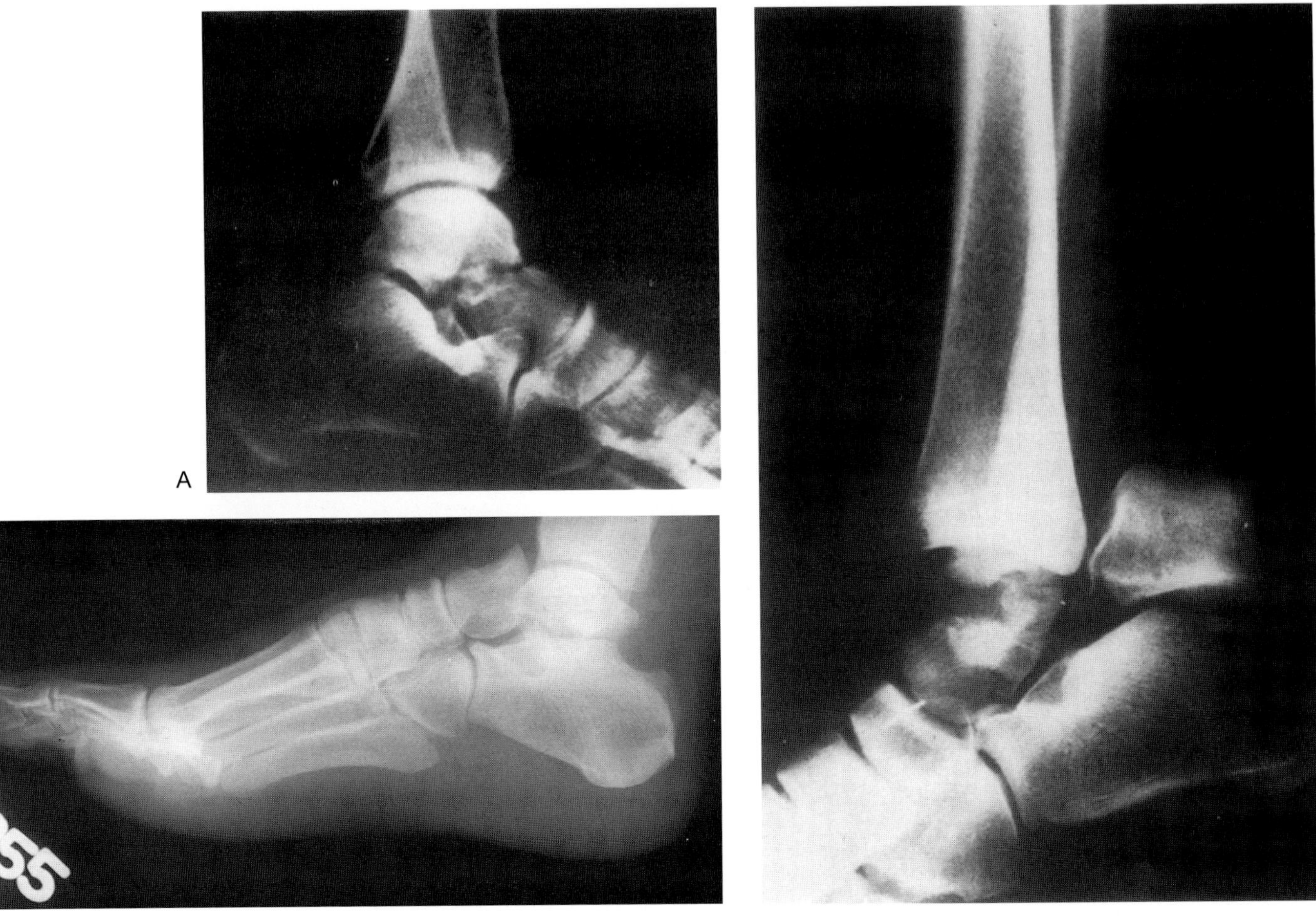

Figure 9. A: Type I Hawkins. **B:** Type II Hawkins. **C:** Radiograph of the class III injury with disruption of the talocalcaneal ligaments and subluxation or frank dislocation of the subtalar and ankle joints.

TALAR NECK MALALIGNMENTS

When reducing talar neck fractures, it is very important to maintain alignment of the talar neck; this is often difficult because of the comminution: the higher grades of injury are associated with a supination mechanism that impacts the talar neck against the medial malleolar and causes comminution on the medial side (18,30). Because the talus articulates with three facets of the calcaneus, a malalignment may alter the mechanical relationships and lead to future degeneration. Alterations in alignment may be responsible for delayed degenerative arthrosis in the subtalar joint and ankle.

To avoid the complications, we advocate the use of anterolateral and anteromedial incisions to address the neck comminution and rotational malalignment. Because supination often plays a role in the higher grades of injury, rotation of the neck will occur. Subtalar instability also occurs and needs to be addressed in the reduction. When using a posterolateral approach, an anteromedial or anterolateral approach is also necessary to achieve temporary reduction and to check alignment. The Canale view provides the best check for neck malalignment; it is often difficult to judge small degrees of malrotation using the image intensifier or routine radiograph. The importance of good talar neck alignment was brought out by a recent laboratory study in which certain degrees of malalignment were fixed into the talar neck reduction and contact stress areas were evaluated. It was found that there was a change in the weight-bearing load pathway and in the contact stresses and peak pressures of the subtalar joint with talar neck malalignment.

Treatment

Class I Injury

Class I injuries occur when there is a minimal displacement of the distal fracture fragment. These injuries can usually be treated by closed means with an anatomic reduction that includes correction of the minimal dorsal displacement and talar neck supination. The incidence of osteonecrosis is low (10%) because the circulation is usually intact (2,3). If an anatomic reduction is obtained, as confirmed by appropriate radiographs, a cast can be used for treatment until trabeculation is demonstrated. Weight bearing is allowed only after trabeculation occurs across the talar neck because of the problem of shear force with weight bearing before trabeculation, particularly with rigid fixation. If anatomic reduction cannot be obtained, or if there is significant comminution, open or percutaneous reduction with screws can be used. An anteromedial or anterolateral approach should be used to achieve provisional K-wire reduction, and it can be combined with a posterolateral approach fire screw insertion for improved fracture mechanics.

The classic approach to the talar neck fracture has been the anteromedial approach (Fig. 10). There is a safe interval adjacent to the anterior tibial tendon. The incision may need to be extended to the ankle joint, and care should be taken to avoid any periosteal stripping. The problem with this approach is the difficulty in obtaining good biomechanical fixation at the fracture site because the talar neck is deviated and shortening in a medial direction. The threads of the screws usually exit the lateral cortex just proximal to the fracture and do not give adequate compression in a axis perpendicular to the fracture site. Although I do not believe there is any place for K-wire

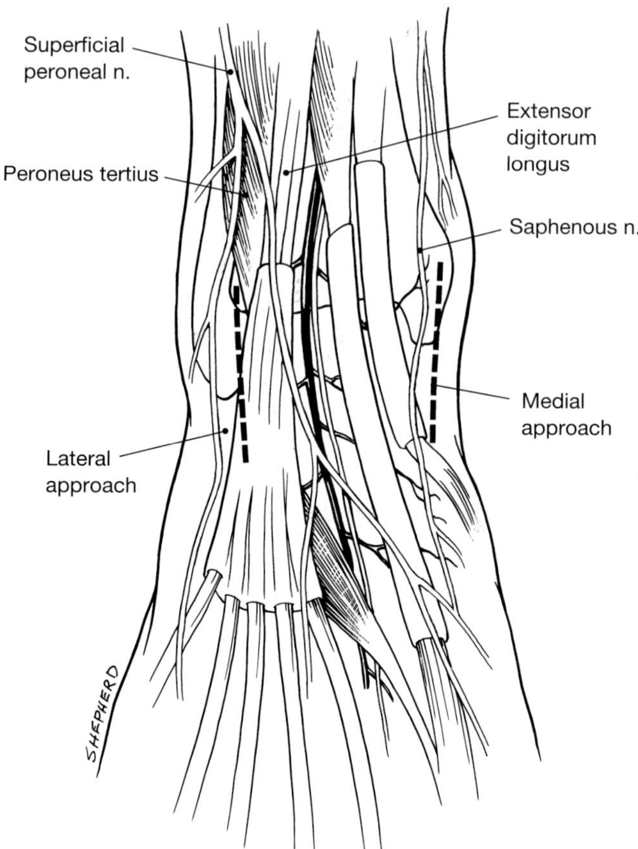

Figure 10. An anteromedial approach to the talar neck fracture through the interval between the anterior tibial and extensor hallucis longus tendons, avoiding neurovascular bundles. Care should be taken not to do a great deal of stripping on the talar neck.

fixation alone in open treatment, K-wires (0.062) can often be used in combination with an appropriate threaded screw to supply some rotational stability (Fig. 11A). At our institution, 4.5- to 6.5-mm titanium cannulated screws have been very helpful. Other centers have felt that fully threaded screws were much stronger, but we have had no problem with breakage. It is important to restate that lateral, anterior, and oblique radiographs with a Canale view should be obtained for each patient at the conclusion of treatment because the image intensifier may often fail to give an accurate picture of the reduction.

The anterolateral approach is a better approach for fixation of the fracture (Fig. 11B). This approach is preferred in higher grades of injury, in which the medial neck is often comminuted and the lateral aspect is not. When there is subtalar injury, the sinus tarsi may have bone fragmentation that needs debridement. The problem with this approach is the risk of causing damage to the anterior tibial perforating vessels and the superficial branch of the peroneal nerve. The anterolateral approach is appropriate for higher grades of injury, particularly when there is medial comminution or sinus tarsi debris.

A posterolateral approach, which was described by Trillat and associates (31), has been used in combination with an anteromedial open or closed manipulation of the fracture site (32,33). In the posterolateral approach (Fig. 12A), using an image intensifier, the patient is placed in the prone or lateral position, and the incision is made lateral to the heel cord. The enlarged lateral posterior process of the talus adjacent to the flexor hallucis muscle mass is identified. After fracture reduction with an anteromedial or anterolateral incision and provisional K-wire fixation, titanium cannulated screws are used (Figs. 12B and 13).

Another technique used is opening the fracture and, with the patient in the lateral position and using the anteromedial approach, passing K-wires retrograde across the proximal fracture and out the posterolateral aspect. The problem with this approach is that the cannulated K-wires are often not directed out the appropriate posterolateral tubercle.

We have found that it is difficult to obtain a good closed reduction. Therefore, a combined anteromedial or anterolateral approach should be used to open the fracture

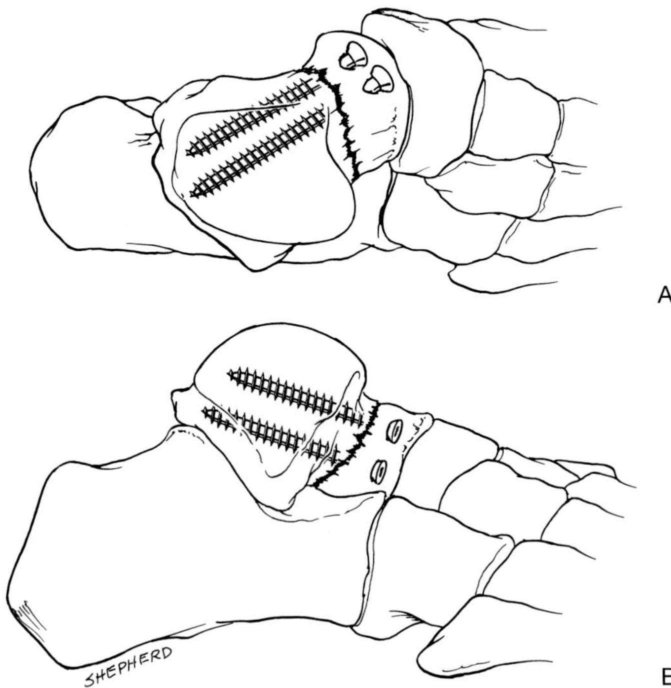

Figure 11. A: Fixation of a talar neck fracture with cannulated screw from the anterolateral approach to the talar neck. **B:** An anterolateral approach to the talar neck.

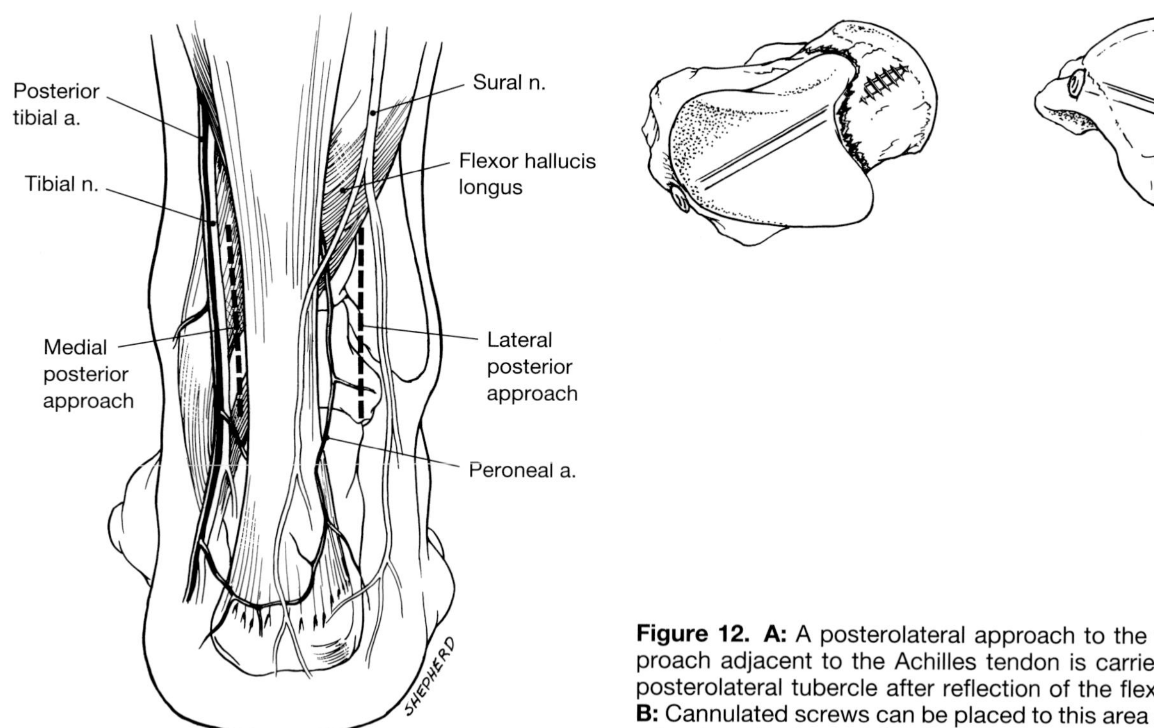

Figure 12. A: A posterolateral approach to the talus. A lateral approach adjacent to the Achilles tendon is carried out down to the posterolateral tubercle after reflection of the flexor hallucis longus. **B:** Cannulated screws can be placed to this area at a biomechanical advantage for fracture fixation.

and hold it anatomically. We believe that no important blood supply is violated by either the anteromedial or the posterolateral approach. Once again, it is important to obtain good radiographs at the conclusion of treatment, particularly an oblique film, as described by Canale and Kelly (12), before accepting a closed or open reduction.

In summary, closed reduction should never be done in displaced injuries. We do not use K-wires as a sole mean of fixation because they have been found to be much weaker than screws. Histomorphic analysis has shown that bone density is greatest in the lateral portion of the head and inferior lateral portion of the body (34). Screws inserted from posterior to anterior provide better biomechanical fixation than those inserted from anterior to posterior (34). We recommend the use of titanium screws (35). The approach depends on the location of the comminution and the fracture type. We feel that a posterolateral approach gives the best biomechanical fixation. An anteromedial or anterolateral approach should accompany this approach to ensure an accurate reduction.

Class II Injury

The disruption of the talocalcaneal ligament in class II injuries makes it difficult to obtain a closed anatomic reduction (Fig. 9). Open reduction is indicated in the presence of 3 mm of dorsal displacement or any rotational deformity that will impede the ability to obtain an accurate closed anatomic reduction. The anteromedial or anterolateral approach is combined with a posterolateral approach for screw fixation. It is critical to obtain an anatomic reduction and to ensure that the subtalar joint has been reduced.

Postoperative care of patients with class II injuries is directly related to the biomechanical rigidity of fixation. With rigid fixation, the patient should be encouraged to immediately start normal motion with action and passive motion, but then a short leg cast should be used. It is important that no weight bearing be allowed for at least 3 months or until trabeculation is demonstrated to avoid shear forces. At 8 weeks, the orthopaedic surgeon should evaluate an anteroposterior (AP) or mortise view to determine signs of vascularization (Hawkins sign) (13) (Fig. 14).

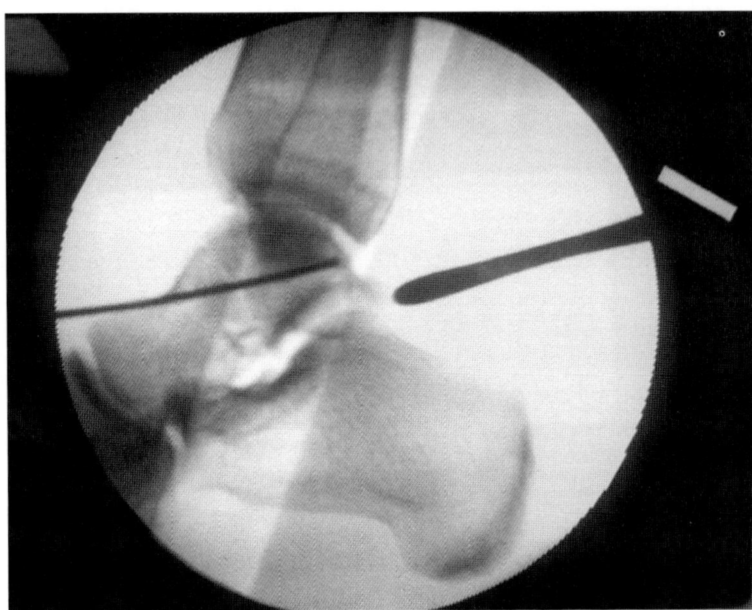
A

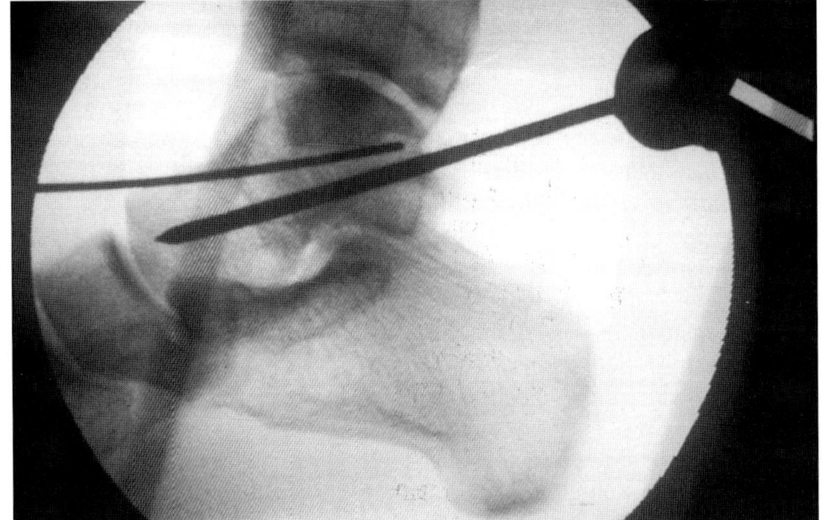
B

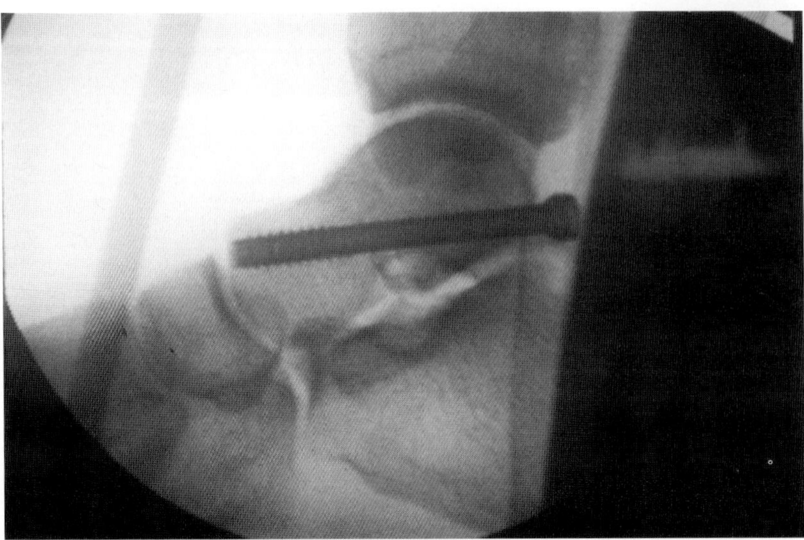
C

Figure 13. Fixation from the posterolateral approach provides the best biomechanical fixation for fractures of the talar neck and body. The screws are usually firmly fixed in the talar head at an angle between 90 degrees and 45 degrees. The posterolateral approach with use of image intensifier and fixation with large titanium cannulated screw. **A:** Position pin near tubercle. **B.** Cannulated pin is placed in from posterior lateral. **C:** Cannulated screw is then placed in.

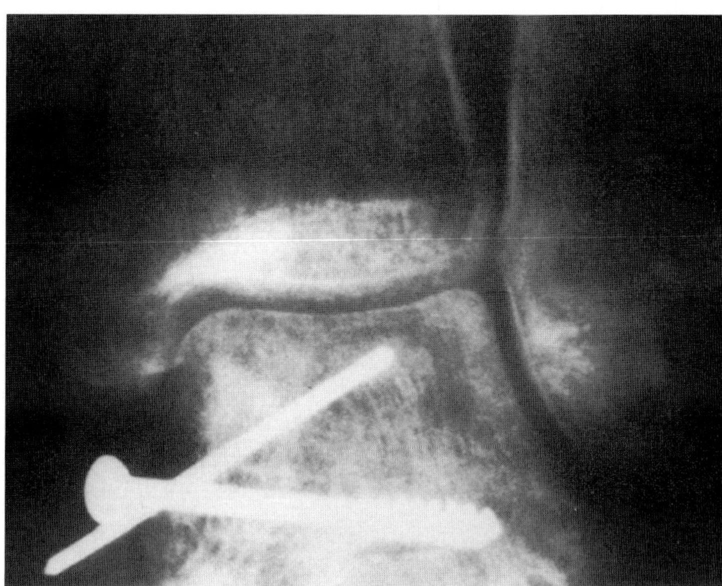

Figure 14. A mortise view of the ankle between 6 and 10 weeks after injury can show evidence of some resorption, which indicates revascularization of the body of the talus (Hawkins sign).

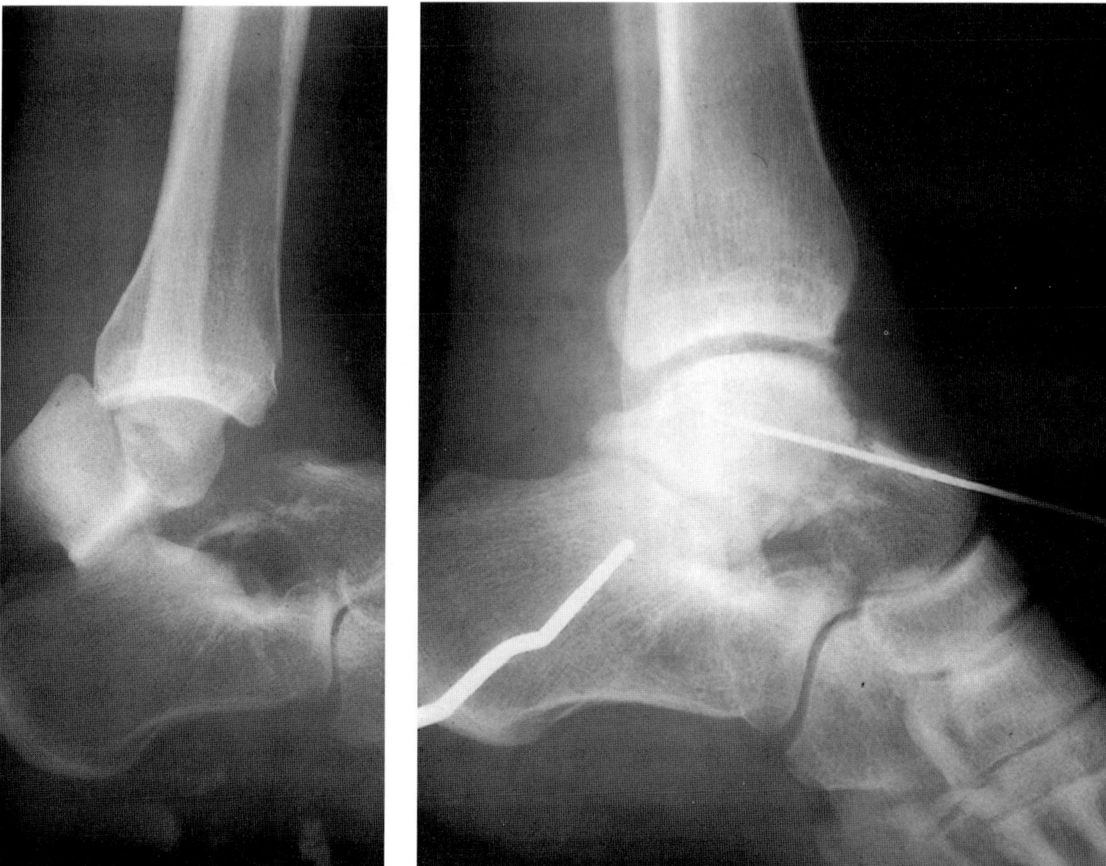

Figure 15. A: Closed reduction techniques are used for initial reduction of a class III injury in which the talus has been dislocated, usually in the medial direction. **B:** Traction is usually applied with a pin through the os calcis in combination with equinus positioning and rotation to allow the talar body to be relocated in the subtalar joint. Getting the body over the posterior articular process is sometimes difficult, and a femoral distractor may be necessary.

Class III Injury

In class III talar neck fractures, the talar body and subtalar joint subluxate or dislocate (Fig. 15). A large percentage of these injuries are open (50%), and the incidence of osteonecrosis has been reported to be greater than 50% (2,3,7). The body of the talus should be reduced by open reduction as soon as possible to decrease the stress on the medial neurovascular bundle. It is important not to injure the deltoid vessels. Manipulation requires the use of an os calcis traction pin and external fixator or femoral distraction (Fig. 15). This reduction can be difficult, requiring traction, equinus, and rotation. The associated soft tissue injuries are usually debrided and left open if they do not violate a joint space or tendons. If the talar body cannot be relocated from its displaced position by closed manipulation, a posterior medial incision is required. The neurovascular bundle is retracted, and direct manipulation of the body of the talus is attempted. K-wires can be used to hold the body of the talus in the mortise temporarily and as a joy stick to reduce it. A femoral distractor is also helpful in cases that resist closed attempts (Fig. 16).

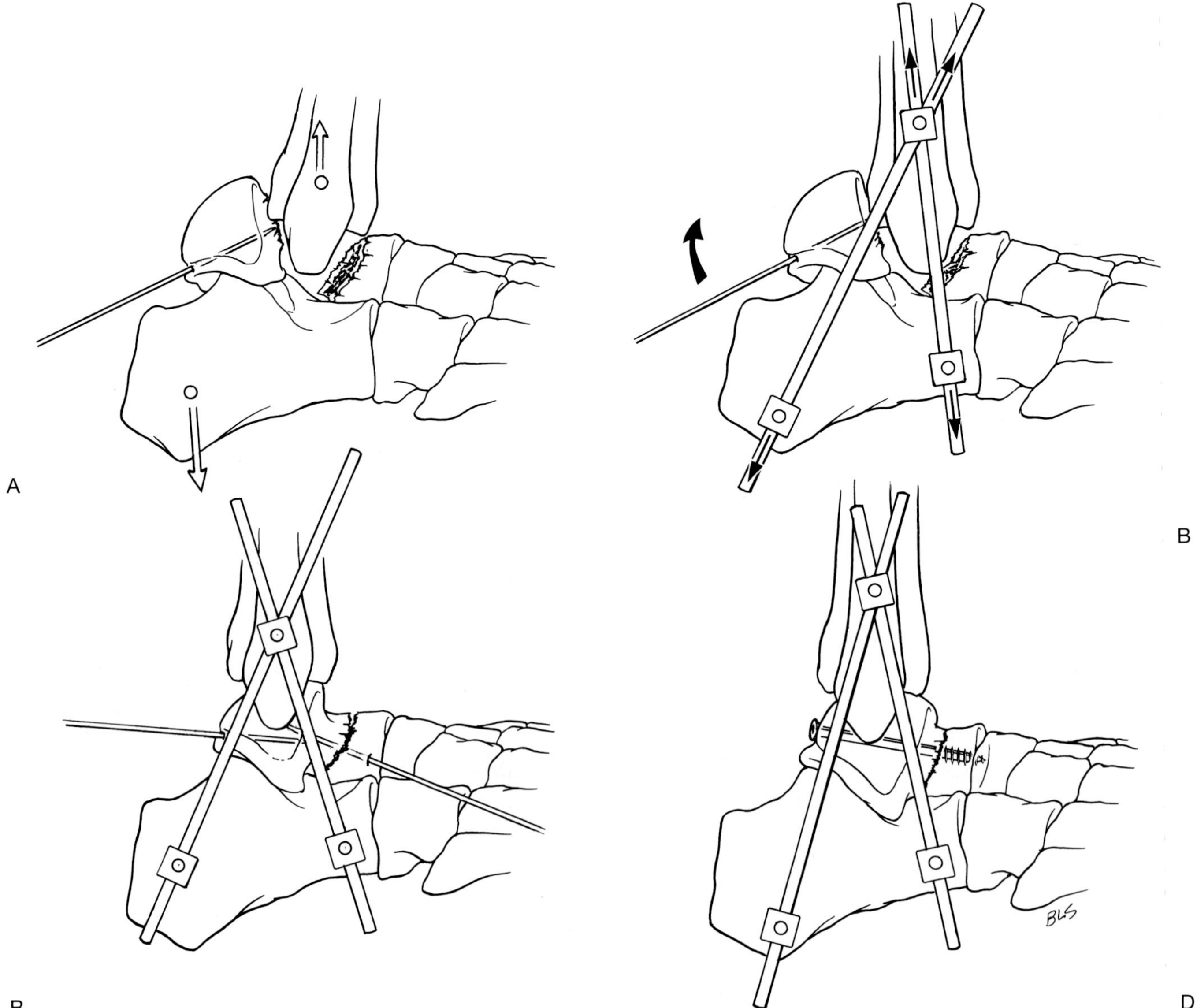

Figure 16. A–D: A femoral distractor is used for difficult class III injuries to hold the anatomic height of the hindfoot. It can be used whether or not the talar body is available for reinsertion into the mortise.

Complications

Complications that occur with talar neck fractures are delayed union, nonunion, malunion, subtalar and ankle arthritis, and osteonecrosis. Reports of long-term complications from this injury (9,15,16,18,28,29,36) indicate that osteonecrosis occurred in only 10% of nondisplaced fracture cases but approached 70% when there was significant displacement. Delayed unions and malunions (Fig. 17A–D) occurred primarily in class II and III injuries, and the incidence of subtalar arthritis (Fig. 17E,F) also became higher as the grade of injury increased. The major morbid complication of a talar neck fracture is osteonecrosis.

Osteonecrosis

Osteonecrosis has been shown to increase with severity of injury (9,29). The Hawkins sign has been described as evidence of revascularization and is felt to be a specific, reliable early indicator of vascular viability with few false negatives. This sign of patchy subchondral osteoporosis usually occurs in 6 to 8 weeks and can be visualized radiographically on the AP or mortise view but not on the lateral view, because it is obscured by the fibula (Fig. 14) (13,37). Magnetic resonance imaging (MRI) has been used to diagnose and quantify the degree of osteonecrosis. We usually recommend waiting at least 3 months until bone healing is present before doing an MRI. MRI has been very sensitive, and few false-negative reports have been published (35). In trabecular bone, the marrow elements are predominantly fat cells. The fat cells are responsible for the strong T_1-weighted images, and MRI is sensitive to altered fat cell signals because marrow necrosis is an early part of osteonecrosis (Fig. 18).

The determination of when to put weight on the talus is made from radiographic evidence of bone healing or trabeculation. The method of weight bearing, whether it is foot flat or associated with a patella tendon brace or with some type of ankle orthosis

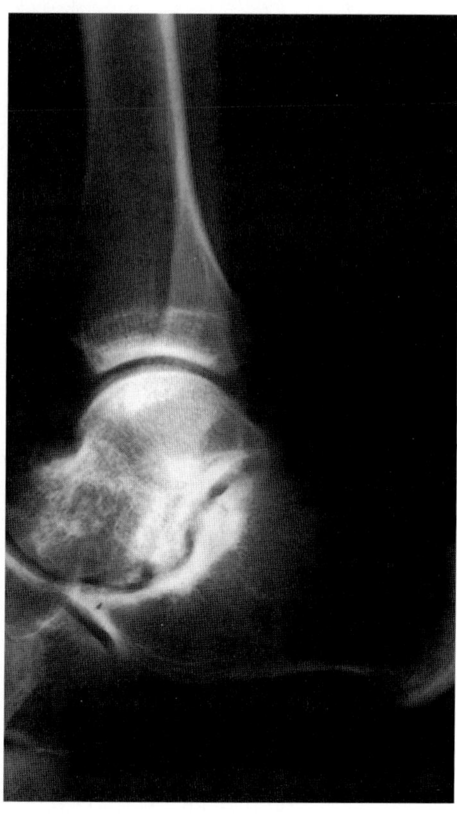

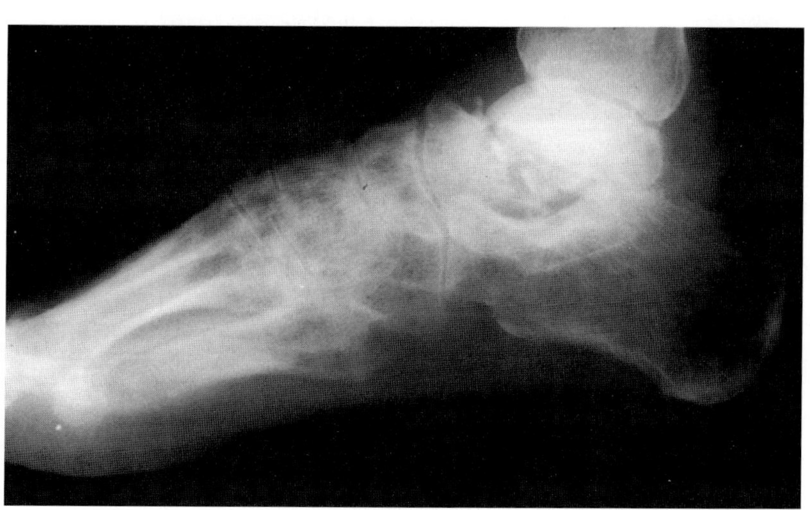

A B

Figure 17. A,B: Malunion of talar neck.

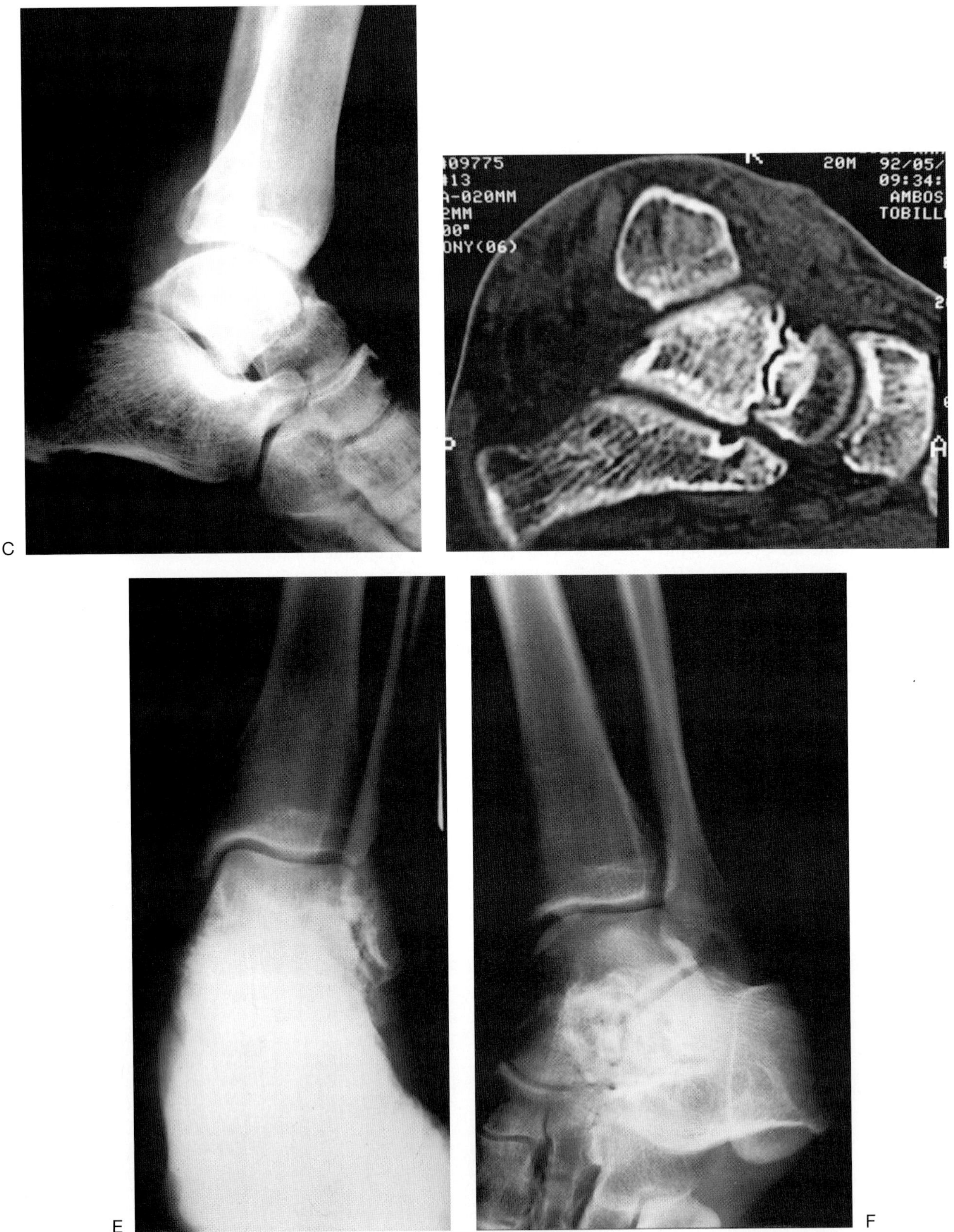

Figure 17. *(Continued.)* **C,D:** Nonunion of talar neck. **E,F:** Subtalar arthritis from fracture or sinus tarsi debris.

Figure 18. **A:** An MRI of the talus demonstrating evidence of segmental osteonecrosis 3 months after a talar neck class II fracture. **B–E:** Type III fracture fixed with appropriate posterior screw. **F:** An avascular talus is present at 3 months.

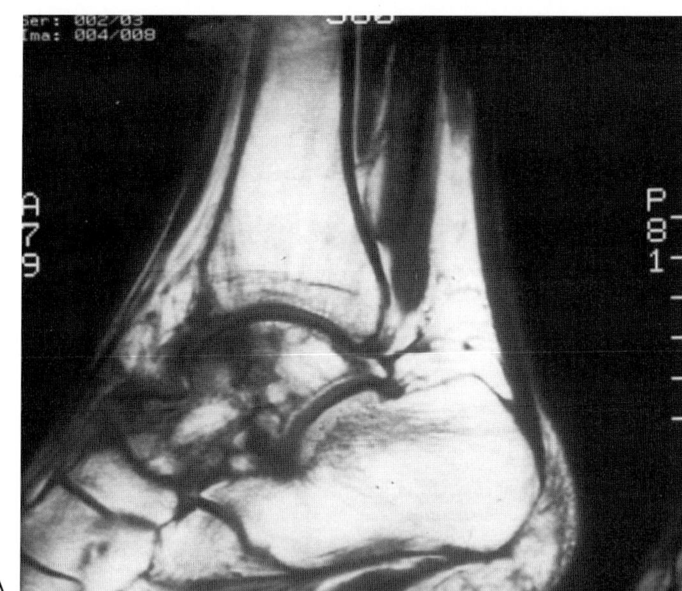

A

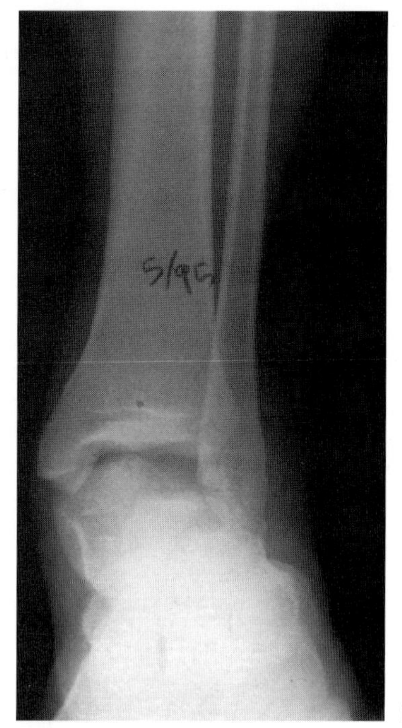
B

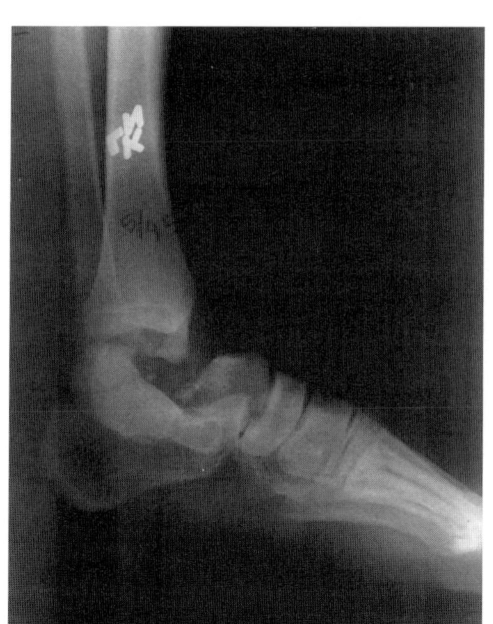
C

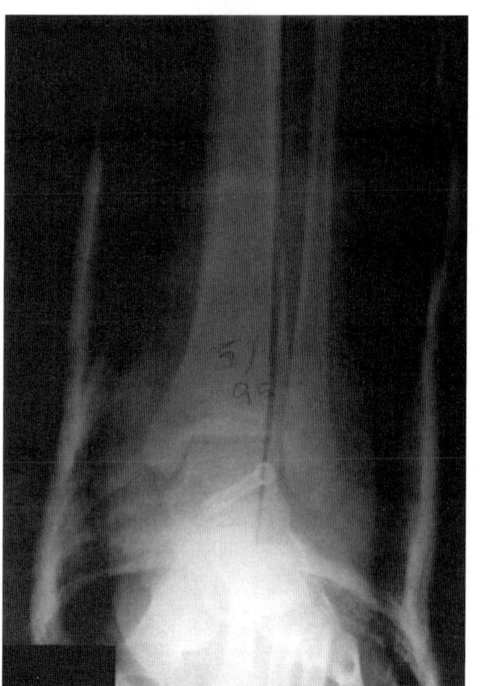
D

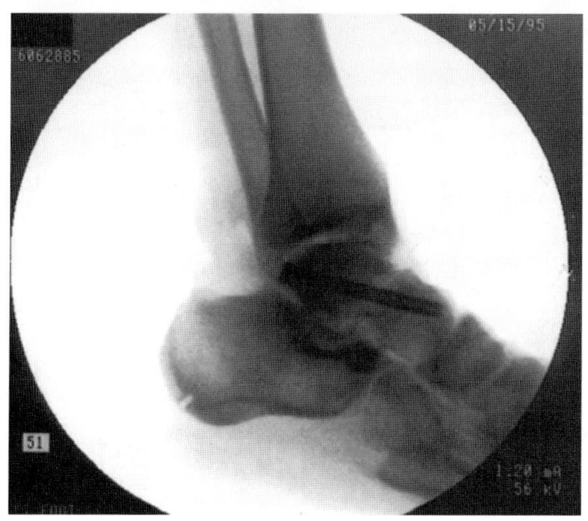

E

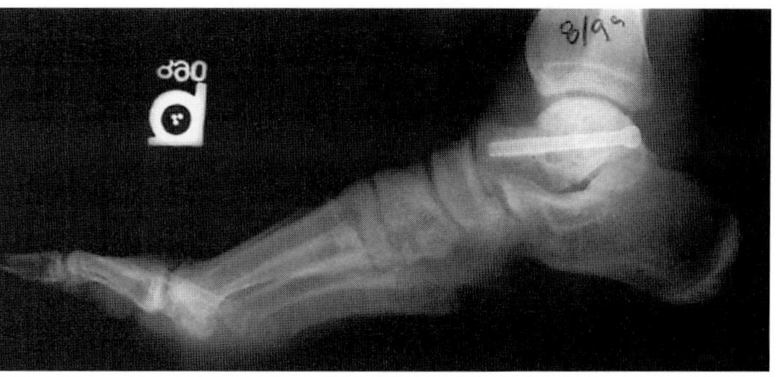
F

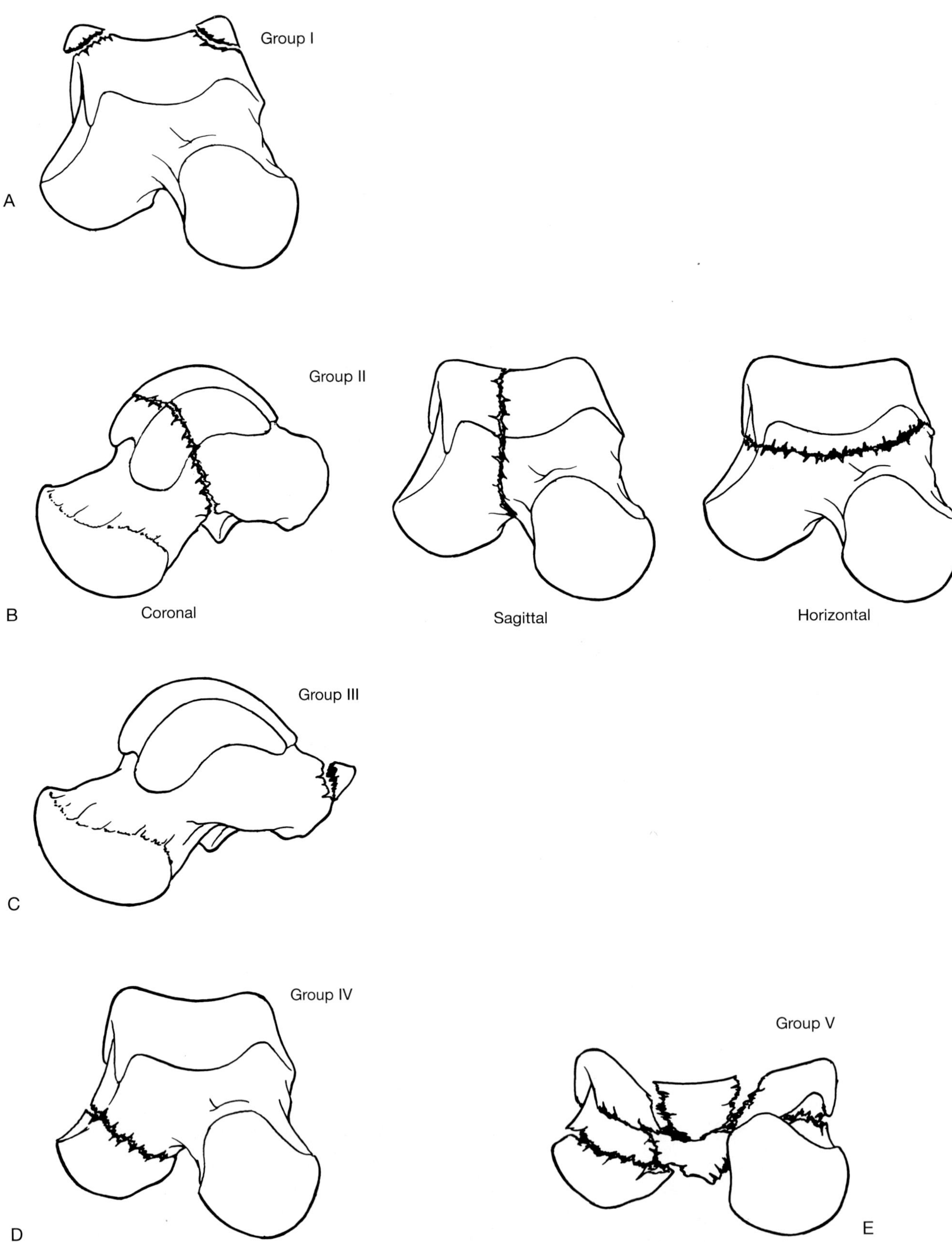

Figure 19. Classification of talar body fractures. **A:** Osteochondral fracture (class I). **B:** Sagittal, vertical, and horizontal talar body injuries (class II). **C:** Posterior process fracture (class III). **D:** Lateral tubercle fracture (class IV). **E:** Crush injury (class V).

to hold the ankle in equinus, is determined by the extent of osteonecrosis. Osteonecrosis may take up to 2 years to heal. There have been no outcome studies done on osteonecrosis of the talus, and it is surprising how well patients do in the face of an avascular talus. We have counseled them as to their disease process and recommend that they not do running athletic events until there is evidence of healing. We do not believe there is any clear evidence that revascularization procedures, subtalar arthrodesis, or core decompressions are of any long-term benefit. It has been recommended that displaced talar fractures or class II and III Hawkins fractures be treated with titanium screws to allow use of MRI in the event of osteonecrosis. Titanium has nonmagnetic properties and creates a signal void, which is only slightly larger than the actual implant. Stainless steel implants, however, have ferromagnetic properties, which cause significant distortion on MRI (35).

TALAR BODY FRACTURES

Fractures of the talar body, constituting about 20% of all talar fractures (Fig. 19), are less common than talar neck fractures; they are classified into five groups. The most common are located in the posterior process and lateral tubercle (2,3). Talar fractures have been classified into group I, the osteochondral fractures; group II, fractures of the body of the talus including coronal, sagittal, horizontal, and shear fractures; group III, posterior process fractures of both the medial and the posterior tubercle; group IV, lateral tubercle fractures; and group V, crush or compression injuries of the talar body. The group II and V fractures of the body of the talus have an osteonecrosis incidence of 25% when no dislocations occur. With dislocation, they have a greater than 50% incidence of osteonecrosis and take an average of 3 to 4 months for bone union. Nonunion and subtalar ankle osteoarthritis are common with these injuries. Group II fractures are body fractures without significant comminution. They are classified with respect to the direction of the fracture—vertical, horizontal, or coronal (Fig. 19) (39,40). It is often necessary to use computed tomography to define fracture pattern and plan surgical strategy (Fig. 20). Because these fractures occur underneath the ankle mortise, exposure is required to perform medial or lateral malleolar osteotomy or to retract the fractures (Fig. 21) (41).

Fixation of talar body fractures involves temporary fixation with K-wires, debridement of small articular fractures that cannot be fixed, and the use of 4.0-mm

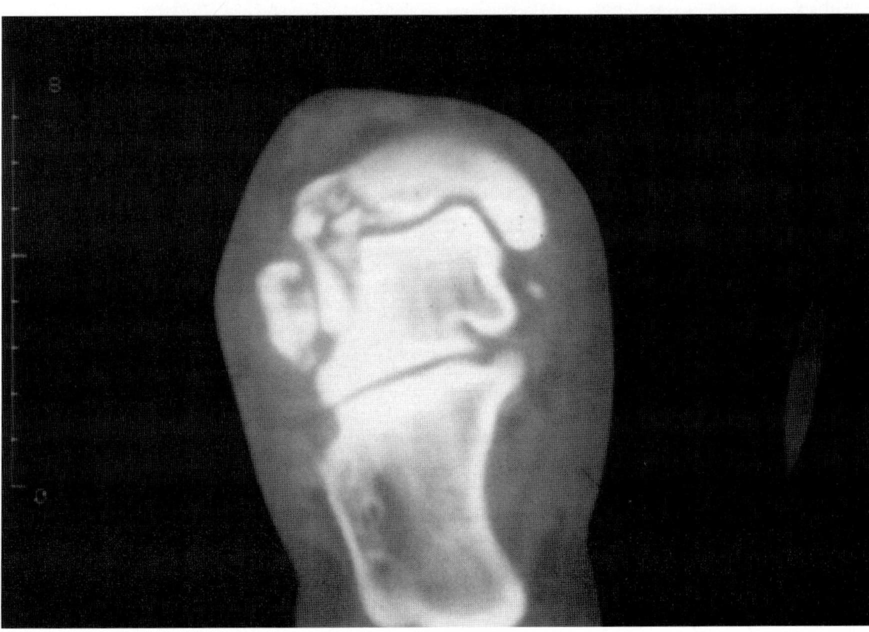

Figure 20. A computed tomographic scan of a crushed or comminuted body of the talus (fracture class V).

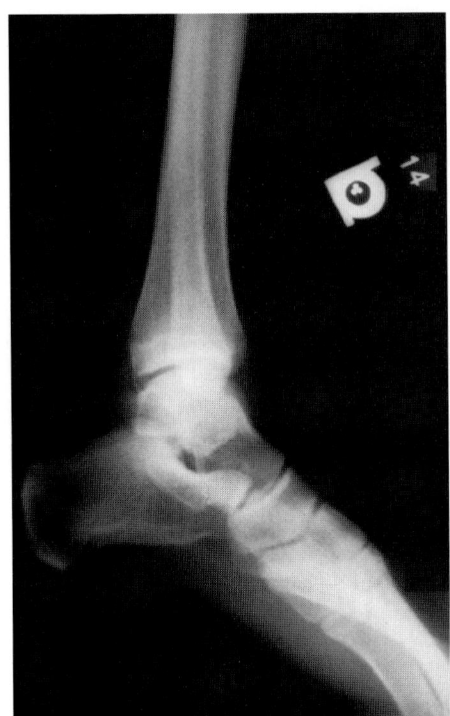

A

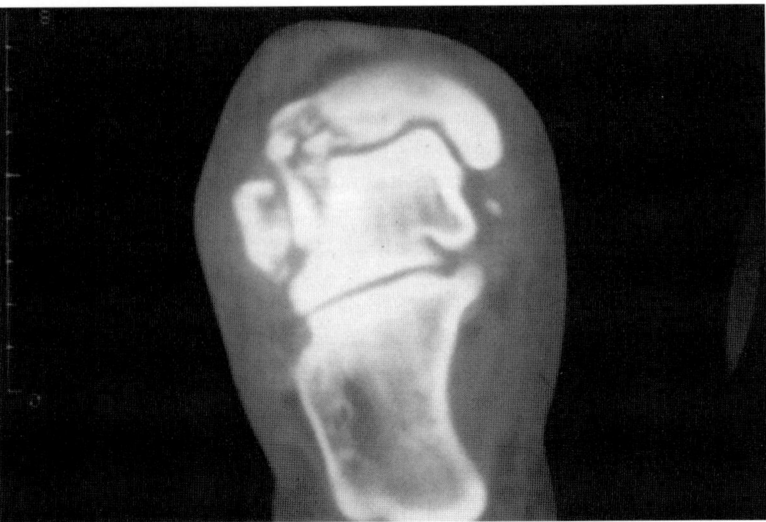

B

C

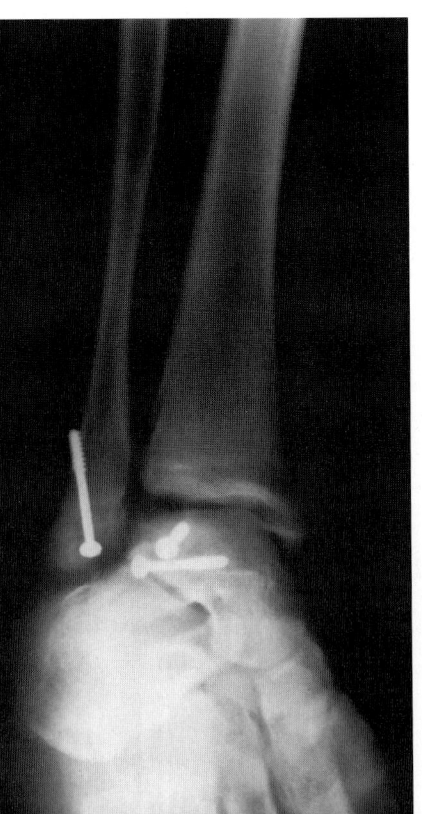

D

Figure 21. A–D: Osteotomy of the lateral malleolus is often needed to treat comminuted fractures of the body of the talus. Care should be taken not to destroy the deltoid ligament.

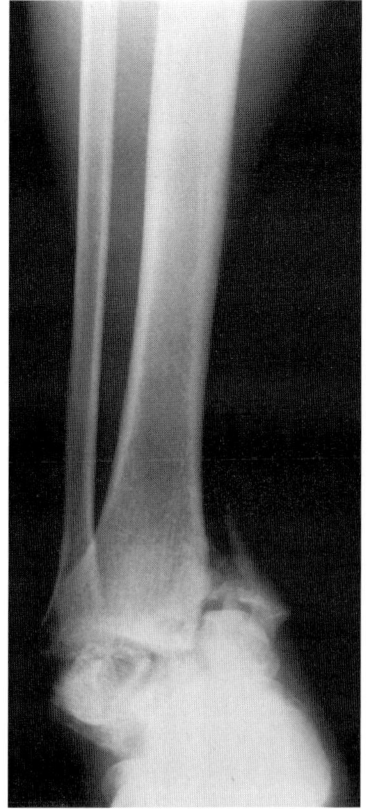
A

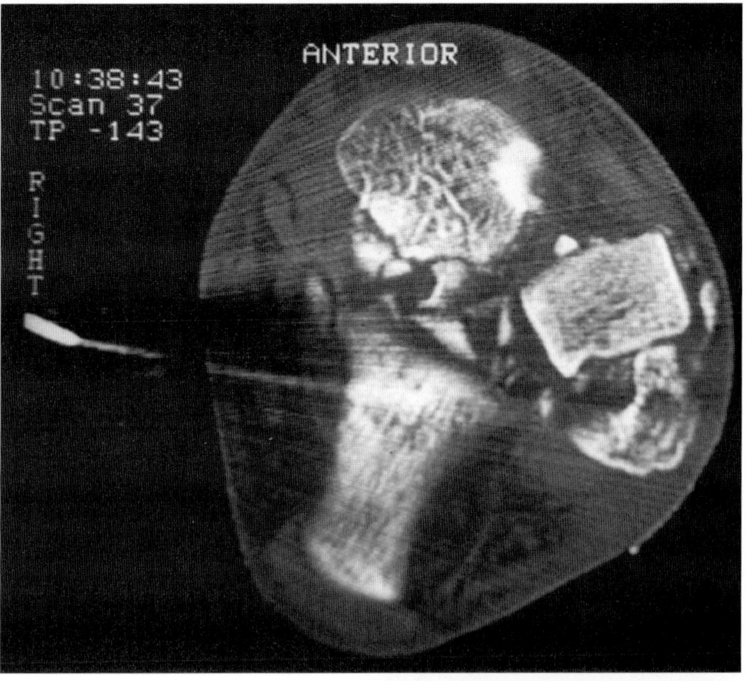

B

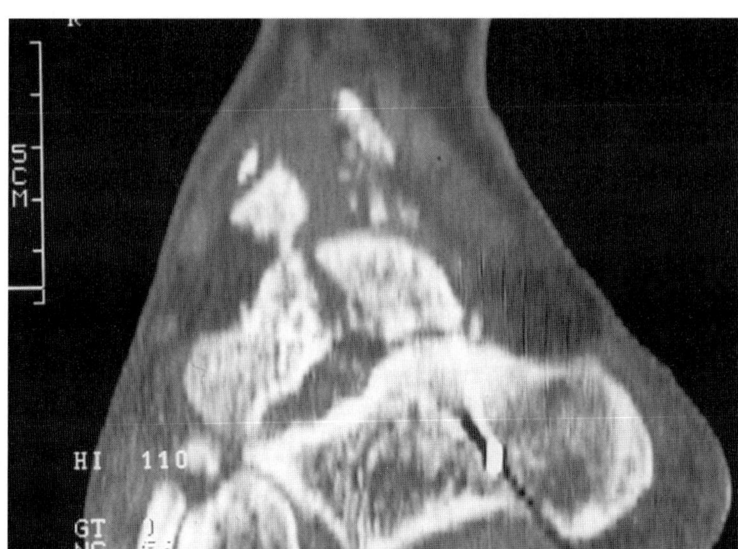

C

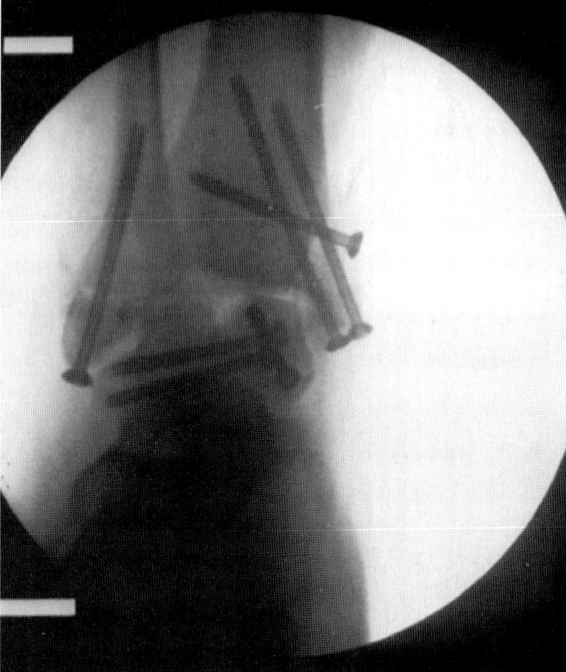
D

Figure 22. A–E: A severely comminuted talar body can still be salvaged with fixation of larger fragments and debridement of smaller fragments.

E 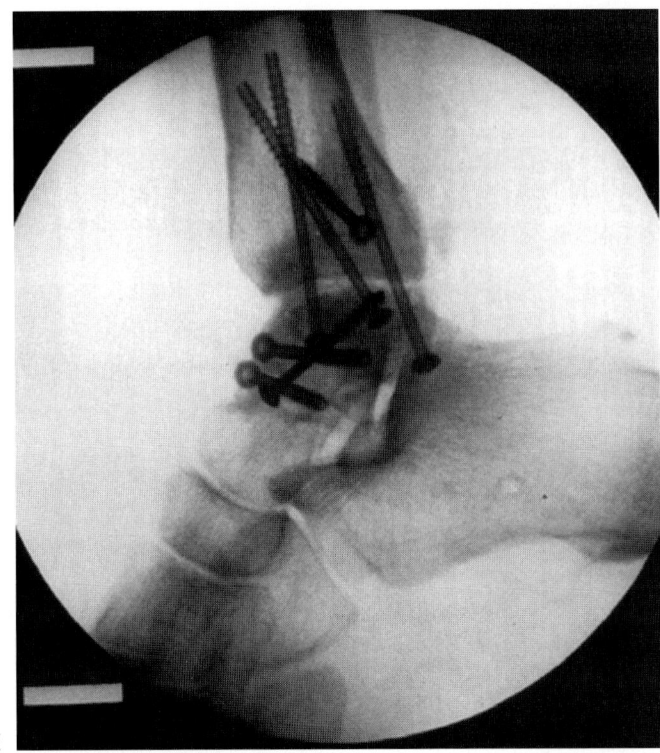

Figure 22. E: See legend on page 87.

titanium cannulated lag screws or subarticular fixation. The small-head subarticular 3.0-mm screws will not be removed. The critical factor is the best possible reconstruction of the body's articular surface. The articular gaps will fill in with fibrous tissue (Fig. 22).

TALAR SALVAGE PROBLEMS

It is important to discuss the severely traumatized avascular or completely detached body of the talus. The goal is to preserve the body of the talus whenever it can be safely reimplanted into the mortise. The body of the talus is used to maintain the hindfoot architecture until soft tissue healing will allow the best reconstructive procedure for the future. We use femoral distractors and external fixators to preserve hindfoot length and achieve soft tissue healing or coverage (Fig. 23).

If the talus is missing or cannot be salvaged, then the best reconstruction is a delayed Blair fusion (Fig. 24) or a tibiocalcaneal arthrodesis with iliac crest distraction grafts (42,43). This is the only salvage procedure that is able to obtain a normal profile of the foot. The Blair procedure is a good reconstructive procedure, but it is difficult to obtain union into the vascularized remaining portion of the talar head (Fig. 24). With this procedure, the tibia is fused to the live portion of the talar neck after excision of the body of the talus. An attempt is made to leave the subtalar joint free to allow some minimal hindfoot motion in the area. It is difficult to obtain good fixation and not to alter the talonavicular articulation.

The tibiocalcaneal arthrodesis is done with the use of large corticocancellous iliac or bank bone grafts, which are implanted in place of the osteonecrotic body of the talus and secured with cannulated screws from the heel to the tibia (Fig. 25). The use of good fixation screws with appropriate bone graft can maintain the anatomic hindfoot architecture; the rigidity of the fixation is important to allow revascularization. A talectomy is the last choice for a salvage procedure. A talectomy gives a severely unstable and noncosmetic shortened hindfoot, which is not tolerated well by the neurologically intact adult patient.

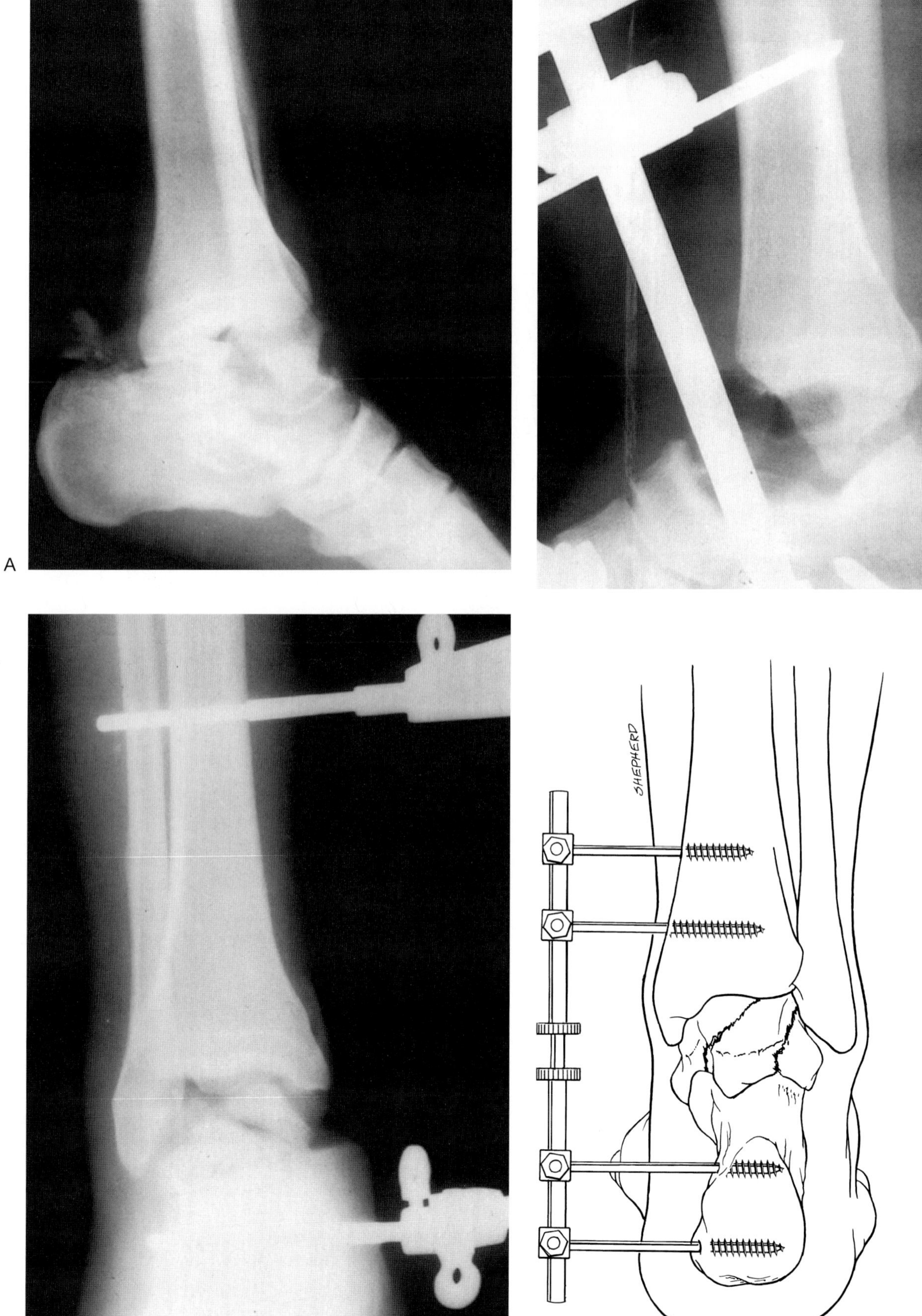

Figure 23. A femoral distractor for an external fixation can maintain the height of the heel in the absence of the body of the talus until a secondary reconstructive procedure can be done (usually 6 to 8 weeks after injury) unless there is a severe soft tissue compromise. **A:** Type III Hawkins fracture dislocation. **B:** AP view of external fixator. **C:** Lateral view of external fixator. **D:** External fixation of talus fracture.

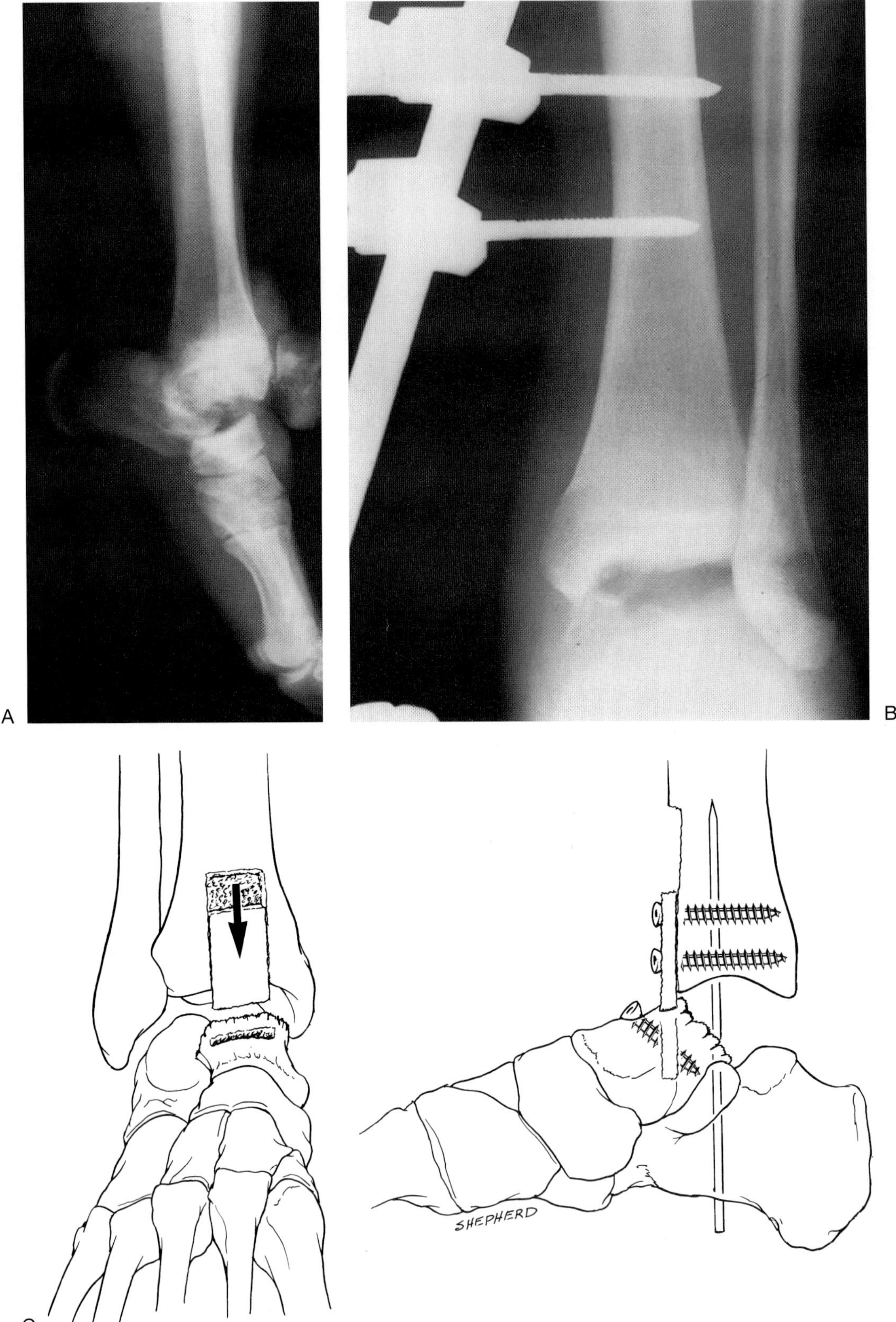

Figure 24. A–E: A Blair-type arthrodesis. **C:** a slot graft from the tibia is fitted into the vascularized talar head and small portion of the neck.

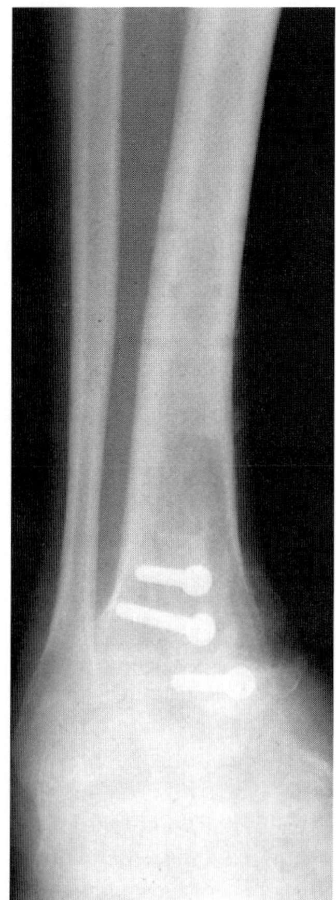

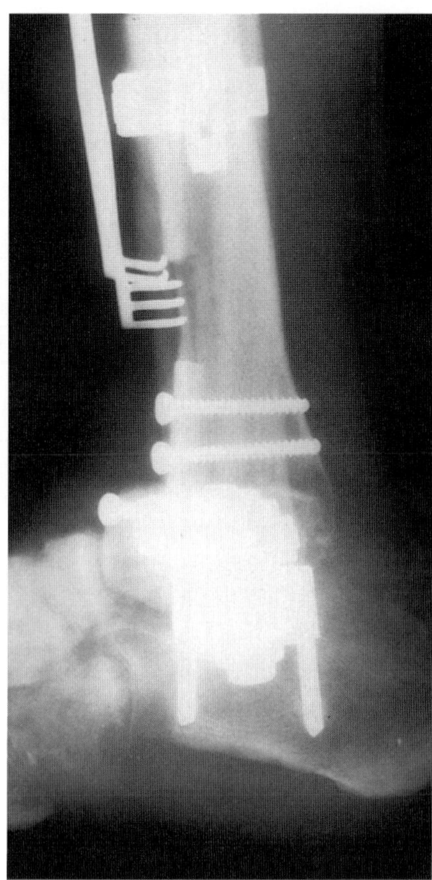

D,E

Figure 24. *(Continued).* **D** and **E:** fixation with screws is recommended.

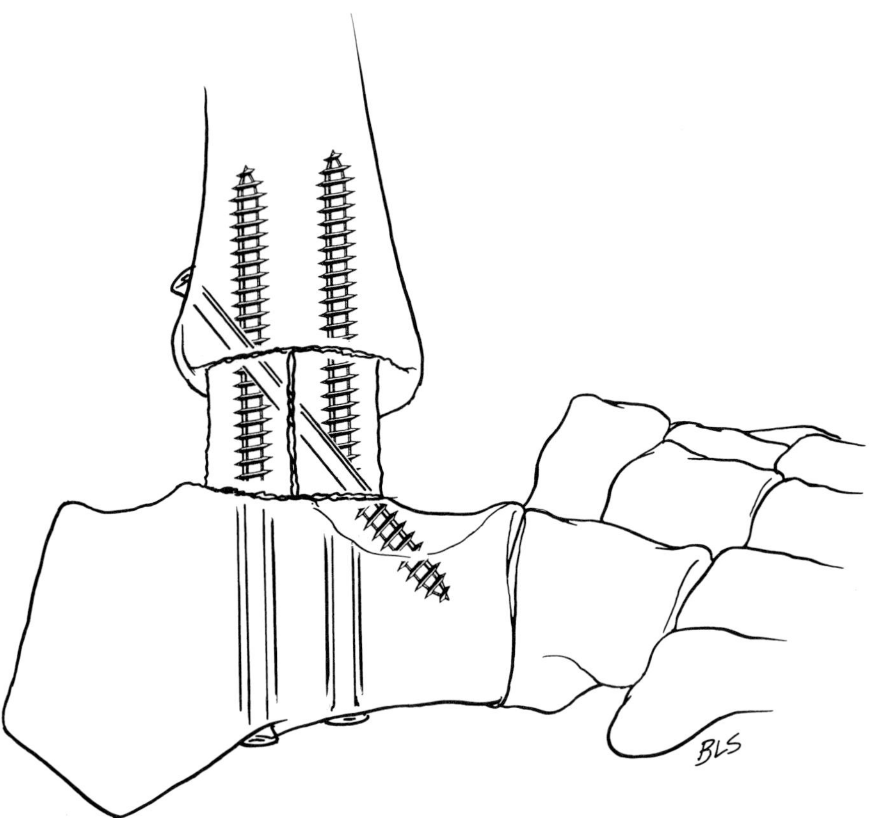

Figure 25. Reconstruction for loss of the body of the talus. When there is insufficient talar head for a Blair fusion, a tibiocalcaneal fusion with a corticocancellous iliac slot graft and cancellous screw fixation from heel to tibia are done.

OPEN FRACTURES OF THE TALUS

Up to 50% of class III Hawkins injuries are open injuries of the talus. These injuries often involved marked fracture displacement, disrupted blood supply, severe soft tissue damage, and contamination. The functional outcome of open injuries has recently been evaluated by Marsh and associates (44). An infection rate of 38% for previously open injuries of the talus is quite high, and it appears higher than that associated with other open lower extremity injuries such as that to the tibia. The high infection rate associated with these open talar injuries was attributed to more skin damage, a larger dead space, and disruption of bone and blood supply. The extruded talus has a particularly high incidence of infection, which has a negative impact on outcome, with many requiring late partial to complete talar body excisions (44). Therefore, if an open injury is associated with an extruded talus and there is significant contamination, it may be more appropriate to maintain hindfoot architecture with an external fixator and perform a late Blair fusion or tibiocalcaneal arthrodesis. This will always remain a judgment call, but I feel it is appropriate to report that there is a higher incidence of late infections with open talar injuries.

OUTCOME

Recent literature has provided evidence of the outcome of talus fractures. The incidence of malunion is related to whether the fracture is opened appropriately for reduction. It is more difficult to determine the accuracy of the reduction in fractures treated closed. Canale views obtained after reduction of talar fractures have revealed incidences of malunion as high as 27%, with varus malunion being the most common deformity (18,28,29,45). The degree of malunion decreases if the fractures were treated with open reduction. A malunion is much less of a problem if two incisions are made to fix an exposed lesion. Appropriate views in the operating room can be taken by image intensifier or by standard radiograph using the Canale technique. Dorsal malunions are usually taken care of by excision of the beak. Varus malunions are more difficult to control, and results of biomechanical studies indicate that they create problems in load transference to the foot (30).

The incidence of posttraumatic arthritis differs depending on whether the injury was to the tibiotalar or the talocalcaneal joint. Subtalar arthrosis depends on degree of injury, with the more severe injuries having increased rates of postinjury arthrosis (18,28,45). In a recent series of 108 patients with a 5-month follow-up (28), the range of motion of the tibiotalar joint was restricted to about half of normal, and inversion/eversion of the subtalar joint also was restricted by 50%. The incidence of arthrosis reached 50% in the highest Hawkins type III fractures. The results in this study paralleled the expected degree of injury. Tibiotalar joint arthrosis does not appear to parallel the degree of injury and stays fairly constant. Some have thought that prolonged periods of immobilization may play a role in the restricted range of motion and arthrosis. The use of more appropriate and early passive ranges of motion after surgery is being stressed to improve the degrees of arthrosis and restriction.

The incidence of osteonecrosis has certainly paralleled the degree of injury, but early appropriate reductions and rigid fixation should help reduce the degree of severity of the osteonecrosis in the talar body. It is much safer to walk on a partially osteonecrotic talus than on a completely osteonecrotic talus. The incidence of osteonecrosis cannot be prevented, but the degree of osteonecrosis may depend on treatment. The morbidity of the osteonecrosis will also depend on the postoperative regimen and clear diagnosis using MRI when appropriate. Decreasing the amount of varus and valgus stresses and loads through the ankle should help decrease the morbidity from osteonecrosis. A higher percentage of excellent and good results has been found in those series in which weight bearing was delayed until there was evidence of bone healing.

SUMMARY

Injuries of the talus make up a significant proportion of complex foot and ankle injuries. The severity of these injuries is increasing because the availability and use of better safety equipment has allowed more people to survive serious accidents. Early rigid and accurate anatomic fixation leads to the best possible outcome for each category of talar injury. If osteonecrosis is suspected, titanium screws should be used for fixation to allow better postoperative follow-up. Treatment of osteonecrosis of the talus still depends mainly on clinical judgment, with the MRI providing more clinical data. The outcome of the osteonecrotic talus has not been established at this point.

The approach to the talus depends on the judgment and skill of the surgeon; two approaches are usually indicated for more severe injuries. A CT scan is quite helpful for fractures of the talar body; preoperative planning and the judicious use of malleolar osteotomy with preservation of the deltoid artery are advocated. Tibiotalar and talocalcaneal motion have been altered as a result of talar fractures. Arthrosis of the subtalar joint depends on the degree of injury.

REFERENCES

1. Bonnin JG. Dislocations and fracture-dislocations of the talus. *Br J Surg* 1940;28:88–100.
2. DeLee JC. Fractures and dislocations of the foot. In: Mann RA, ed. *Surgery of the foot,* 5th ed. St Louis, MO: CV Mosby, 1986:592–808.
3. Heckman JD. Fractures and dislocations of the foot. In: Rockwood CA Jr, Green DP, eds. *Fractures in adults,* vol 2. Philadelphia: JB Lippincott, 1984:1703–1832.
4. Anderson HG, Flack MW, Gotch OH, eds. *The medical and surgical aspects of aviation.* London: H Frowde, 1919.
5. Coltart WD. "Aviator's astragalus." *J Bone Joint Surg [Br]* 1952;34:545–566.
6. Pennal GF. Fractures of the talus. *Clin Orthop* 1963;30:53–63.
7. Dunn AR, Jacobs B, Campbell RD Jr. Fractures of the talus. *J Trauma* 1966;6:443–468.
8. Penny JN, Davis LA. Fractures and fracture-dislocations of the neck of the talus. *J Trauma* 1980;20:1029–1037.
9. Gilquist J, Oretop N, Stenstrom A, et al. Late results after vertical fracture of the talus. *Injury* 1974;6:173–179.
10. Mindell ER, Cisek EE, Kartalian G, et al. Late results of injuries to the talus: analysis of forty cases. *J Bone Joint Surg [Am]* 1963;45:221–245.
11. Kenwright J, Taylor RG. Major injuries of the talus. *J Bone Joint Surg [Br]* 1970;52:36–48.
12. Canale ST, Kelly FB Jr. Fractures of the neck of the talus: long-term evaluation of seventy-one cases. *J Bone Joint Surg [Am]* 1978;60:143–156.
13. Hawkins LG. Fractures of the neck of the talus. *J Bone Joint Surg [Am]* 1970;52:991–1002.
14. Kleiger B. Fractures of the talus. *J Bone Joint Surg [Am]* 1948;30:735–744.
15. Lorentzen JE, Christensen SB, Krogsoe O, et al. Fractures of the neck of the talus. *Acta Orthop Scand* 1977;48:115–120.
16. Pantazopoulos T, Galanos P, Vayanos E, et al. Fractures of the neck of the talus. *Acta Orthop Scand* 1974;45:296–306.
17. Zwipp H. Severe foot trauma in combination with talar injuries. In: Tscherne H, Schatzker J, eds. *Major fractures of the pilon, the talus, and the calcaneus: current concepts of treatment.* Berlin: Springer-Verlag, 1993:123–135.
18. Daniels TR, Smith JW. Talar neck fractures. *Foot Ankle* 1993;14:225–234.
19. Hawkins LG. Fracture of the lateral process of the talus: a review of thirteen cases. *J Bone Joint Surg [Am]* 1965;47:1170–1175.
20. Heckman JD, McLean MR. Fractures of the lateral process of the talus. *Clin Orthop* 1985;199:108–113.
21. Mukherjee SK, Pringle RM, Baxter AD. Fracture of the lateral process of the talus: a report of thirteen cases. *J Bone Joint Surg [Br]* 1974;56:263–273.
22. Haliburton RA, Sullivan CR, Kelly PJ, et al. The extra-osseous and intra-osseous blood supply of the talus. *J Bone Joint Surg [Am]* 1958;40:1115–1120.
23. Kelly PJ, Sullivan CR. Blood supply of the talus. *Clin Orthop* 1963;30:37–44.
24. Mulfinger GL, Trueta J. The blood supply of the talus. *J Bone Joint Surg [Br]* 1970;52:160–167.
25. Wildenaur E. Die Blutversorgung des Talus. *Z Anat Entwicklungsgesch* 1950;115:32–36.
26. Larson RL, Sullivan CR, Janes JM. Trauma, surgery, and circulation of the talus: what are the risks of avascular necrosis? *J Trauma* 1961;1:13–21.
27. Peterson L, Romanus B, Dahlberg E. Fracture of the collum tali: an experimental study. *J Biomech* 1976;9:277–279.
28. Szyszkowitz R, Seggl W, Wildburger R. Late results of fractures and fracture-dislocation after ORIF. In: Tscherne H, Schatzker J, eds. *Major fractures of the pilon, the talus, and the calcaneus: current concepts of treatment.* Berlin: Springer-Verlag, 1993:105–112.
29. Behrens F. Long-term results of displaced talar neck fractures. In: Tscherne H, Schatzker J, eds. *Major fractures of the pilon, the talus, and the calcaneus: current concepts of treatment.* Berlin: Springer-Verlag, 1993:113–121.

30. Sangeorzan BJ, Wagner UA, Harrington RM, et al. Contact characteristics of the subtalar joint: the effect of talar neck misalignment. *J Orthop Res* 1992;10:544–551.
31. Trillat A, Bousquet G, Lapeyre B. Displaced fractures of the neck or of the body of the talus: value of screwing by posterior surgical approach. *Rev Chir Orthop Reparatrice Appar Mot* 1970;56:529–536.
32. Gatellier J. The juxtoretroperoneal route in the operative treatment of fracture of the malleolus with posterior marginal fragment. *Surg Gynecol Obstet* 1931;52:67–70.
33. Lemaire RG, Bustin W. Screw fixation of fractures of the neck of the talus using a posterior approach. *J Trauma* 1980;20:669–673.
34. Swanson T, Bray T. Talar neck fractures: a mechanical and histomorphometric study of fixation. *Orthop Trans* 1989;13:762.
35. Thordarson DB. MRI imaging of AVN of the talus following displaced talus fractures. Presented at the AAOS Annual Meeting, February, 1995.
36. Comfort TH, Behrens F, Gaither DW, et al. Long-term results of displaced talar neck fractures. *Clin Orthop* 1985;199:81–87.
37. Henderson RC. Posttraumatic necrosis of the talus: the Hawkins sign versus magnetic resonance imaging. *J Orthop Trauma* 1991;5:96–99.
38. Bobechko WP, Harris WR. The radiographic density of avascular bone. *J Bone Joint Surg [Br]* 1960;42:626–632.
39. Alexander AH, Lichtman DM. Surgical treatment of transchondral talar-dome fractures (ostochondritis dissecans): long-term follow-up. *J Bone Joint Surg [Am]* 1980;62:646–652.
40. Sneppen O, Christensen SB, Krogsoe O, et al. Fracture of the body of the talus. *Acta Orthop Scand* 1977;48:317–324.
41. Deyerle WM, Burkhardt B, Comfort T, et al. Displaced fractures of the talus: an aggressive approach. *Orthop Trans* 1981;5:465.
42. Dennis MD, Tullos HS. Blair tibiotalar arthrodesis for injuries to the talus. *J Bone Joint Surg [Am]* 1980;62:103–107.
43. Ries M, Healy WA Jr. Total dislocation of the talus: case report with a 13-year follow up and review of the literature. *Orthop Rev* 1988;17:76–80.
44. Marsh JL, Iverson M, Shapiro D, et al. Major open injuries of the talus. *Orthop Trans* 1994;18:720–721.
45. Jensen I, Wester JU, Rasmussen F, et al. Prognosis of fracture of the talus in children: 21 (7–34)-year follow-up of 14 cases. *Acta Orthop Scand* 1994;65:398–400.

Complex Foot and Ankle Trauma,
edited by Robert S. Adelaar,
Lippincott–Raven Publishers, Philadelphia © 1999.

8

Occult Injuries of the Talus

Robert S. Adelaar

In the previous chapter, we discussed primarily talar neck and body fractures, which are usually due to high-energy injuries. However, several injuries to the talus that are often missed can create disabling situations. In the following sections, we discuss osteochondral injuries to the talar dome, posterior process fractures, and injuries to the lateral and (less often) medial tubercle of the talus. These injuries are often missed on routine screening views in primary care or emergency room situations. They require further clinical suspicion, intricate knowledge of the anatomy, and appropriate radiographic and imaging studies when the diagnoses are suspected.

FRACTURES OF THE POSTERIOR PROCESS

Fractures of the body of the talus comprise 15% to 20% of all talar injuries. The most common injuries in this group are fractures of the posterior processes and the lateral tubercle. Fractures of the body of the talus are classified into five groups (1,2) (Fig. 1). Group I includes osteochondral fractures, group II fractures of the body of the talus including the coronal, sagittal, and horizontal shear fractures, group III posterior process fractures of both the medial and lateral process, group IV fractures of the lateral tubercle, and group V crush or compression injuries of the talar body. Groups II and V injuries have been discussed in previous chapters and do not represent diagnostic dilemmas, only treatment and reduction dilemmas.

Posterior process fractures make up the largest number (20%) of body fractures of the talus. The lateral posterior process is larger than the medial and often represents an accessory bone; the incidence of such fractures has been reported to be from 3% to 30% (3). It should be noted that the blood supply to the lateral portion of the body of

R. S. Adelaar: Department of Orthopaedics, Medical College of Virginia/Virginia Commonwealth University, Richmond, Virginia 23298.

I. Osteochondral fracture

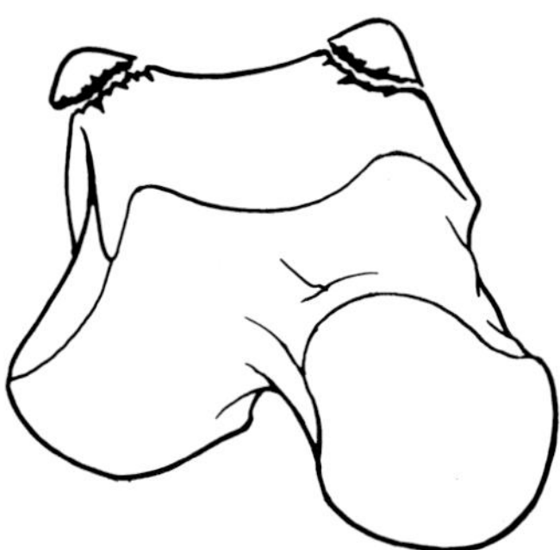

IIa. Sagittal body fracture

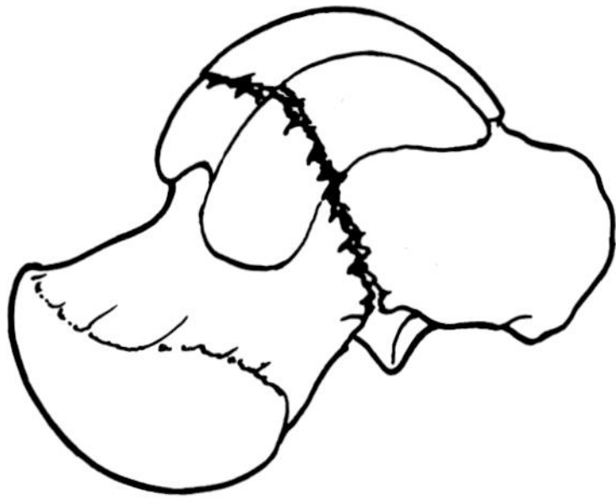

IIb. Coronal body fracture

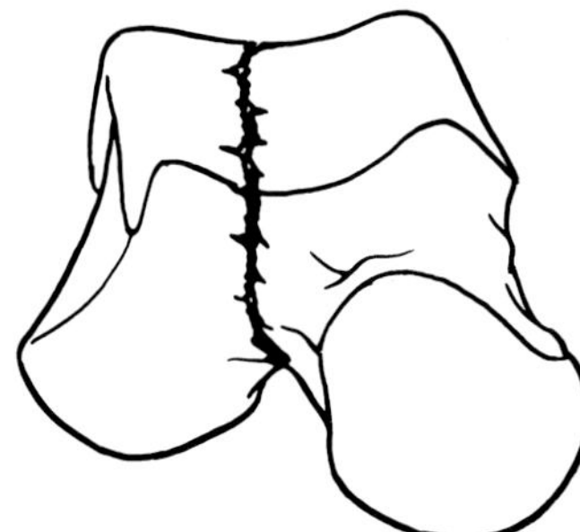

IIc. Horizontal body fracture

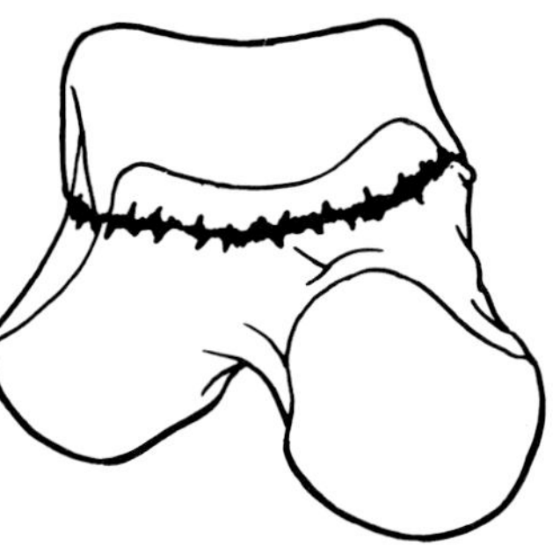

III. Posterior process fracture

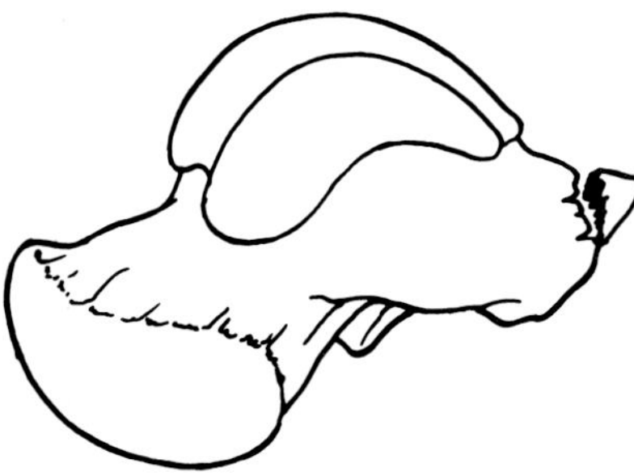

IV. Lateral and medial tubercle fracture

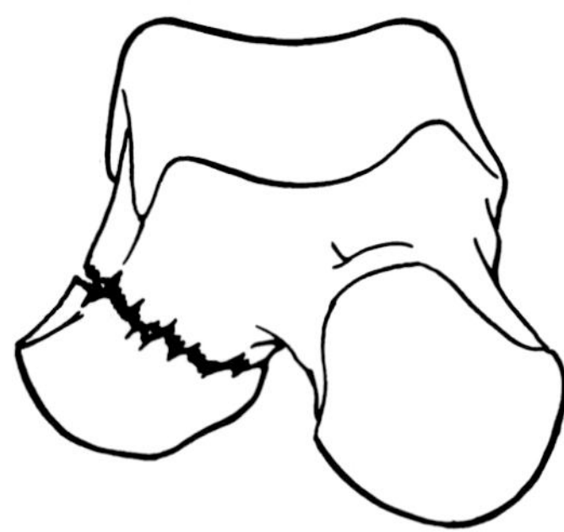

V. Crush fracture of talus

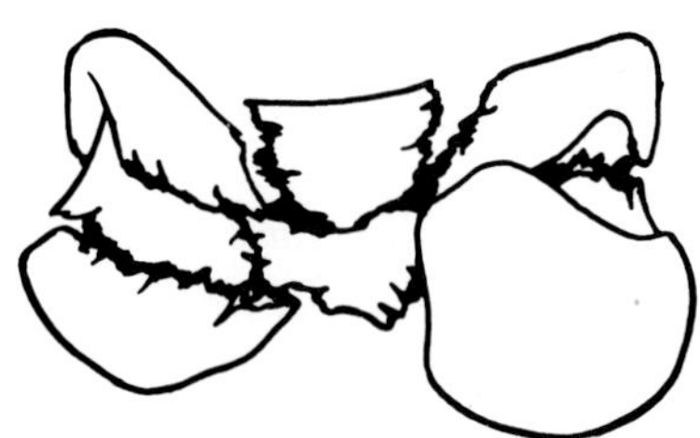

Figure 1. Classification of fractures of talar body.

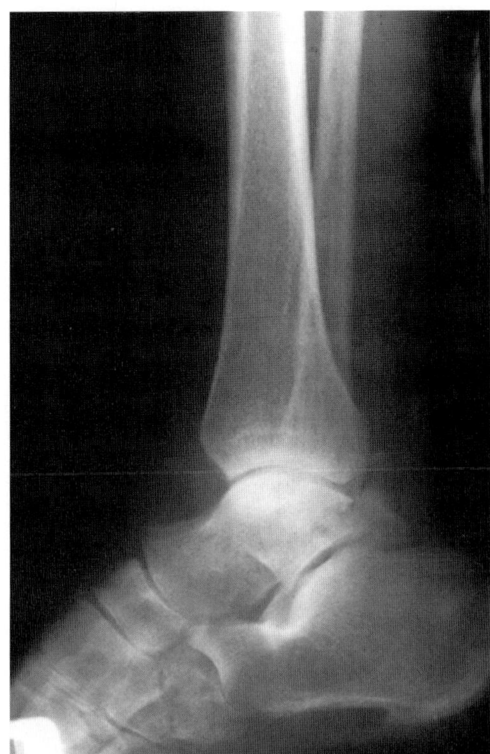

A

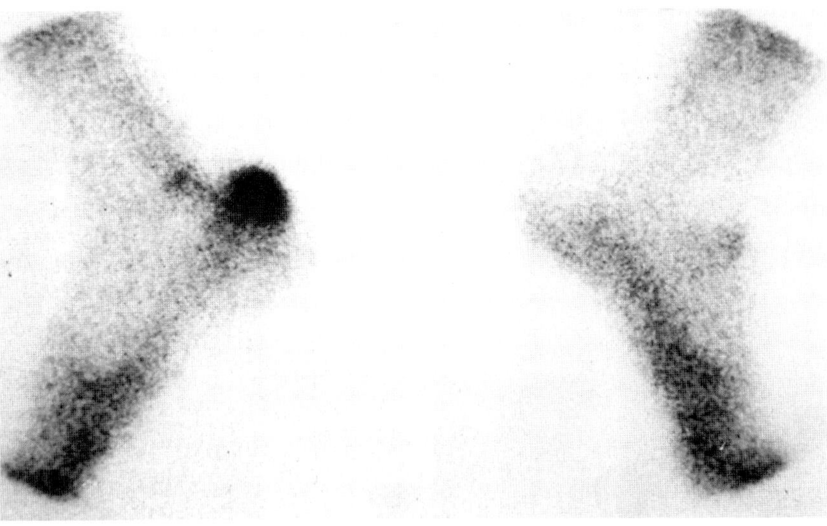

B

Figure 2. A: A posterior process fracture of undetermined age of the lateral process. **B:** Bone scan was positive, confirming an ongoing reactive process near the posterior process compared to normal on the opposite side.

the talus and the posterior process, particularly the lateral posterior process, is low. Nonunions are often seen with fractures involving the lateral posterior process, due to lack of blood supply. It is often difficult to distinguish an os trigonum from a fracture of the posterior lateral process, and a bone scan may be needed for differentiation (Fig. 2A,B). Between the medial and lateral processes, there is a tunnel for the flexor hallucis longus tendon. Up to a point, the flexor hallucis longus muscle is quite muscular and

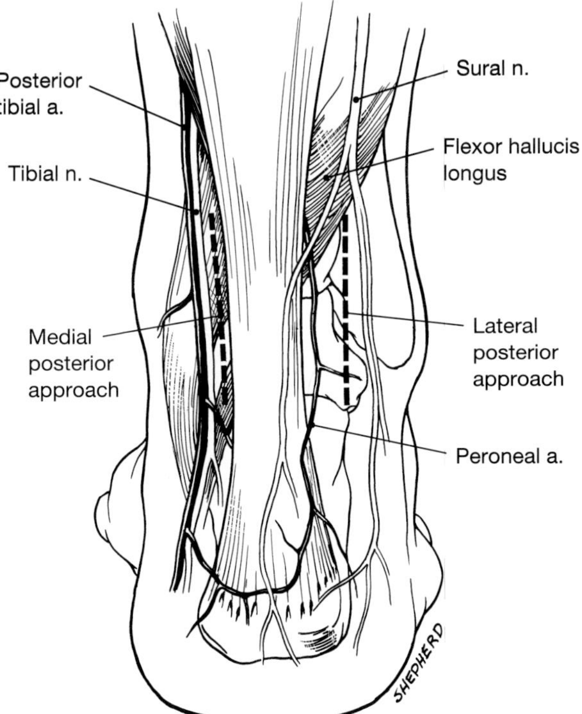

A

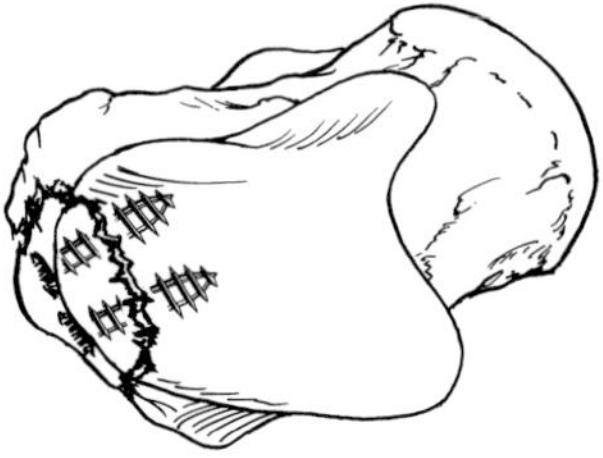

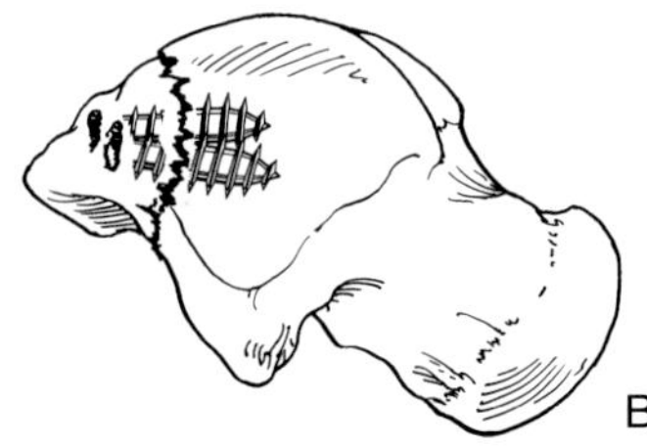

B

Figure 3. A: Posterior lateral approach to posterior process. **B:** Posterior process fracture approached from posterior lateral and articular screws.

forms a very narrow tendon that passes through the processes and into a sheath, which travels on the medial side of the os calcis. The flexor hallucis longus often becomes trapped or triggers in this area, preventing the first toe from flexing as the forefoot is pushed up to allow for the normal tenodesis mechanism. This usually implies an entrapment at this point. The tendon can often be tender in this area and can be mistaken for a posterior process injury.

If a posterior process fracture is suspected, then a bone scan would usually be necessary for differentiation in an acute situation (Fig. 2A,B). Routine x-ray film shot on the lateral projection and specialized axial views similar to sesamoid views of the

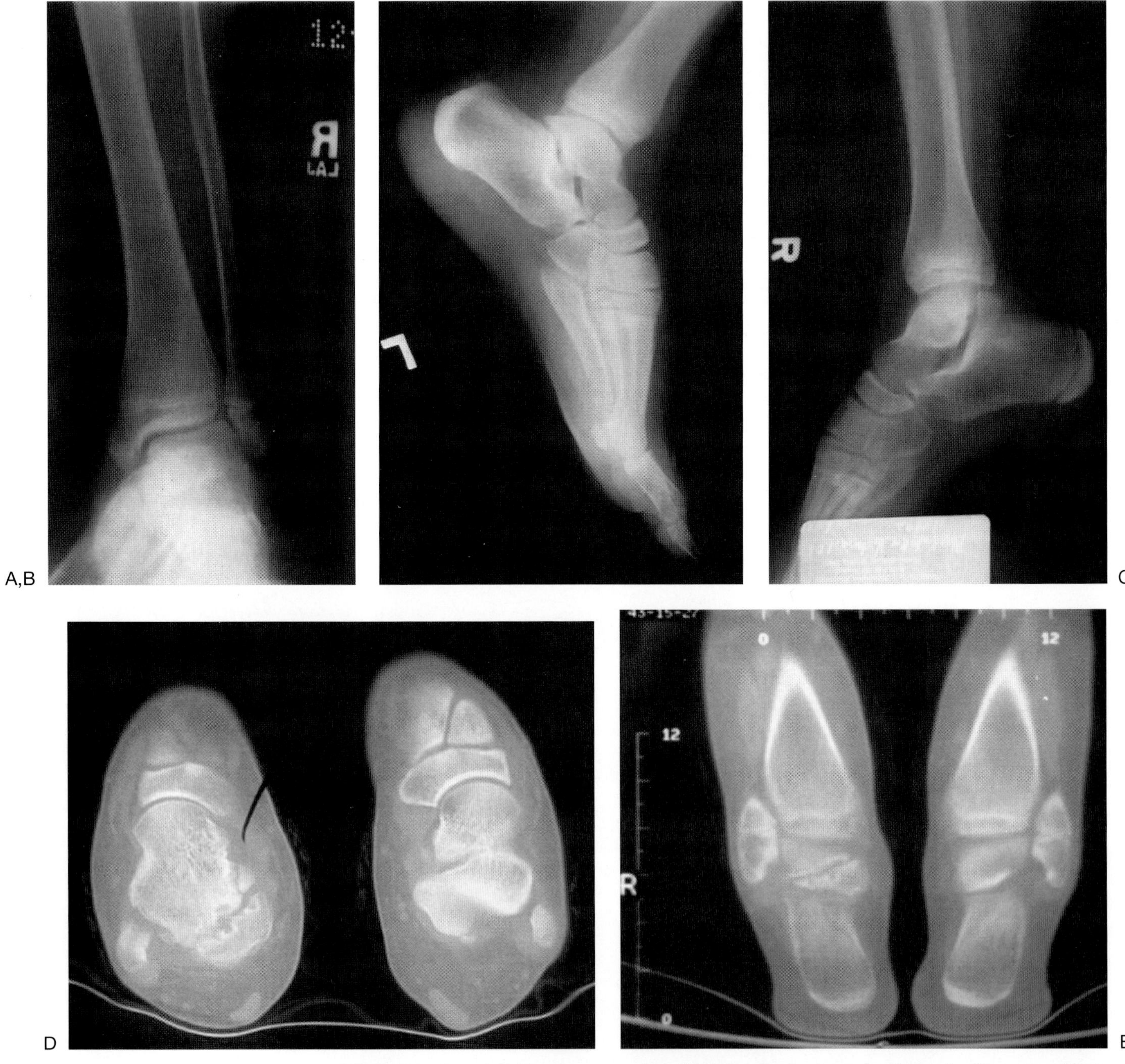

Figure 4. A and **B:** Twelve-year-old girl with posterior lateral ankle pain. The x-ray film is interpreted as negative. **C:** Lateral x-ray film 2 months after A and B. **D** and **E:** CT scan showing large posterior lateral posterior process fracture.

posterior processes can be obtained, particularly if one has a portable fluoroscope in the office. Fractures of the posterior processes do not always require treatment. If the diagnosis is made early, treatment is usually a cast, initially in slight equinus, applied for 6 to 8 weeks because of the poor vascularity and slow healing. There are subtalar capsular attachments to the posterior process. If the injury is chronically symptomatic, a surgical procedure should be considered for improvement of symptoms (2–4).

The surgical procedure of choice is excision of either the symptomatic os trigonum or the posterior process nonunion. The usual approach is posterior lateral, coming behind the peroneal tendons and identifying the muscle of the flexor hallucis longus (Fig. 3A). The flexor hallucis muscle is then traced out to its tendinous origin; at that point, one can palpate the lateral process, which is the larger of the two processes, and an excision can be made. One should know ahead of time how far the process fracture extends into the body of the talus. A computed tomography (CT) scan is frequently necessary to identify these larger posterior process with extension to the body, which often may not be excised due to instability and involvement of posterior articular facet (Fig. 4). The larger injuries can be reduced with cannulated-type screws of smaller caliber (Fig. 3B). It should be remembered that the smaller steel cannulated screws tend to strip more easily than solid core screws and that the head should be countersunk.

In summary, a posterior process injury is usually occult, requiring diagnostic studies and clinical suspicion. Treatment is usually by excision if the injury is symptomatic, but the larger lesions require an attempt at fixation.

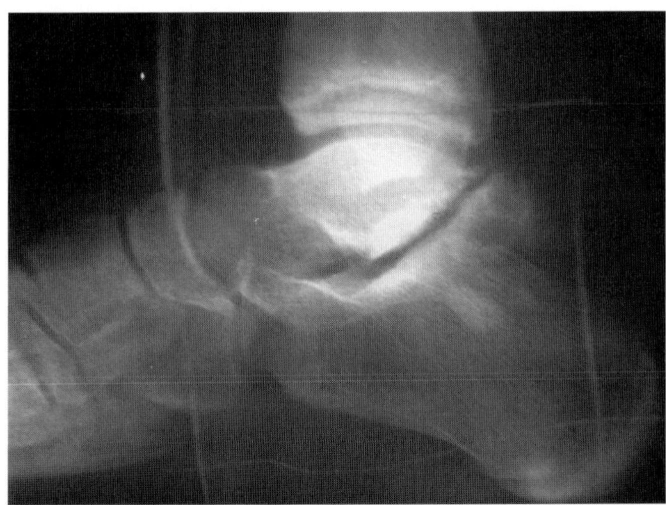
F

Figure 4. (*Continued*). **F:** Lateral x-ray film 6 months after A and B. **G:** Fracture fragment isolated at surgery by fluoroscopy. **H:** At surgery after exclusion of fragment.

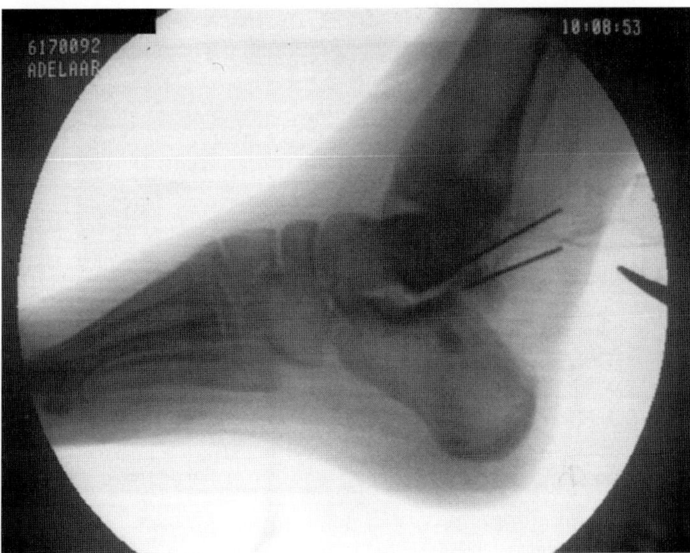

G

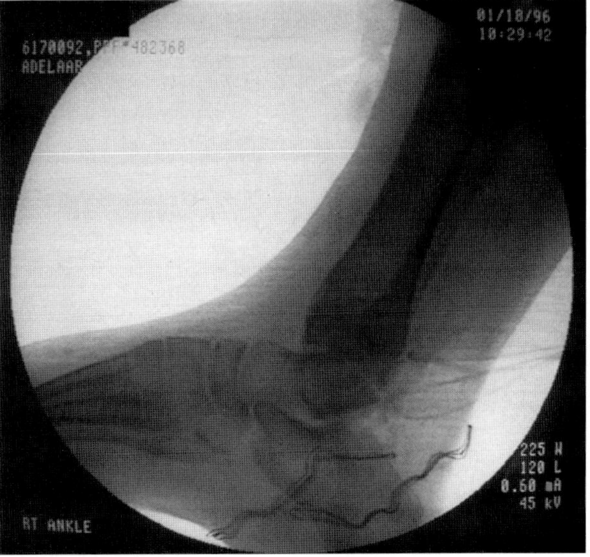

H

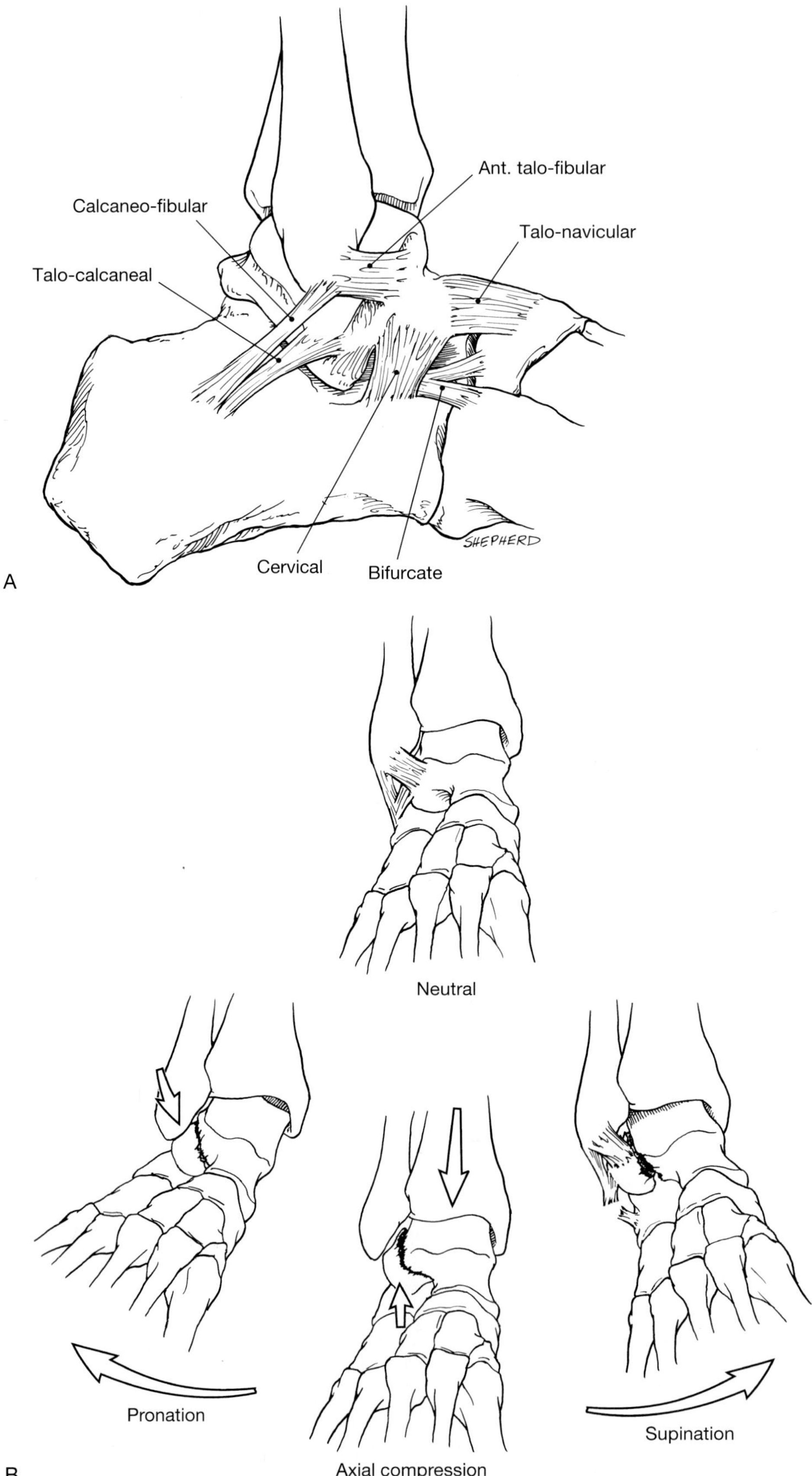

Figure 5. A: Lateral ligament attachments near the lateral tubercle of the talus. **B:** Mechanism of injury to the lateral tubercle of talus.

A

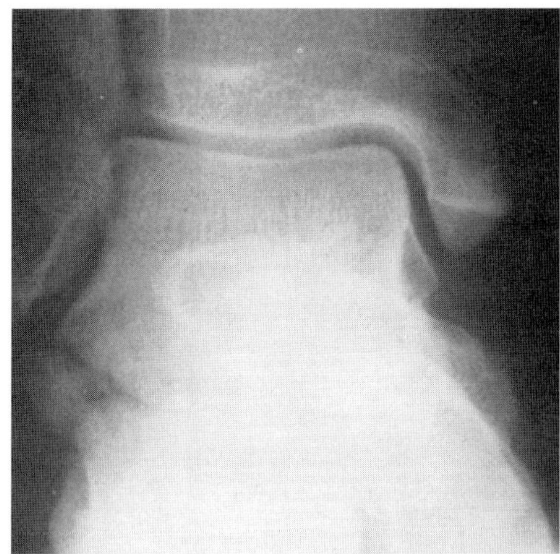

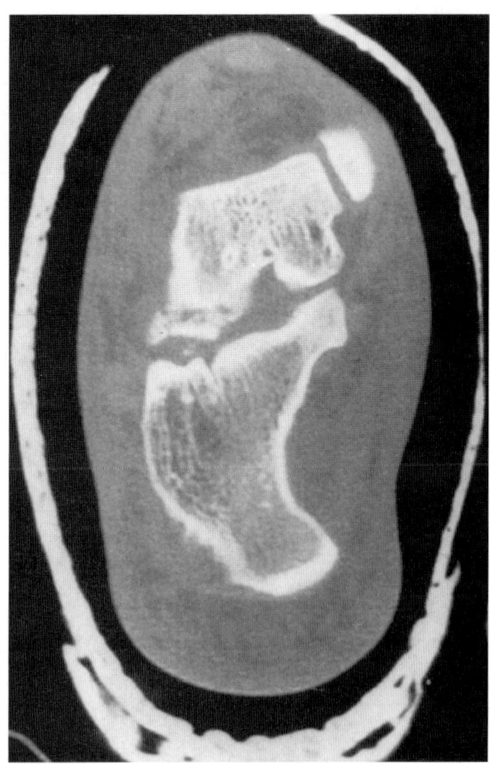

B

Figure 6. A: Inversion injury with radiograph of lateral tubercle indicating injury. **B:** CT scan of lateral tubercle fracture with multiple fragments, which will require debridement of sinus tarsi.

LATERAL TUBERCLE FRACTURES

Fractures of the lateral tubercle make up 24% of all talar body fractures. The talofibular and talocalcaneal ligaments are usually involved with the fragments (Fig. 5A). Of the several possible mechanisms for the lateral process fracture (1,5–9) (Fig. 5B), axial compression with dorsiflexion and external rotation is the most common. Inversion stress can cause avulsion of this area or eversion with the lateral and posterior tubercle of the talus being sheared off by the lateral malleolus. The treatment depends on the symptoms and the size of the fragment. Usually, the diagnosis is missed on routine anterior posterior views but can be seen in retrospect as comminution in the lateral tubercle area (Figs. 6 and 7). It should be noted that medial tubercle fractures have also been diagnosed, but these are very rare (10) (Fig. 7).

The treatment depends on when this diagnosis is made. If it is diagnosed acutely or relatively acutely within the first 3 to 4 weeks, a cast in slight equinus with no weight bearing for 6 to 8 weeks would be appropriate. If the fragment is large, it needs to be fixed by open reduction and internal fixation; a CT scan would be appropriate to define how large the fragment is and what is the best method of positioning the screw. The smaller fragments can be debrided if symptomatic. The lateral tubercle, like the posterior process, does not have an abundant blood supply. Healing of these lesions takes a great deal of time, firm fixation, and patience.

OSTEOCHONDRAL LESIONS OF THE TALUS

Osteochondral lesions of the talus were first described by Monroe in 1738, Konning in 1887, and then Rendu in 1932. These are often classified as osteochondroses (11–19). There is usually a delay in diagnosis, with the most common presenting symptoms being ankle pain, swelling, and occasionally locking. Joint laxity or a

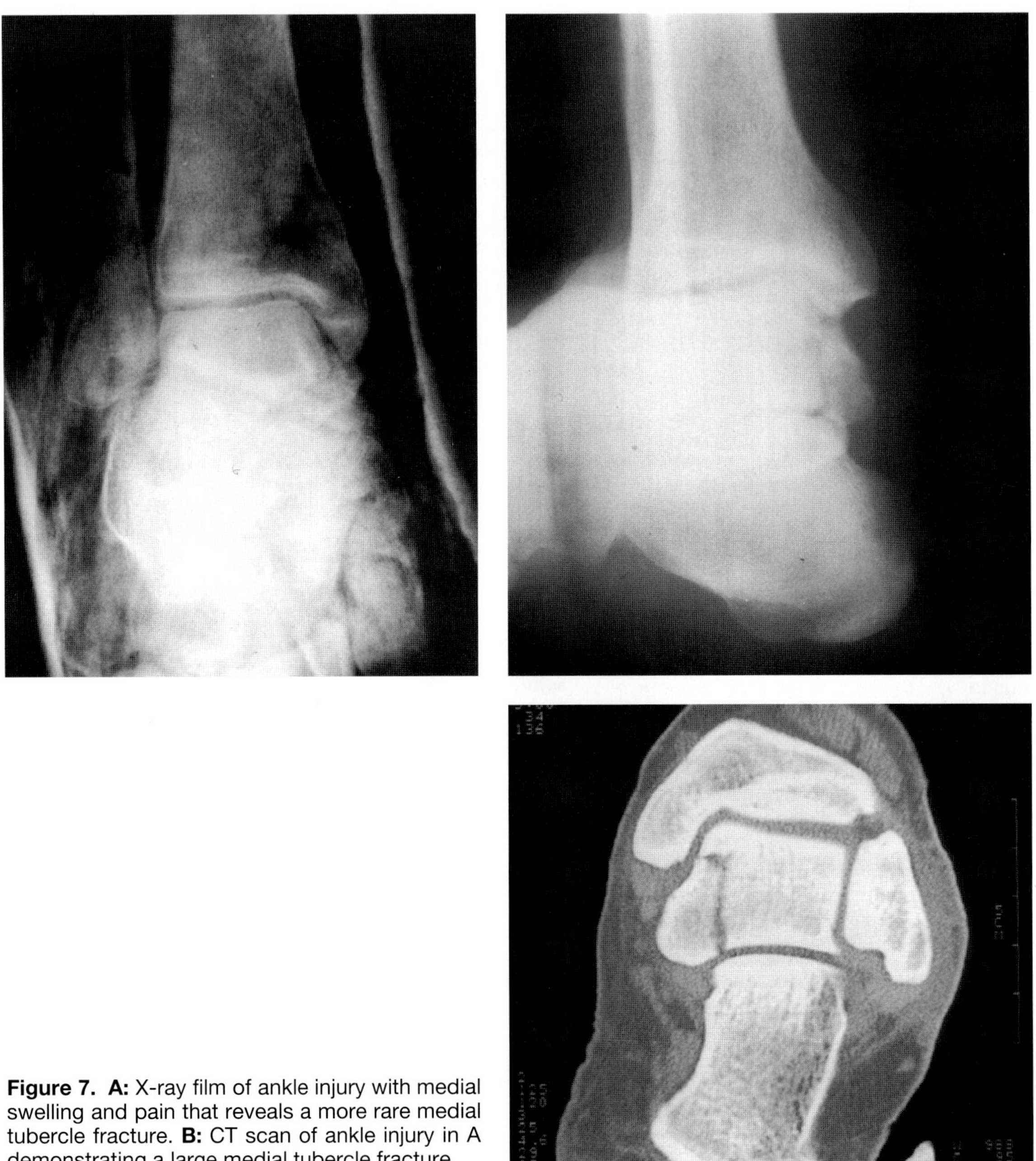

Figure 7. A: X-ray film of ankle injury with medial swelling and pain that reveals a more rare medial tubercle fracture. **B:** CT scan of ankle injury in A demonstrating a large medial tubercle fracture.

history of recurrent inversion injuries may coexist with osteochondral fractures. The lesions have been grouped in two basic types (Fig. 8C). The medial lesion, which is usually more posterior, can be associated with osteochondritis (Fig. 8A). The lateral lesions are thought to be secondary to trauma, and they are located more anterior (Fig. 8C). The lesions have been staged by Brendt and Harty (12) as follows: stage I, compression of the subchondral bone without break of the cartilage; stage II, an incomplete lesion with no cartilage flap tear; stage III, a lesion that is partly detached with the cartilage flap; and stage IV, a totally detached lesion associated with arthritic degeneration (Fig. 9).

The mechanism of injuries for osteochondral lesions is usually associated with traumatic inversion, anterior subluxation, with or without dorsiflexion (12,13) (Fig. 10). Because the blood supply to the talus is relatively poor, particularly on the lateral side,

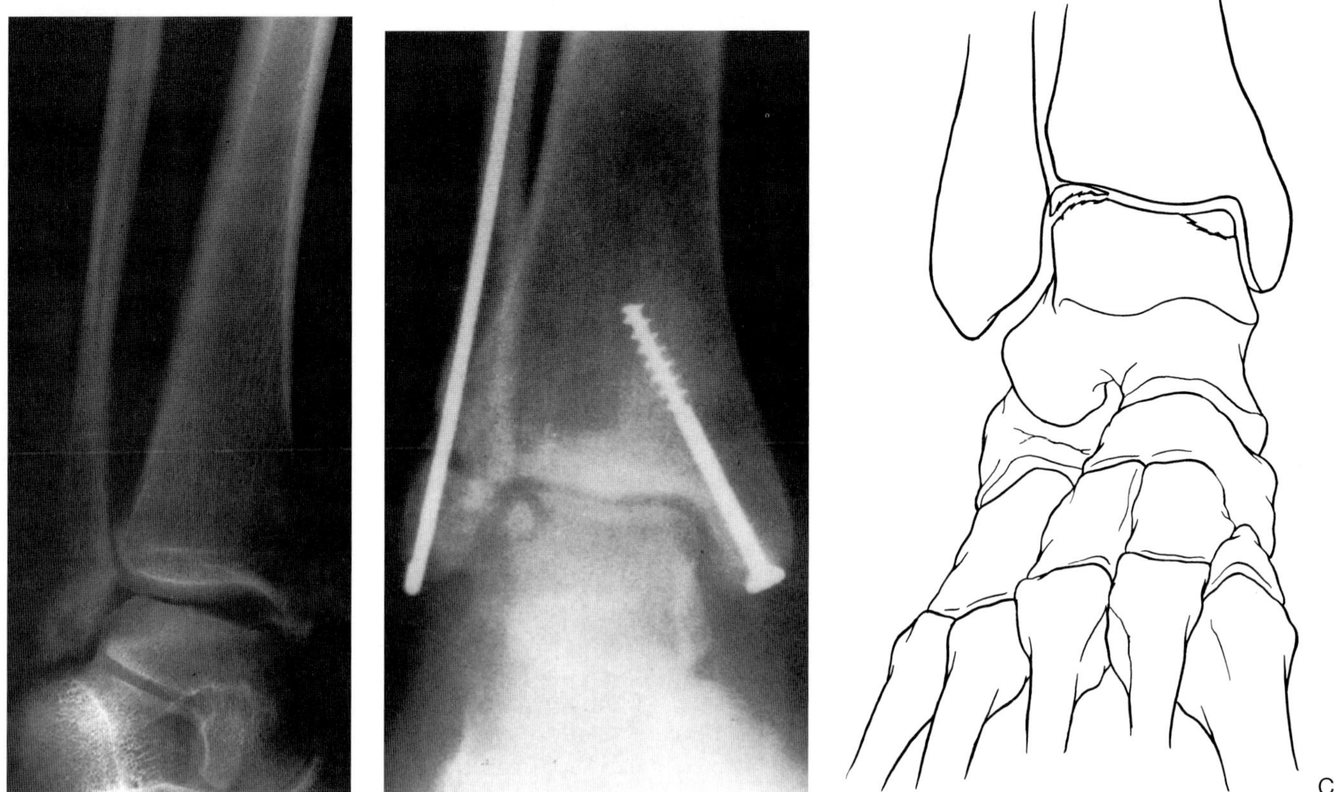

Figure 8. Osteochondral lesions of the talus. **A:** Medial osteochondral talus lesion. **B:** Lateral osteochondral lesion. **C:** Lateral and medial osteochondral talus fragment.

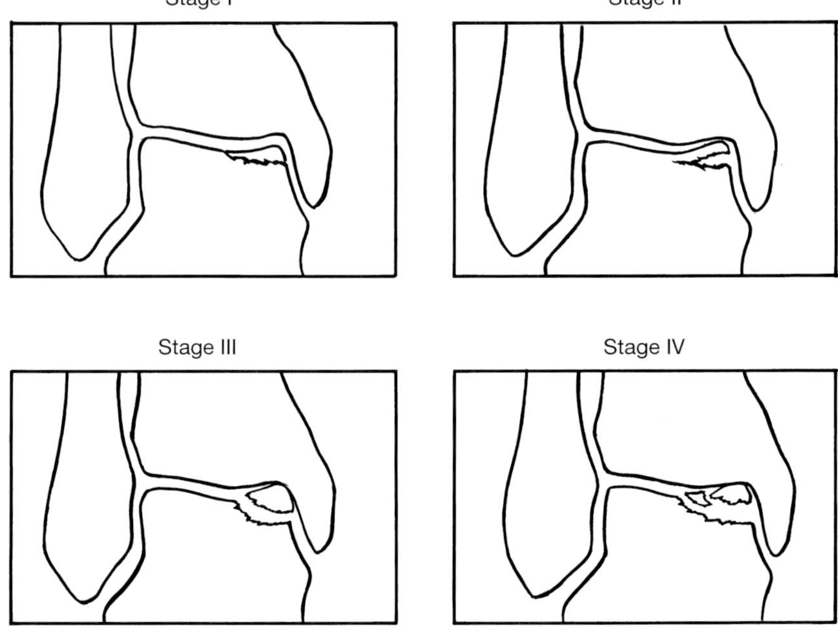

Figure 9. Stages of osteochondral injuries. (From ref. 12, with permission.)

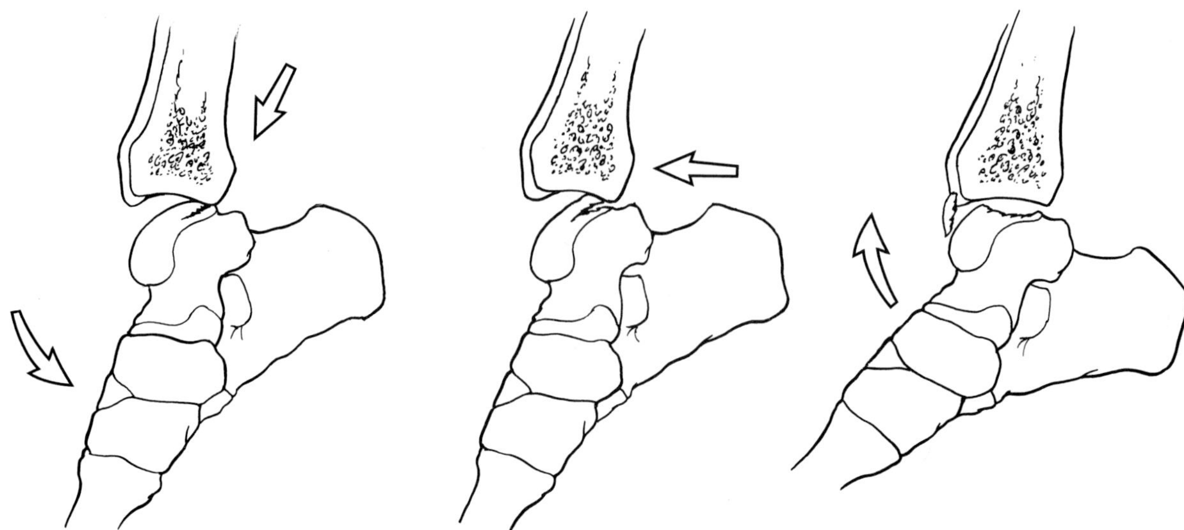

Figure 10. Mechanisms of injury of medial osteochondral lesions of the talus.

these lesions frequently do not unite. If a lesion is found acutely, then a cast would be appropriate unless evidence of cartilage detachment is present; we would then advocate an early arthroscopic procedure. The long-term prognosis is that few lesions unite when treated nonoperatively and that arthritic changes occur in a large percentage of cases, regardless of the type of treatment (11). Fortunately, this gloomy prognosis existed prior to the advent of arthroscopic treatment. It is felt that the lateral lesions are more wafer shaped and the medial lesions cup shaped. A CT scan is often helpful to locate the exact area of the lesion and the amount of subchondral collapse. Magnetic resonance imaging is helpful to determine how extensive the lesion is in the talar body (Fig. 11). The approach to these lesions (if symptomatic) is usually surgical and should be arthroscopic, since the lateral anterior lesion can be easily reached with the arthroscope. The medial lesion tends to be more of a technical problem with the arthroscope, but with the combined posterior lateral approach, most of the posterior medial portion of the talus can be evaluated and debrided if necessary (Fig. 12A). Recently, transtalar drilling in a retrograde fashion has been advocated (20) (Fig. 12B). With the advent of better arthroscopic skills, I see no reason to consider any type of malleolar osteotomy in the treatment of these disorders.

The problem with this fracture is how to treat it when a soft lesion is present under the cartilage or when there is an actual flap tear. Such a tear should be debrided unless it is very large. With large lesions, pinning and drilling may be appropriate. It may also be appropriate to consider the use of bioabsorbable pins, particularly the 2-mm variety, but it is difficult to get these into the hard talus. If the lesion is found by palpation to represent soft cartilage only, then drilling is sometimes recommended, but we do not recommend scooping out the cartilage lesion if there has been no breach in the cartilage. An anterior cruciate ligament (ACL) type guide can be used to drill the pins through the malleolar area (Fig. 12A). A new technique of drilling through the body of the talus to prevent articular damage was discussed by Dr. Stephen Conti (20) at a recent symposium on talar injuries (Fig. 12B). A retrograde drilling process is utilized through the medial or lateral tubercle of the talus under fluoroscopic control with arthroscopic evaluation of drill direction. Bone grafting can also be carried out by impacting small portions of cancellous bone up through the hole drilled into the talar lesion. Although there is no outcome study of this technique, it appears to make the most sense at this time. Cartilage grafting may also apply in these disorders in the future.

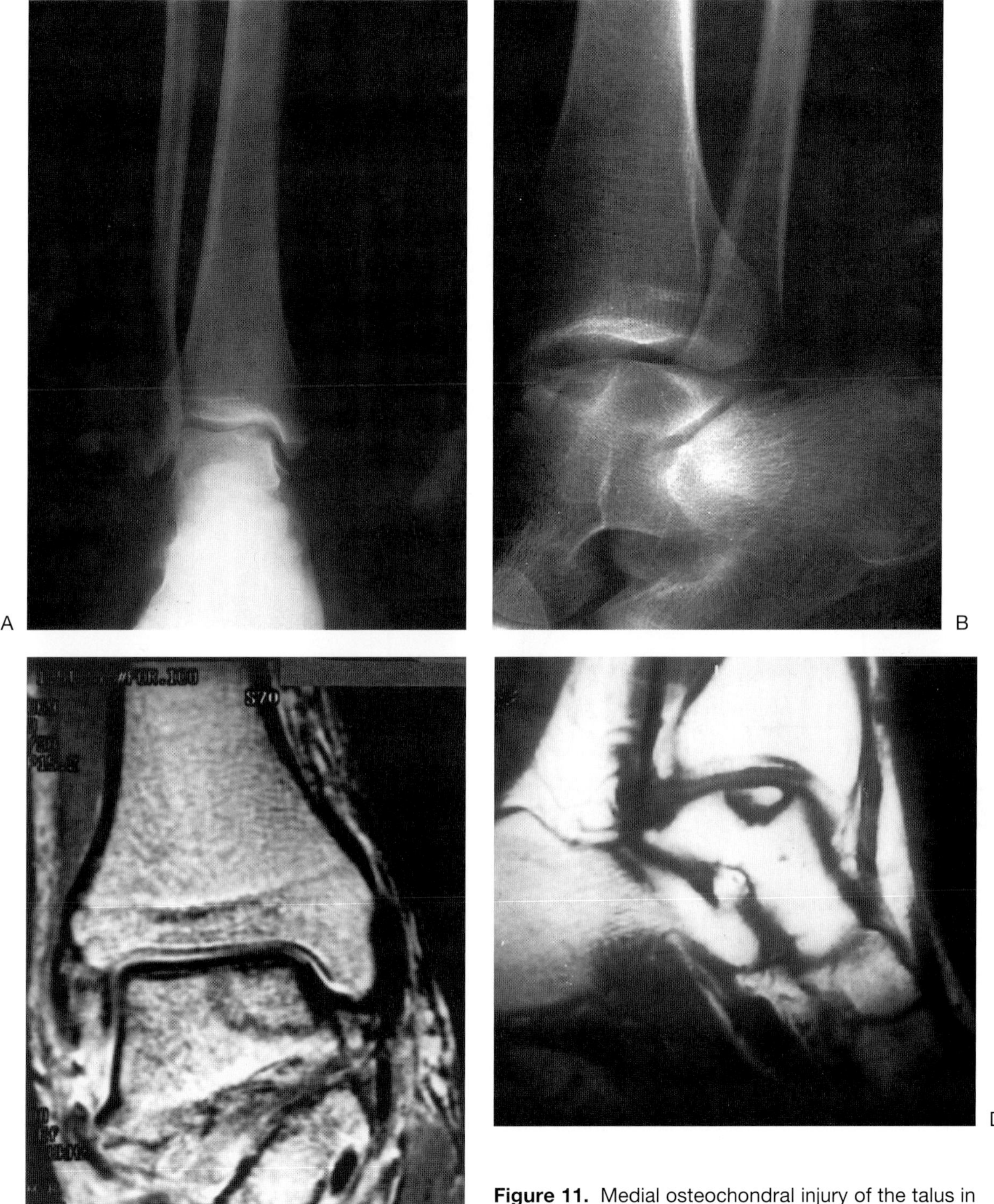

Figure 11. Medial osteochondral injury of the talus in 40-year-old secretary with ankle pain and swelling. **A,B:** Anterior posterior lateral radiograph showing a medial posterior lesion. **C,D:** Anterior posterior and lateral magnetic resonance imaging views.

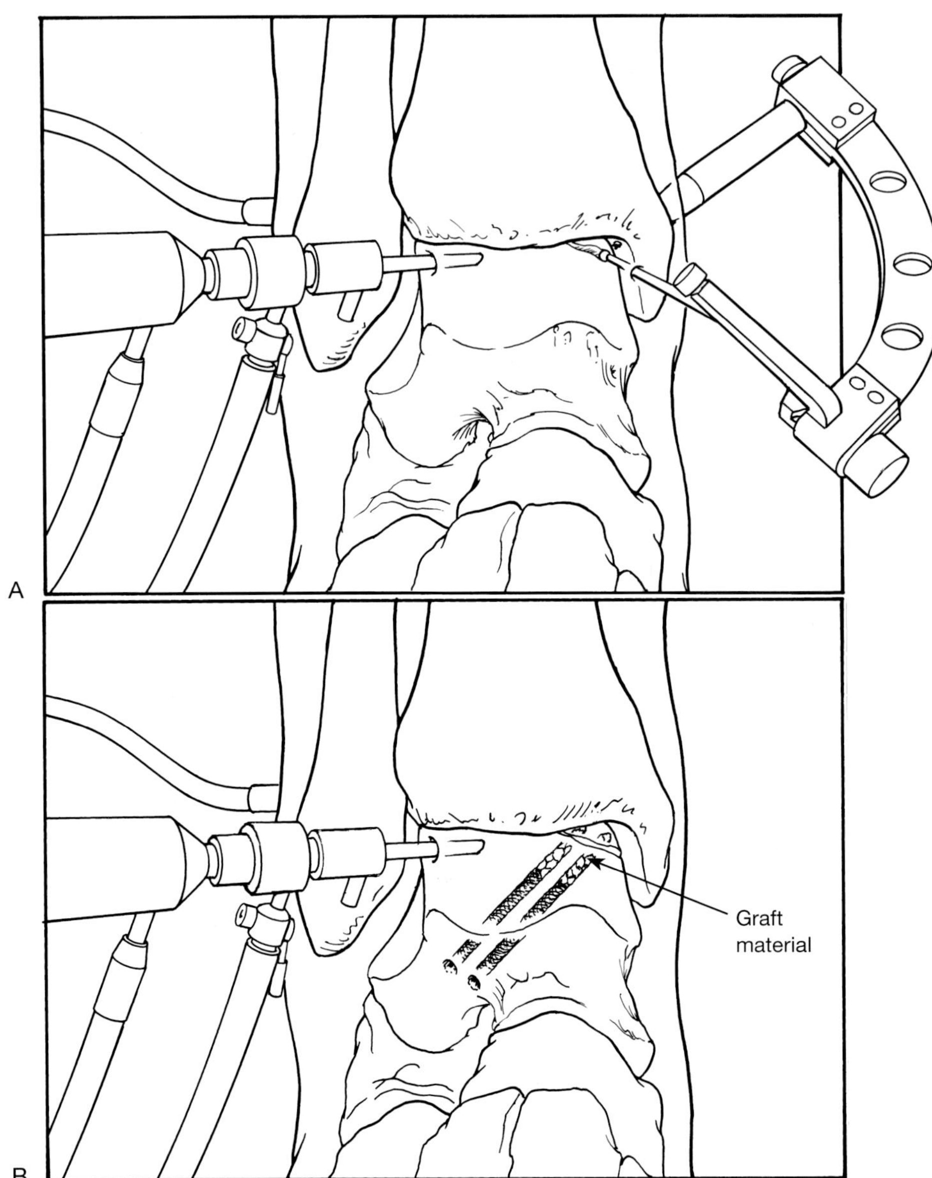

Figure 12. A: Arthroscopy evaluation and treatment of a medial osteochondral lesion. **B:** Transchondral drilling and bone graft of osteochondral lesions of the talus.

CONCLUSION

In summary, it is important to remember that because the talus has such a poor blood supply and so much articular cartilage, these lesions can give rise to long-term symptoms. It is often necessary to check the talus carefully for nonhealing or malunited posterior process, tubercle, or osteochondral lesions; excision is usually the treatment of choice when indicated. Treatment of these problem areas of the talus requires an early diagnosis, proper diagnostic imaging, and long-term stable treatment, either closed or open.

REFERENCES

1. Kleiger B. Fracture of the talus. *J Bone Joint Surg [Am]* 1948;30:735–744.
2. Sneppen O, Christiansen SB, Krogsoe O, et al. Fractures of the body of the talus. *Acta Orthop Scand* 1977;48:214–217.
3. Dimon JH. Isolated displaced fractures of the posterior facet of the talus. *J Bone Joint Surg [Am]* 1961;43:275–281.
4. Gatellier J. Juxtorectro-peritoneal root—operative treatment of fracture of the malleolus with posterior marginal fracture. *Surg Gynecol Obstet* 1931;52:67–70.

5. Hawkins LG. Fracture of the lateral process of the talus. *J Bone Joint Surg [Am]* 1965;47:1170–1175.
6. Heckman JD. Fracture of the lateral process of the talus. *Clin Orthop* 1985;199:108–113.
7. Mukherjee SK, Pringle RM. Fracture of the lateral process of the talus. *J Bone Joint Surg [Br]* 1974;56:263–273.
8. Fjeldborg O. Fracture of the lateral process of talus. *Acta Orthop Scand* 1968;39:407–412.
9. Deyrele M, Burhardt B. Displaced fractures of the talus: an aggressive approach. *Orthop Trans* 1981;5:465.
10. Kim DH, Hrutkay JM, Samson MM. Fracture of medial tubercle of posterior process of talus: a case report. *Foot Ankle Int* 1996;17:186.
11. Alexander AH, Lichtman DM. Surgical treatment of transchondral talar-dome fractures. *J Bone Joint Surg [Am]* 1980;62:646–652.
12. Brendt AL, Harty M. Transchondral fracture of the talus. *J Bone Joint Surg [Am]* 1959;41:988–1029.
13. Canale ST, Belding RH. Osteochondral lesions of the talus. *J Bone Joint Surg [Am]* 1980;62:92–102.
14. Davidson AM, Steele HD, MacKenzie DA, et al. A review of twenty-one cases of transchondral fractures of the talus. *J Trauma* 1967;7:378–415.
15. McCullough CJ. Osteochondritis dissecans of the talus. *Clin Orthop* 1979;144:24–268.
16. O'Farrell TA. Osteochondritis dissecans of the talus. *J Bone Joint Surg [Br]* 1982;64:494–497.
17. Ray R, Coughlan EJ. Osteochondritis dissecans of the talus. *J Bone Joint Surg* 1947;29:697–706.
18. Scharling M. Osteochondritis dissecans of the talus. *Acta Orthop Scand* 1978;49:89–94.
19. Yvars MF. Osteochondral fractures of the dome of the talus. *Clin Orthop* 1976;114:185–191.
20. Conti S, Taranow W. Retrograde drilling with bone grafting of talar dome osteochondral lesions. *Operative Tech Ortho* 1996; May.

Complex Foot and Ankle Trauma,
edited by Robert S. Adelaar,
Lippincott–Raven Publishers, Philadelphia © 1999.

9

Subtalar Dislocations

Michael J. Brennan

Simultaneous dislocation of both the talocalcaneal and talonavicular joints is referred to as a subtalar dislocation. This injury occurs because the weaker talonavicular and talocalcaneal ligaments and capsules rupture, while the strong calcaneonavicular ligament remains intact. This causes the midfoot to displace as a unit. Although this injury is rare enough that few series in the literature have more than ten patients, it is important to recognize the potential problems in treating it.

Most of these injuries occur as a result of high-energy impact, as in a motor vehicle accident or a fall from a height, but some happen simply as a result of stumbling on the basketball court. About 10% of these injuries are open, and all have some degree of soft tissue compromise (Fig. 1); a few cases of neurovascular compromise have been reported in closed injuries. Extensive swelling can mask the deformity, making diagnosis more difficult. If only ankle radiographs are obtained, the diagnosis can be missed and the appropriate treatment delayed. Figure 2 is part of an ankle series that was interpreted as normal until additional radiographs of the foot, shown in Fig. 3, clearly demonstrated the medial subtalar dislocation. The postreduction view (Fig. 4) shows the normal anatomic alignment.

Classifying the dislocation by the displacement of the distal part, 80% of subtalar dislocations are considered medial, and 20% have the foot displaced lateral to the talus. Associated fractures are present in about one-half of these injuries. Avulsions from the talar head or body of the calcaneus may block concentric reduction. Impaction of the talar head and navicular may prevent closed reduction. Fractures of the navicular, fibula, or base of the fifth metatarsal may require further care.

M. J. Brennan: Arizona State University, Phoenix, Arizona 85016.

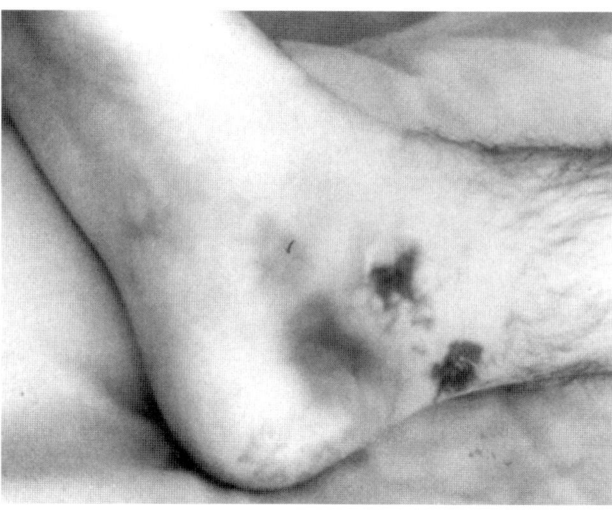

Figure 1. Medial soft tissue damage associated with lateral subtalar dislocation.

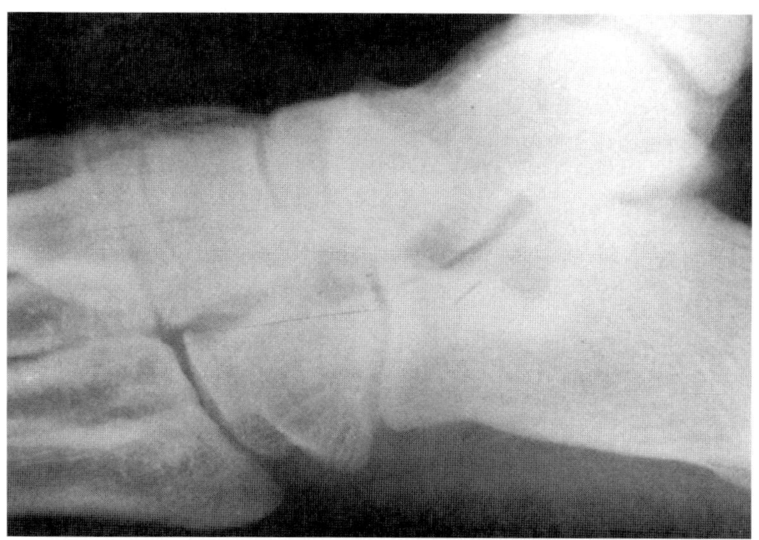

Figure 2. Medial subtalar dislocation. Note talar head overriding navicular.

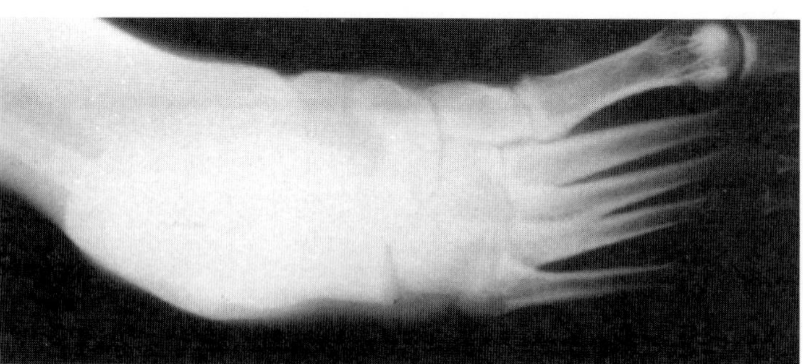

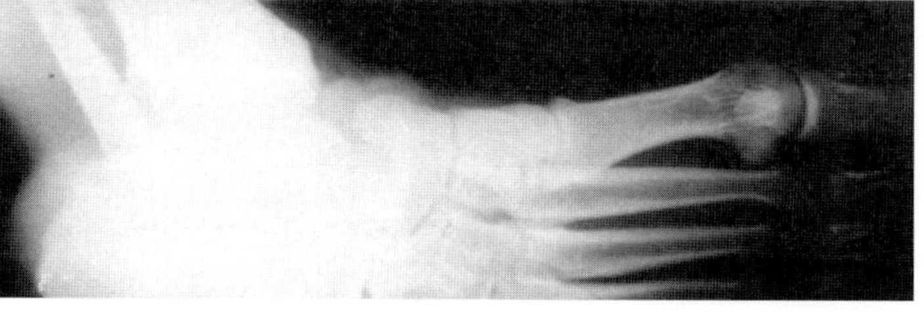

Figure 3. Anterior and oblique radiographs of foot confirm diagnosis of medial subtalar dislocation.

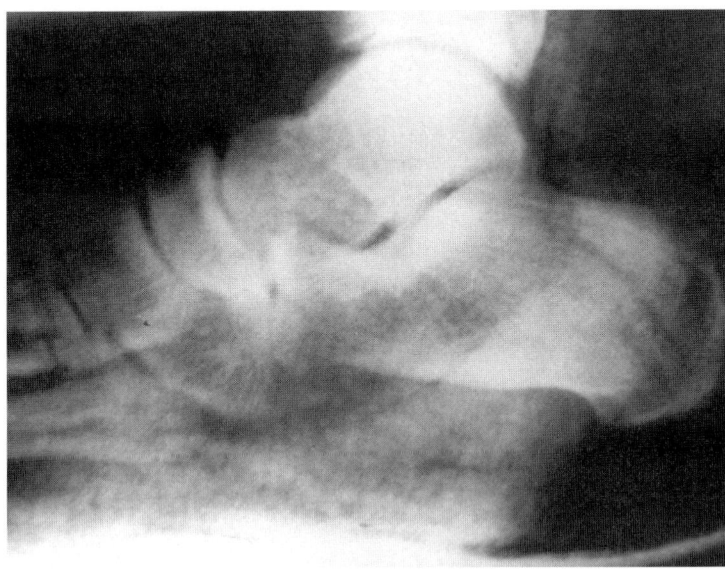

Figure 4. Postreduction view.

REDUCTION

Closed reduction is commonly performed with the patient under intravenous sedation, but I prefer to attempt closed reduction with the patient under general anesthesia, because I believe that muscle relaxation decreases the potential of articular cartilage damage and increases the likelihood of a successful closed reduction. If the attempted closed reduction is unsuccessful, I am prepared for immediate open reduction of the dislocation. To perform a closed reduction, use the following maneuver. Flex the knee and the forefoot. Apply gentle traction. Accentuate and then reverse the deformity, with digital pressure over the talar head. The surgeon can usually feel the dislocated part return to its normal position. The range of motion returns to normal with intrinsic bony stability, rarely requiring internal fixation.

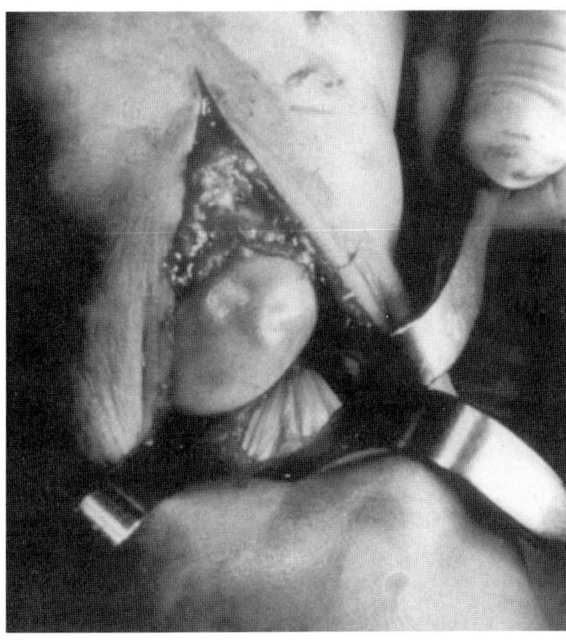

Figure 5. Extensor tendons block reduction of talar head.

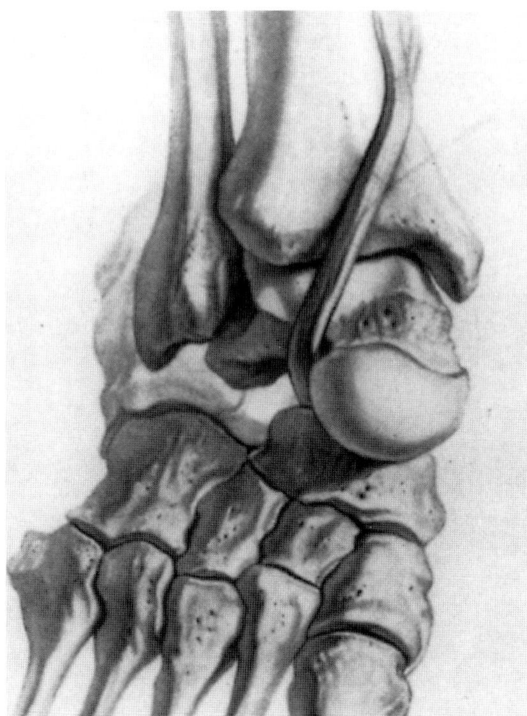

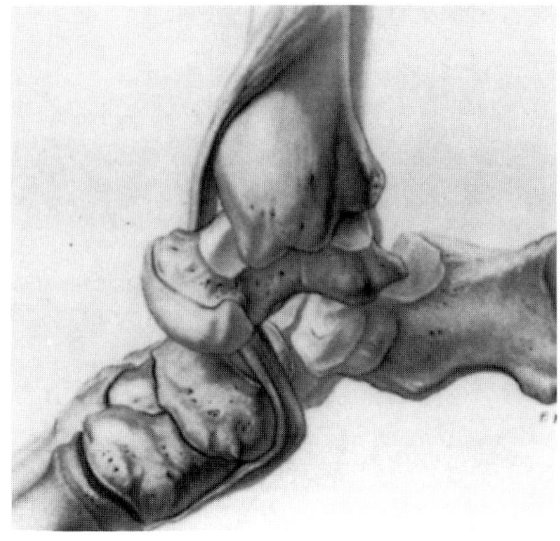

Figure 6. Posterior tibialis tendon blocks reduction of talar head. (From ref. 5, with permission.)

IRREDUCIBLE DISLOCATIONS

An irreducible subtalar dislocation is usually caused by the talar head being buttonholed through the surrounding longitudinally directed anatomic structures. To achieve reduction, make a longitudinal incision over the protruding talar head, avoiding compromised skin. Subsequent osteonecrosis of the talus is rare, occurring in only 5% to 10% of cases, but the blood supply should be preserved when possible. For this reason, soft tissue should not be stripped from the talar neck. Reduction of medial dislocations may be blocked by the extensor or anterior tibial tendons (Fig. 5). In the case of a lateral dislocation, the posterior tibialis tendon can prevent reduction and will require mobilization (Fig. 6). If the tendon must be transsected to allow reduction, it should be repaired. Locked impaction fractures may also hinder reduction. Avulsion or osteochondral fragments that can prevent a concentric reduction should be cleared from the joint or, if large enough, reduced and fixed in place (Fig. 7).

OPEN DISLOCATIONS

Goldner et al. (1) reported long-term results in 15 patients treated for open subtalar dislocations. There were ten lateral and five medial dislocations. Of the ten lateral dislocations, nine had associated osteochondral fractures, four had disruptions of the posterior tibial nerve, five had ruptures of the posterior tibial tendon, and five had lacerations of the posterior tibial artery. Of these ten, three were managed with a myocutaneous flap, four were managed with a split-thickness skin graft, and three had healing by secondary intention.

All the patients in this series developed posttraumatic arthritis. Osteonecrosis of the talus with segmental collapse of the talar body developed in five of the 15 patients at an average of 2 years after the injury. All five of these patients underwent arthrodesis surgery within 5 years of the injury. All 15 patients had decreased motion of the ankle, subtalar joint, and midfoot. Seven of the 15 had been stabilized initially with internal fixation. The overall results were judged as only fair to poor.

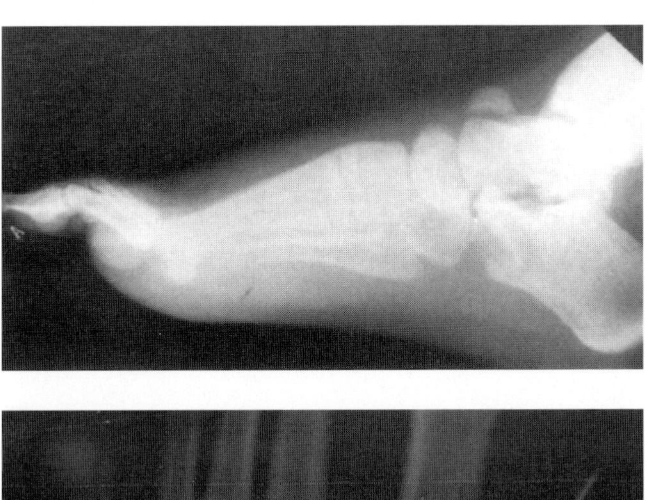

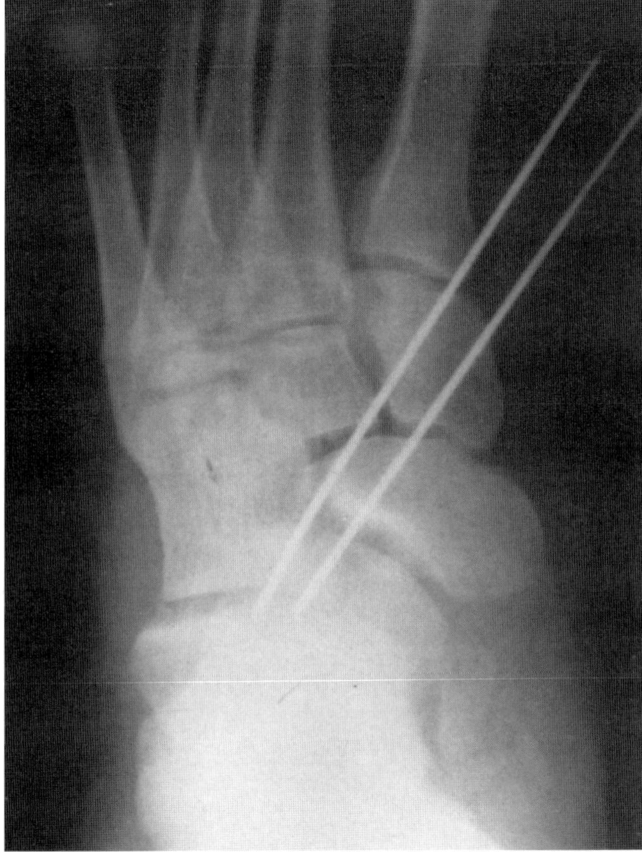

Figure 7. Top: Unstable reduction with osteochondral fragment. **Bottom:** Status after open reduction and internal fixation.

TREATMENT

I immobilize patients in a short leg cast for at least 4 weeks, increasing this period to 6 weeks for patients who are young or loose-jointed or who have associated fractures. Historically, the concern has been for loss of subtalar motion after this injury. Some loss of motion is detected in nearly all patients; however, few complain of stiffness. Stiffness may be less functionally impairing than subtalar instability. Zimmer and Johnson (2) reported that five of eight patients treated described problems of instability. These patients tended to be younger and had an average period of immobilization of only 4.4 weeks. Larsen (3) described a patient with recurrent subtalar dislocation. Heppenstall and associates (4) described the loss of reduction of a subtalar dislocation while it was in a cast. For these reasons, the trend to a shorter period of immobilization and early range of motion may be inappropriate for this injury.

REFERENCES

1. Goldner JL, Poletti SC, Gates HS, Richardson WJ. Severe open subtalar dislocations. *J Bone Joint Surg [Am]* 1996;77:1075–1079.
2. Zimmer TJ, Johnson KA. Subtalar dislocations. *Clin Orthop* 1989;238:190–194.
3. Larsen HW. Subastragalar dislocation (luxatio pedis sub talo): a follow-up report of eight cases. *Acta Chir Scand* 1957;113:380–392.
4. Heppenstall RB, Farahvar H, Balderston R, et al. Evaluation and management of subtalar dislocations. *J Trauma* 1980;20:494–497.
5. Leitner B. Obstacles to reduction in subtalar dislocations. *J Bone Joint Surg [Am]* 1954;36:304.

EDITORIAL COMMENTS

Subtalar Dislocations

Michael J. Brennan

Subtalar or peritalar dislocations are uncommon injuries. They have been reported to account for only about 1% of all traumatic dislocations in various texts. Sixty percent of these unusual dislocations are medial and 24% are lateral. The mechanism of injury usually involves forceful inversion of the forefoot with the head and neck of the talus pivoting on the sustentaculum tali and causing a talonavicular dislocation followed by the subtalar dislocation in the more common medial dislocations. Poor results have been associated with open injury and associated fractures at the time of dislocation. Avascular necrosis has not been reported in these injuries. In the long term, patients do lose some motion, but this loss of motion in the subtalar joint may not be detectable clinically and is usually associated with prolonged immobilization, open, more high-energy injuries, or associated fractures.

A good clinical examination and appropriate x-rays including oblique views should be done to rule out the more subtle subluxations. General anesthesia is certainly preferred for full reduction, but one could consider sciatic nerve blocks or other forms of regional anesthesia. Subtalar dislocations are usually stable after reduction, and they should be stressed if they tend to be unstable. If fractures are associated, then pinning may be appropriate for short periods. One should look for irreducible dislocations, particularly on the medial side, with entrapment of the short extensor, extensor retinaculum, or anterior tibialis.

Robert S. Adelaar, M.D.

Complex Foot and Ankle Trauma,
edited by Robert S. Adelaar,
Lippincott–Raven Publishers, Philadelphia © 1999.

10

Intraarticular Calcaneal Fractures: A Basic Science Update with Clinical Correlations

James B. Carr

The intraarticular calcaneal fracture remains ''unsolved,'' and too many patients continue to experience poor results. Enthusiasm for the operative treatment of this fracture has recently been renewed. A historical inspection reveals a literature full of pessimism and controversy. In 1942 Bankhart (1) stated that ''the results of os calcis fractures are terrible.'' The calcaneus fracture has been subjected to many diverse treatments (2–10): the Cotton mallet, the Harris triradiate traction, percutaneous pins, open reduction, primary fusion, and total excision. No other articular fracture in the body has been treated so variously with such seemingly similar results. The calcaneus fracture seems to defy common sense—why is this? These apparent mysteries spur us onward in the search for better solutions. The purpose of this chapter is to present an update on recent advances in the basic science of such fractures and to provide clinical correlations. We begin with anatomic considerations.

ANATOMY

Although it is doubtful whether any new gross anatomic aspects of the calcaneus have been discovered lately, it is useful from a surgical standpoint to review the

J. B. Carr: Department of Orthopaedic Surgery, Medical College of Virginia, Richmond, Virginia 23298; Department of Orthopaedic Surgery, MCV Hospitals, Richmond, Virginia 23298.

gross anatomy. The calcaneus supports four articular facets and has a complex trabecular structure (12,13) (Fig. 1). It forms an integral link to the motion of the subtalar and transverse tarsal joints. From a surgical standpoint, the posterior facet is best visualized from a lateral approach; the middle and anterior facets remain hidden behind stout interosseous and talocalcaneal ligaments. The cuboid facet can be visualized via a lateral approach, but its complex saddle shape make full visualization difficult. Fortunately, these latter three articulations often reduce indirectly when the other components of this fracture are reduced anatomically (5,10).

One of the hindrances to the operative treatment of this injury is the development of wound complications. Deep infection following surgical treatment is a disaster, inevitably leading to poor results. These complications seem particularly problematic for incisions parallel to the peroneal tendons (5). Benirschke et al. (5) have recently modified the lateral approach to allow extensile exposure (Fig. 2). This incision parallels the border of the Achilles tendon and curves anteriorly to parallel the plantar surfaces. This incision ''outlines'' the cutaneous arterial distribution of the peroneal artery (14). Thus, the Benirschke incision essentially develops a deep fascial cutaneous flap based on the peroneal artery, which probably explains its success. This flap also avoids the sural nerve, except in its most proximal and distal limits of exposure. Wound complications have been reported in approximately 5% of patients with this incision (5).

Medial approaches are hindered by interference with the cutaneous sensory nerves and the posterior tibial nerve vascular bundle (6,10). The medial approach does allow direct access to the superomedial fragment, a key component of fracture pathology.

Regarding the cortical and trabecular structures of the calcaneus, a complex situation exists. There are four trabecular systems of the calcaneus, thalamic, anterior apophyseal, anterior plantar, and posterior plantar (15) (Fig. 3). The thalamic radiation is a direct continuation of the weight-bearing trabeculae from the distal tibia and talus. It is best developed beneath the posterior facet. The anterior apophyseal trabeculae function as a strut from the cuboid to the posterior facet. The confluences of these four systems outline a fatty filled neutral triangle nearly devoid of trabeculae (12). Examined by optical density scanning, the values range from 0.8 in the thalamic radiation to 0.02 in the neutral triangle (1.0 equals cortical bone) (15). Thus, depending on location, there is a 40-fold difference in trabecular density. Measuring cortical density, the thickest bone is observed medially and superiorly; the thinnest bone is consistently seen along the lateral wall and plantar surfaces. Medial wall thickness can approach 4 mm in the confluences of the sustentaculum tali (15) (Fig. 4). The thickest lateral bone is represented by the strut of cortex running

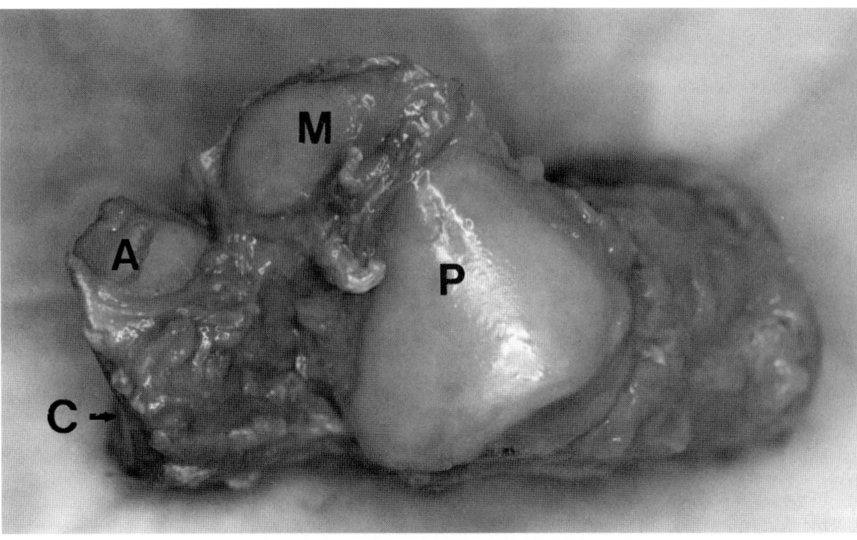

Figure 1. The calcaneus, demonstrating the four articular facets. *P,* posterior facet; *M,* middle facet; *A,* anterior facet; *C,* cuboid facet. Note that the middle facet lies anterior and superior to the posterior facet. This becomes important when aiming screws into the sustentacular region.

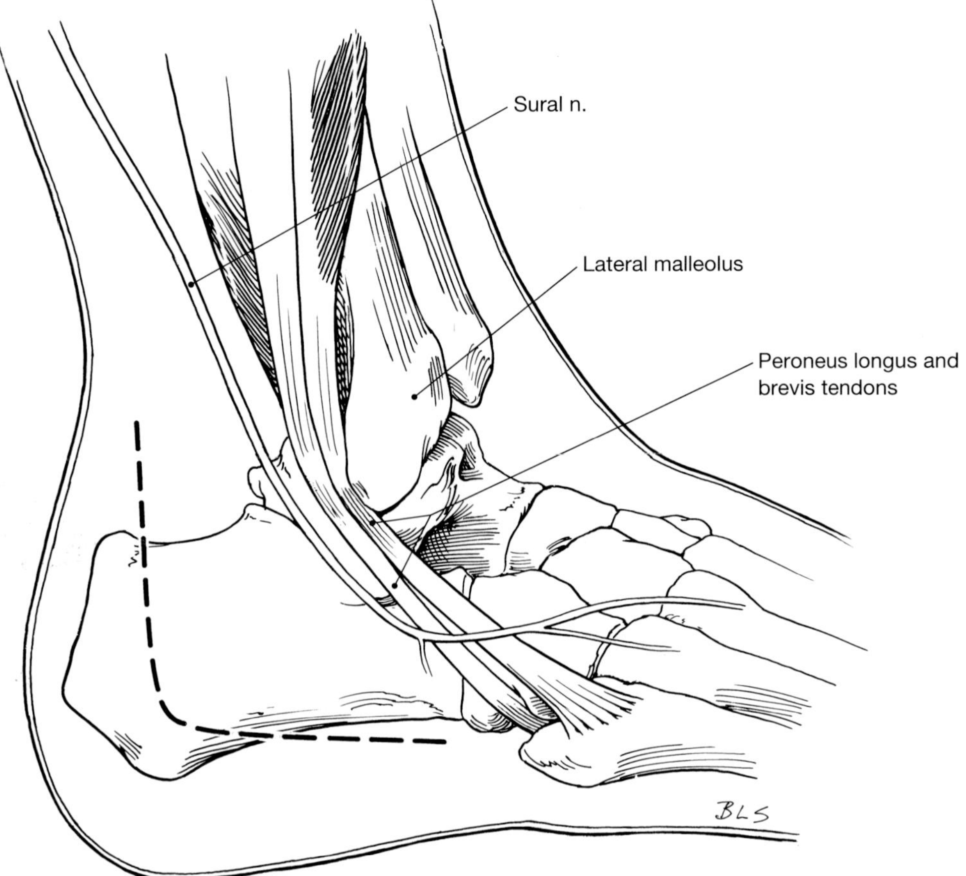

Figure 2. The lateral extensile approach of Benirschke is based on the cutaneous distribution of the peroneal artery (*dotted line*). It thus creates a deep fasciocutaneous flap.

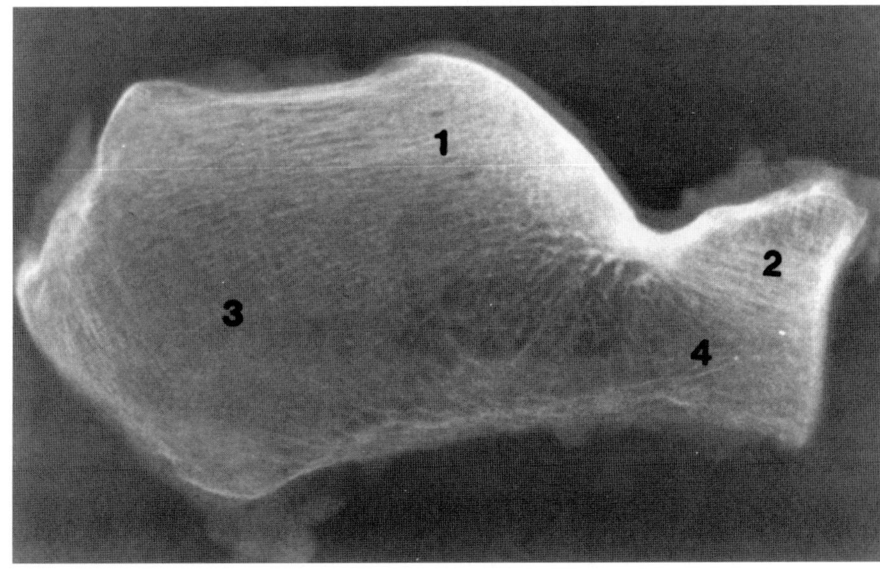

Figure 3. The trabecular anatomy of the calcaneus consists of the following: *1*, thalamic; *2*, anterior apophyseal; *3*, posterior plantar; and *4*, anterior plantar systems. The densest bone is consistently juxtarticular and superior within the calcaneus.

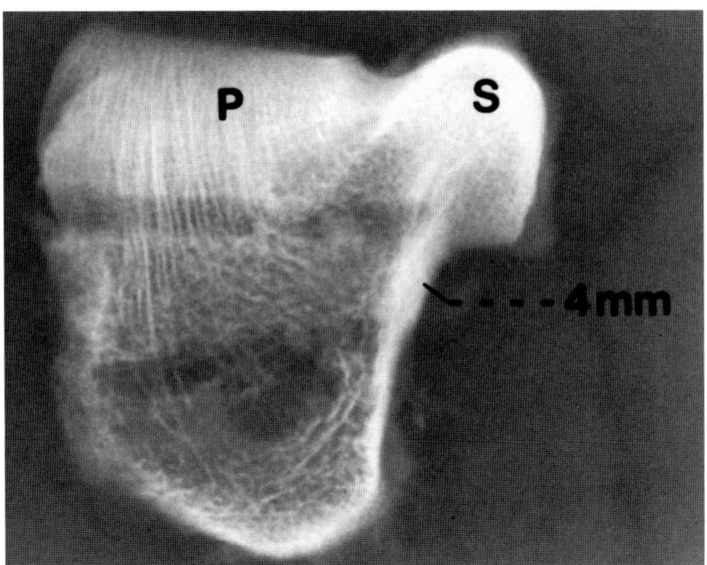

Figure 4. The coronal cut demonstrates the thick confluence of bone beneath the sustentaculum tali (*S*) and the posterior facet (*P*). Here the medial wall measures 4 mm in thickness.

between the posterior and cuboid facets. The clinical correlation of this histomorphometry is evident when one examines screw purchase in the calcaneus. Using lateral to medially directed screws in an intact calcaneus, the consistently best screw purchase is found in the superior regions of the calcaneus and juxtaarticular locations (15). Medial bone stock would thus appear critical for adequate screw purchase. This medial bone stock is represented by the superomedial fragment (7). As Burdeaux (7) pointed out, this fragment is a consistent finding, although the size and comminution may vary from case to case. The superomedial fragment can be assessed preoperatively with the use of computed tomography (CT) (16). Conversely, lack of an intact medial bone stock, or improper placement of a screw, may result in fixation of approximating the proverbial custard pie to which McLaughlin referred.

MECHANISM AND PATHOANATOMY

It is intuitive that a complete knowledge of the mechanism and pathoanatomy would aid in the surgical treatment of the calcaneus fracture. A historical review questions whether or not understanding of this fracture anatomy is possible. As Cotton (2) stated, "the x-ray shows an unintelligible confusion of lines which mean nothing." However, numerous authors have noted two consistent fracture patterns: the joint depression and the tongue

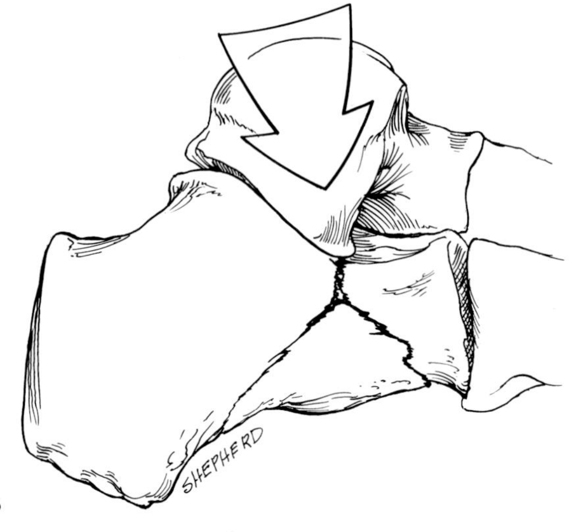

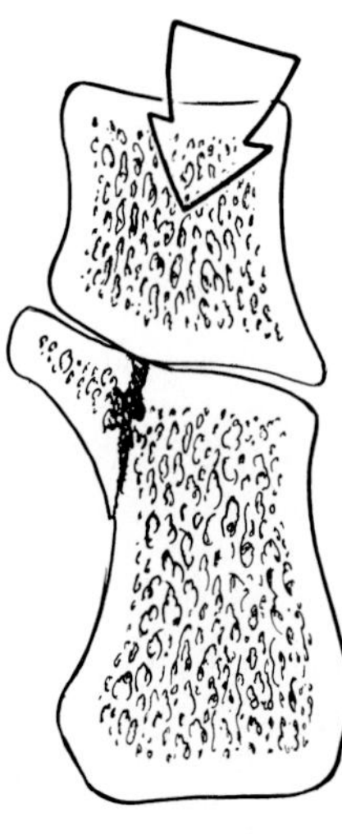

A,B

Figure 5. A: On the lateral view, the wedge-like process of the talus is driven into the angle of Gissane. **B:** On the axial view, the talus sits eccentrically. It shears the calcaneus into medial and lateral portions.

fracture of Essex-Lopresti (7). The concept of the *primary fracture line* developed to explain the split depression of the posterior facet commonly observed in the injury. In 1953, Warrick and Bremner (17) derived "An Atlas of Calcaneal Fractures," based on x-ray study of 350 cases. Their illustration and concept of the primary fracture line has appeared in numerous publications since that time. Notably lacking in their atlas is detail of the anterior fracture anatomy. It was McReynolds (26) and Burdeaux (7) who called attention to the superomedial fragment and its key role in pathoanatomy and subsequent

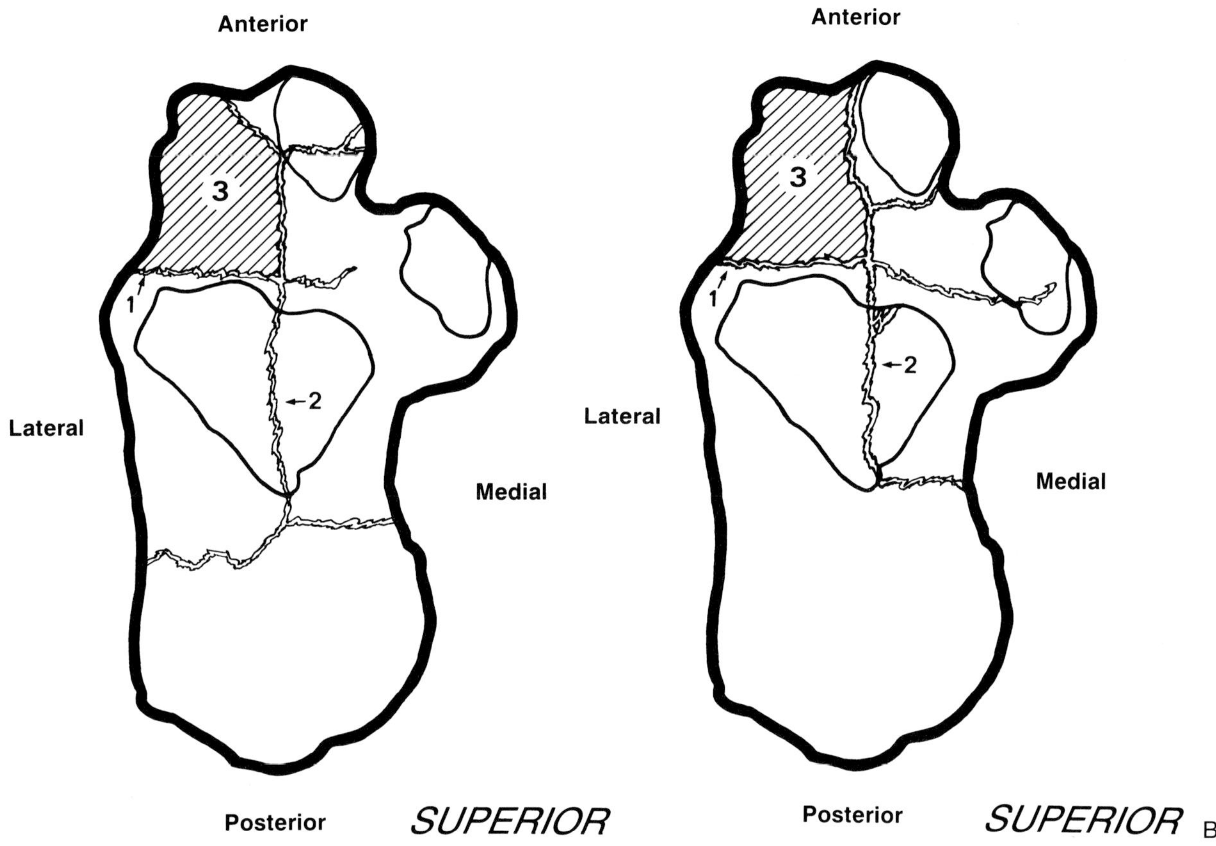

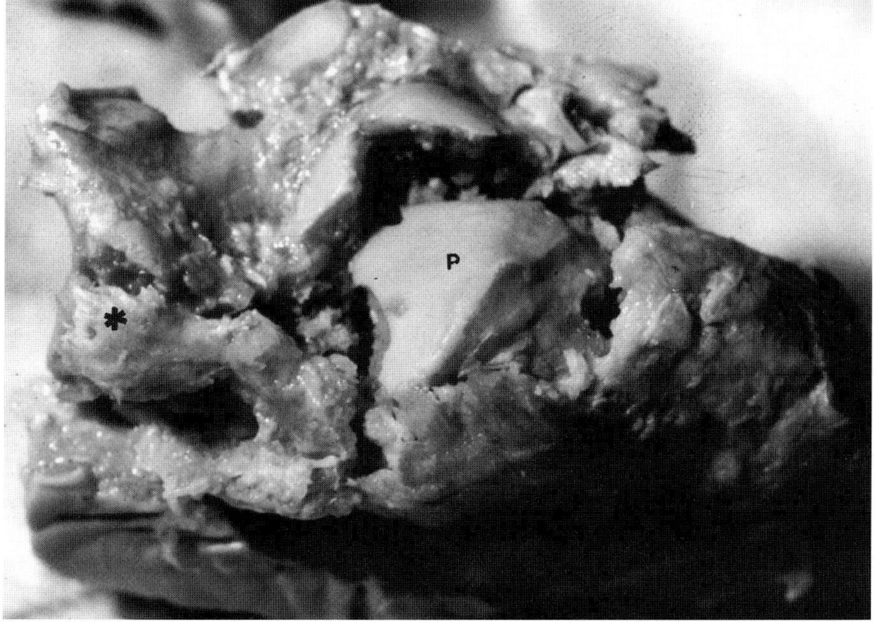

Figure 6. Dorsal view of the primary fracture lines producing a joint depression (**A**) and tongue-type (**B**) fracture. *1,* primary fracture line dividing in the coronal plane; *2,* primary fracture line dividing in the sagittal plane; *3,* anterolateral fragment. **C:** Lateral view depicting a left specimen with a joint depression fracture. Note the split stepoff in the posterior facet (*P*). The anterolateral fragment (*) is present. Lateral wall expansion occurs in the region of the coronal primary fracture line.

treatment. Based on experimental data, literature review, and clinical observations, I have synthesized these concepts into a mechanism that, I believe explains comprehensively the pathoanatomy observed in most cases (18). This description refers to injuries produced by axial loading. Obviously, as the energy levels and force vectors increase, it becomes very difficult to discern recognizable fracture pieces and patterns.

A key to the understanding of the fracture mechanism is an appreciation of the unique relationship of the talus to the calcaneus (12). Firmly bonded by the thick medial and central interosseous ligaments, the talus sits slightly medial to the midaxis of the calcaneus when viewed from the axial projection. Laterally, the wedge-like anterolateral process of the talus is poised over the angle of Gissane (Fig. 5). Axial loading produces a stereotypical fracture pattern. Shear forces split the calcaneus into medial and lateral portions (17). Since this split occurs early in the genesis of the fracture, it has been termed the primary fracture line (4). This line splits the posterior facet and then runs anteriorly to dissipate into the body, where it can produce fractures of the anterior and cuboid facet. If the foot is in valgus at the time of loading, the line tends to occur in the lateral portion of the posterior facet. Conversely, a varus position tends to produce a fracture line more medially.

The second primary fracture line is produced by the anterolateral process of the talus, which crushes the angle of Gissane and divides the calcaneus into anterior and posterior portions (4, 18). This fracture line can course medially to split the middle facet, unless it dissipates into the sagittal primary fracture line previously described. Laterally, the fracture line continues in an inverted Y-configuration of varying directions. This produces the anterolateral fragment (18,19). The lateral wall is crushed outward, producing characteristic peroneal tendon impingement (Fig. 6).

As the talus recoils upward, it carries the superomedial fragment with it. The split-off lateral piece of the posterior facet remains buried in the body of the calcaneus, producing a characteristic stepoff of up to 1 cm. The tuberosity fragment is typically translated laterally and angulated into varus. The tuberosity is driven up between the split posterior facet fragments. It must be pulled from this position before an anatomic reduction of the posterior facet can be obtained (Fig. 7). *This critical step cannot be overemphasized* (5,20). The calcaneal body loses height, and the longitudinal shape is altered.

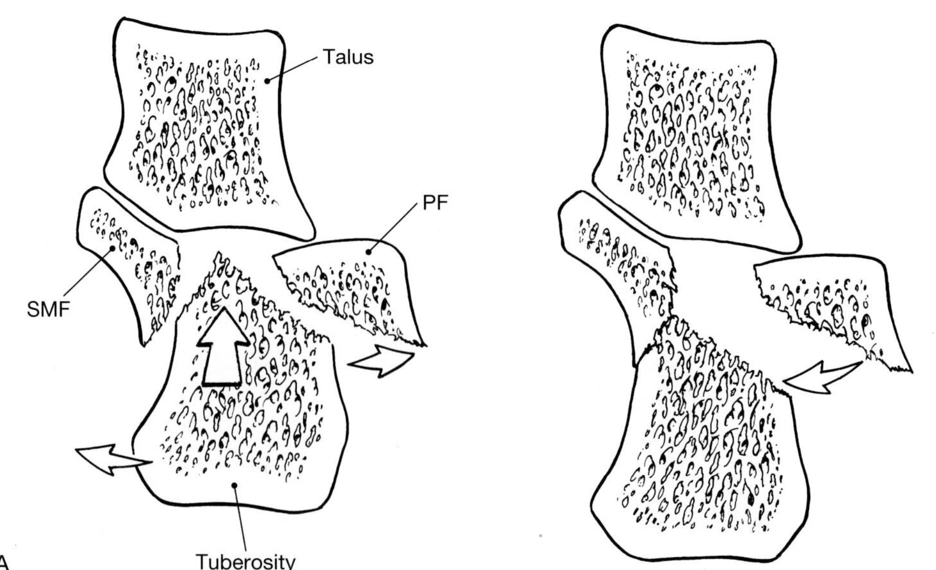

Figure 7. A: The tuberosity is driven and impacted in the gap between the posterior facet (*PF*) and the superomedial fragment (*SMF*). **B:** Reduction of the posterior facet is impossible until the tuberosity is anatomically reduced to the SMF. This concept is the keystone of the McReynolds medial approach. It is also applicable to the extensile lateral approach. *Arrows* represent the direction of fracture fragment movement.

In addition to the ''two-piece split'' of the posterior facet, three major pieces may be encountered in the posterior facet. It is hypothesized that the middle piece is produced by the talus fracturing off the lateral portion of the superomedial fragment as it descends into the plantar aspect of the foot. Thus, this middle piece tends to be displaced on the order of 1 to 2 mm and is commonly tilted downward on its lateral side.

Finally, the cuboid facet can be split by the sagittal 1-degree fracture line (17). As in the posterior facet, a single or double split can occur. Occasionally, an anterolateral process type of fracture is observed, which breaks off a portion of the upper lateral cuboid facet.

NATURAL HISTORY

To appreciate the effects of intervention, one must know the natural history of the displaced intraarticular calcaneal fracture. This section refers to fractures treated without operative or nonoperative manipulation of any type. The information presented is based on numerous series, as well as the author's own experience (6,8,21–24).

The typical fracture results from a fall onto a hard surface. Severe heel pain is immediately experienced. Assuming the absence of foot compartment syndrome or other complications, this pain gradually subsides over 7 to 14 days. If the patient is kept non-weight-bearing, the heel becomes relatively painless. At 8 to 12 weeks, when weight bearing is instituted, pain develops in one or more of four locations (8): (a) the lateral tip of the fibula, (b) the medial ankle, (c) the anterior ankle, and (d) the plantar surface. The lateral heel pain is the most common. Interestingly, it has been observed in patients treated with and without immediate subtalar fusion (23). This lateral pain is probably produced by peroneal/fibular impingement and/or subtalar arthritis. Swelling is common, tends to be worse at the end of the day, and accompanies the pain. The patient will experience a limp and impaired functional abilities. Over time (sometimes as long as 2 years), the pain improves to a stable state. Rare cases continue to improve slowly beyond that time. In one series, the average time off work was 6 months, with approximately 20% unable to perform ''heavy work'' (23). Overall, only 17% of patients in the same series had no complaints related to their fractures (23).

CLASSIFICATION

Historically, classification systems have focused on the appearance of the lateral radiograph or the amount of displacement, as well as the important distinction between intra- and extraarticular fractures. The widely used Essex–Lopresti *tongue* and *joint depression* types remain useful descriptive terms (4). A problem with these pre-CT-scan systems is the failure to identify factors relevant to treatment and prognosis on a consistent basis.

The current trend is toward a CT scan-based classification focusing on displacement and fragmentation of the posterior facet. In 1987, Carr et al. (18) proposed a column classification, in an attempt to correlate the displacement observed with a surgical approach and also to provide a language and framework to discuss the pathoanatomy observed on a CT scan. Important deficiencies of this classification include lack of treatment correlations and determination of prognosis.

In 1992, Crosby and Fitzgibbons (21) proposed three types of calcaneal fractures, based on displacement of the posterior facet: type I, with the posterior facet minimally displaced; type II, greater than 2 mm displacement of the posterior facet; and type III, comminuted displaced injuries involving the posterior facet. Although this was not strictly a natural history study, since percutaneous reductions and manipulations were included in the nonoperatively treated group, it is important in that posterior facet displacement of more than 2 mm did correlate with a poor prognosis.

Sanders et al. (9) have proposed a classification based on CT scanning that focuses on the number of fragments in the posterior facet as well as the displacements (Fig. 8): type I, undisplaced fracture; type II, two major fragments in the posterior facet;

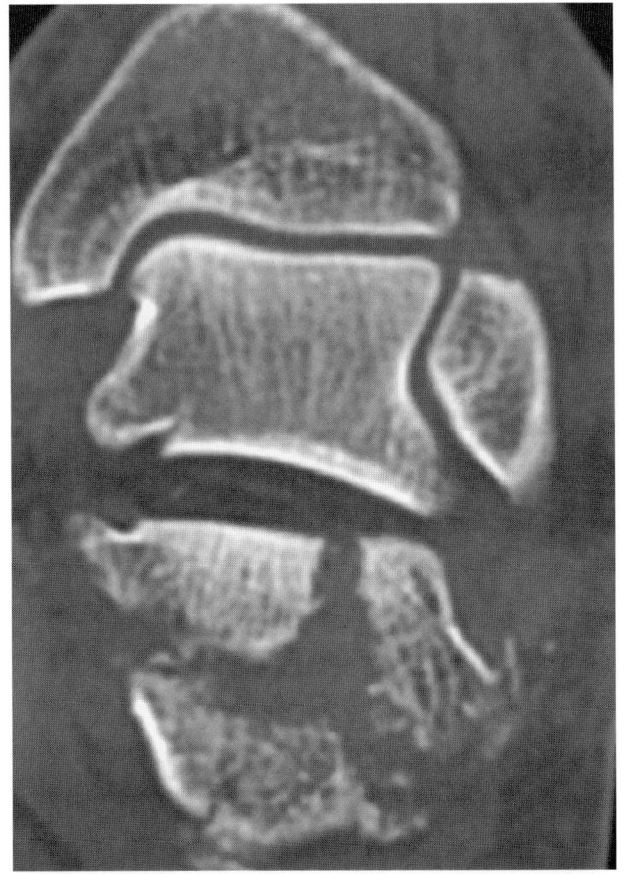

A

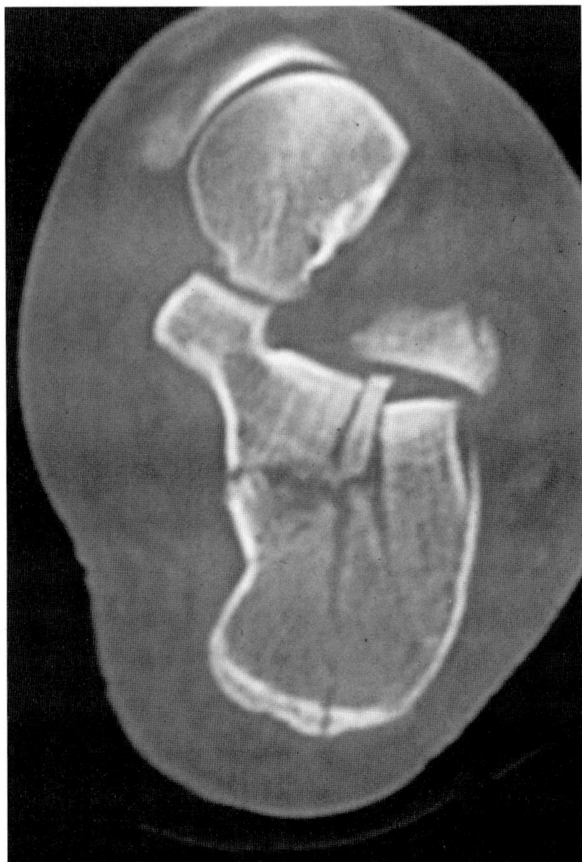

B

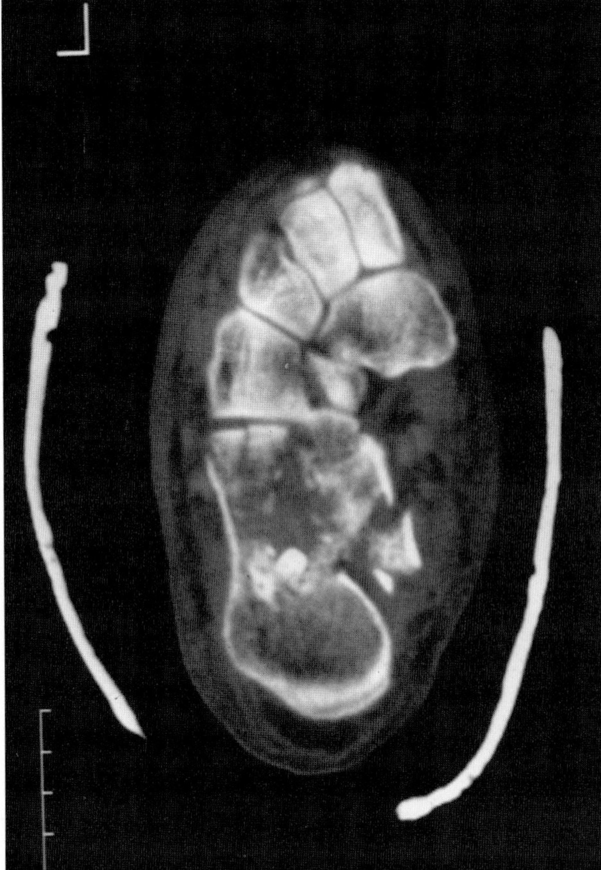

C

Figure 8. The Sanders classification is based on the number of major fragments (*arrows*) in the posterior facet. **A:** Type II. **B:** Type III. **C:** Type IV.

type III, three major fragments in the posterior facet; and type IV, posterior facet comminuted into more than three major pieces. These groups are additionally divided by location of the primary fracture line, but it is not clear whether this further subdivision is necessary for clinical decisions. In Sanders et al.'s (9) study, type I fractures were treated nonoperatively, and 85% good and excellent results were obtained. For type II fractures, if an anatomic reduction was obtained, 85% good and excellent results were obtained. Type III fractures represented a more difficult surgical challenge and had a higher percentage of poor results despite anatomic reduction. In type IV fractures it was the most difficult to obtain an anatomic reduction, and 73% of patients treated surgically experienced poor results.

The use of 2 mm as a threshold for fixating these fractures has recently been studied by Sangeorzan and Tencer (25). They noted a significant increase in joint contact stresses if a 2 mm displacement was produced in the posterior facet.

CLINICAL CORRELATIONS

In the past, the calcaneus fracture has defied surgeons' attempts to improve on its natural history. Indeed, numerous surgeons would state that we only impair the outcome of its natural history by our attempts to manipulate this fracture. A comparative literature review is difficult for obvious reasons. Only now are randomized, prospective studies in progress that compare operative and nonoperative treatment. Foot rating scales provide more objective information than "good and excellent." To paraphrase McReynolds (26), the good result of a triple arthrodesis is not the same as the good result of successful open reduction and internal fixation. Patient-based outcome studies will be another important advance. Given these deficiencies of the literature, some observations relevant to treatment can still be made.

It does appear that posterior facet displacement is important in determining the prognosis (21,25). Experimentally and clinically, 2 mm is a useful guideline for significant displacement. Thus, while a seemingly minor fracture can result in poor results, the prognosis is generally good if there is minimal posterior facet displacement (22–24). Conversely, posterior facet displacement greater than 2 mm carries a higher chance of a poor result if nonoperative treatment is chosen (21). Importantly, the prognosis remains poor if surgical treatment is chosen but a less than exact anatomic result is obtained. A study by Buckley and Meek (6) suggests that the margin for error may be as small as 1 mm of residual articular incongruity. In my opinion, this may explain why comparative studies in the past have failed to demonstrate a clear superiority for operative treatment (6,8). Conversely, demonstrating the disadvantages of operative treatment has been relatively easy given the high incidence of complications. The soft tissues must also be kept in mind. Manoli and Weber (27) have called attention to the possibility of calcaneal compartment syndrome. This may also explain late findings such as claw toes.

To synthesize this information into useful clinical algorithms, treatment can be selected on the basis of posterior facet displacement and the degree of comminution present. Minimally displaced fractures are best treated with early motion and weight bearing initiated at 6 to 8 weeks as pain allows. Displaced fractures with two to three major posterior facet fragments are suitable candidates for open reduction and internal fixation. Contraindications would include comminution of the medial column and poor underlying bone stock or metabolic deficiencies, e.g., diabetes. A displaced fracture with extensive posterior facet comminution remains a dilemma and perhaps is a candidate for primary fusion.

SURGICAL TREATMENT

Whichever surgical approach or fixation is chosen, an exact anatomic reduction of the entire calcaneus should be the goal. If one chooses a single approach, some type of indirect reduction of the opposite column will be required. Combined approaches allow for direct visualization of medial and lateral columns simultaneously (7,10,20).

The primary drawbacks of the medial approach are the neurovascular bundle and the cutaneous sensory branches. Laterally, the sural nerve is at risk, and incisions parallel to the peroneal tendons are at risk for wound complications (5,9).

As previously stated, the reduction of the posterior facet should be as accurate as possible. Since it is difficult to visualize this facet once it is reduced, intraoperative Broden and axial views with fluoroscopy are recommended (9,16) (Fig. 9). We have also found a small (2.7-mm) arthroscope useful as an adjunct to visualize reduction directly with the goal of perfect restoration of the posterior articular facet.

From the histomorphometry data, excellent screw purchase may be obtained in the medial column and juxtaarticular regions (15). In my practice, this boils down to lateral to medially directed screws with a lateral plate placement. In my opinion, one only needs a low-profile plate, such as a flattened out one-third tubular small-fragment plate or one-third 3.5-mm reconstructive plate, to obtain sufficient fixation for the ''large piece'' fractures. Highly comminuted patterns may require a more complex fixation montage, e.g., reconstruction Y-plate (Synthes, Paoli, PA). Other surgeons have recommended thicker plates, and still others have used devices such as staples or screws (7,10,20).

Other intraoperative guidelines include accurate reduction of the anterolateral fragment and the angle of Gissane (5,19). This should help restore lateral length and alignment. The superomedial fragment needs to be reduced anatomically to the tuberosity. Importantly, unless this piece is anatomically reduced, posterior facet reduction is extremely difficult (7,10,20). This may be done either indirectly with distraction via a temporary external fixator applied on the medial side of the tibia and calcaneus, or with manipulation through a Shanz screw inserted in the tuberosity. I find axial fluoroscopy imaging indispensable for determining alignment (16). Once the medial wall is reduced, it can be temporarily fixated with an axially directed Steinman pin, or held in place until buttressed by the lateral plate. Importantly, the contouring of this plate must be straight in order not to displace the tuberosity into varus.

Finally, the calcaneocuboid joint commonly reduces indirectly when other fracture components are reduced (10).

Regarding the issue of bone grafting, histomorphometry data and clinical experience provide some insight. Since the inferior central region is normally devoid of trabeculae (12,13,15), bone grafting to ''fill the void of the posterior facet'' is not indicated. Bone

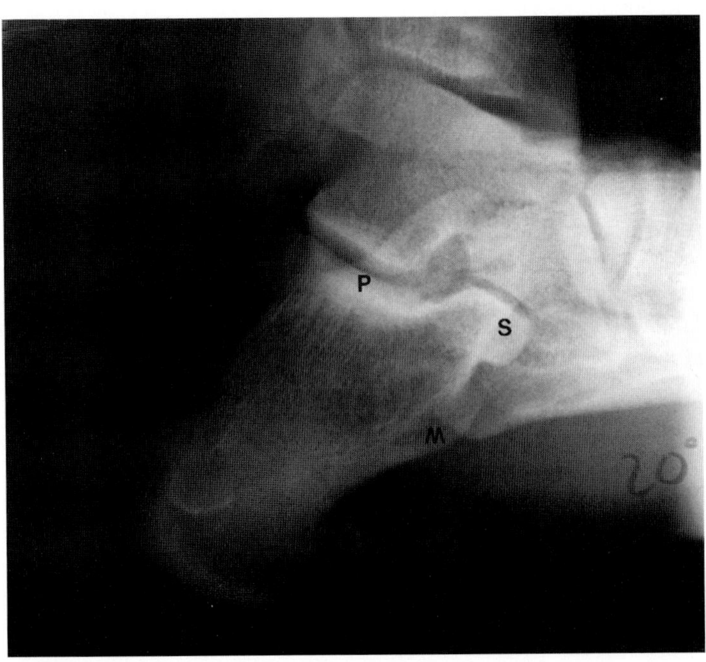

Figure 9. The intraoperative Broden view is useful in imaging the posterior facet. As the beam is angled cephalad, more anterior portions of the posterior facet (*P*) are visualized. Also note that the medial (*M*) wall and sustentaculum (*S*) is well visualized.

grafting may be of some value to speed healing or support extremely comminuted patterns, but clinical data are lacking. A large clinical series supports the omission of bone grafting on a routine basis (9). Since bone grafting adds to the morbidity of the surgery in a predictable manner, and thus detracts from operative treatment, I feel it is desirable to avoid its use, if at all possible.

SUMMARY

When compared with other articular fractures, the calcaneus fracture, even today, remains ''the fracture of mystery.'' Unlike injuries such as the Galeazi fracture (aptly named ''the fracture of necessity''), it does not seem to make much sense. A review of the literature suggests that diverse treatments will arrive at a common clinical result, with some authors even recommending excision of the bone. Hopefully, analysis of the basic science data, which are now being applied to the clinical treatment, will help resolve some of the open questions. Importantly, it appears that the calcaneus can respond favorably to an accurate anatomic reduction and internal fixation. It also appears that stable internal fixation is possible. Conversely, if one does not achieve these goals, the patient is probably better off treated nonoperatively, which makes intuitive sense. For those fractures with a poor result despite an exact surgical fixation, perhaps factors such as avascular necrosis of the cartilage surface are to blame. In the final analysis, success with this injury can best be obtained by matching the appropriate treatment with the pathoanatomy at hand.

REFERENCES

1. Bankart AS. Fractures of the os calcis. *Lancet* 1942;11:171–180.
2. Cotton FJ. Os calcis fracture. *Ann Surg* 1916;64:480.
3. Harris RI. Fractures of the os calcis. Their treatment by tri-radiate traction and subastragalar fusion. *Ann Surg* 1946;124:1082–1101.
4. Essex-Lopresti P. The mechanism, reduction technique, and results in fractures of the os calcis. *Br J Surg* 1952;39:395–419.
5. Benirschke SK, Mayo DA, Sangeorzan BJ, et al. Results of operative treatment of os calcis fractures. Presented at the AAOS 57th Annual Meeting, New Orleans, LA, February 8–13, 1990.
6. Buckley RE, Meek RN. Comparison of open versus closed reduction of intraarticular calaneal fractures: a matched cohort in workmen. *J Orthop Trauma* 1992;6:216–222.
7. Burdeaux BD. Reduction of calcaneal fracture by the McReynolds medial approach, technique and its experimental basis. *Clin Orthop* 1983;177:87–103.
8. Jarvholm V, Korner L, Thoren O, Wiklund LM. Fractures of the calcaneus. A comparison of open and closed treatment. *Acta Orthop Scand* 1984;55:652–656.
9. Sanders R, Fortin P, Dipasquale T, et al. Operative treatment in 120 displaced calcaneal fractures: results using a prognostic computed tomography scan classification. *Clin Orthop* 1993;290:87–95.
10. Stephenson JR. Treatment of displaced intra-articular fractures of the calcaneus using medial and lateral approaches, internal fixation and early motion. *J Bone Joint Surg [Am]* 1987;69:115–130.
11. Pridie KH. A new method of treatment for severe fractures of the os calcis. *Surg Gynecol Obstet* 1946;82:671–675.
12. Harty M. Anatomic considerations in injuries of the calcaneus. *Orthop Clin North Am* 1973;4:179–183.
13. Sarrafian SK. *Anatomy of the foot and ankle: descriptive, topographic, functional,* 2nd ed. Philadelphia: JB Lippincott, 1993.
14. Hall RL, Shereff MJ. Anatomy of the calcaneus. *Clin Orthop* 1993;290:27–35.
15. Carr JB, Beaudoin AR, Bear LS. Histomorphometry and screw pull-out loads in the calcaneus. Presented at the Orthopaedic Trauma Association: Annual Meeting, Toronto, Canada, 1990.
16. Koval KJ, Sanders R. The radiologic evaluation of calcaneal fractures. *Clin Orthop* 1993;290:41–46.
17. Warrick CK, Bremmer AE. Fractures of the calcaneum. *J Bone Joint Surg [Br]* 1953;45:33–45.
18. Carr JB, Hamilton JJ, Bear LS. Experimental intra-articular calcaneus fractures: anatomic basis for a new classification. *Foot Ankle* 1989;10:81–87.
19. Langdon IJ, Kerr PS, Atkins RM. Fractures of the calcaneum. The anteriorlateral fragment. *J Bone Joint Surg [Br]* 1994;76:303–305.
20. Stephenson JR. Displaced fractures of the os calcis involving the subtalar joint: the key role of the superomedial fragment. *Foot Ankle* 1983;4:91–101.
21. Crosby LA, Fitzgibbons T. Computed tomographic scanning of acute intra-articular calcaneus fractures. A new classification system. *J Bone Joint Surg [Am]* 1990;72:852–859.
22. Day FG. Treatment of fractures of the os calcis. *Can Med Assoc J* 1950;63:373–376.
23. Lindsey WRN, Dewar FP. Fractures of the os calcis. *Am J Surg* 1958;95A:555–576.
24. Pozo JL, Kirwan EO, Jackson AM. The long-term results of conservative management of severely displaced fractures of the calcaneus. *J Bone Joint Surg [Br]* 1984;66:386–390.

25. Sangeorzan B, Tencer AF. Contact stresses in the posterior facet in an experimentally produced calcaneal fracture model. Presented at the Annual Meeting of the Foot and Ankle Society, Asheville, NC, 1993.
26. McReynolds IS. The case for operative treatment of fractures of the os calcis. In: Leach RE, Hoaglund FT, Riseborough EJ, eds. *Controversies in orthopaedic surgery.* Philadelphia: WB Saunders, 1982.
27. Manolli A, II, Weber TG. Fasciotomy of the foot: an anatomical study with special reference to release of the calcaneal compartment. *Foot Ankle* 1990; 10:267–275.

EDITORIAL COMMENTS

Intraarticular Calcaneal Fractures: A Basic Science Update with Clinical Correlations

James B. Carr

Dr. James B. Carr has given us a synopsis of the new basic science knowledge available for developing a treatment plan for calcaneal fractures. Much of this work has been done by him, and his quest to develop a rational approach to the treatment of this very difficult injury is ongoing. The modern approach to this injury involves proper classification, which can only be done by appropriate CT views to develop knowledge of the number of articular fragments and comminution throughout the calcaneus and the lateral cuboid articulation. With this knowledge one can determine which fracture treatment is necessary and how to approach accurate and stable reduction scientifically. The goal in the treatment of calcaneal fractures is to reconstruct the hindfoot to prevent salvage complications of untreated calcaneus such as fibular impingement, loss of lateral or medial height, axial malalignment, loss of proper talar inclination by loss of angle of Gussane support, and articular restoration. Even in the most severe cases, the goal should be restoration of the basic hindfoot architecture to make reconstructive surgery at a later time more technically feasible.

Using the arterial supply of the peroneal artery, a lateral extensile approach has been developed that is now used as the utility approach to all calcaneal open reductions. If done appropriately, there are few significant complications in the flap reconstruction, although tip necrosis is still a minor complication. Use of the lateral approach is based on the premise that there is an intact sustenacular superior–medial fragment that is anatomic. If this is not the case, then the superior–medial fragment must be made anatomic by an accessory medial approach. Reconstruction of the calcaneus depends on where the histomorphic strength in the bone is, with initial screw placements to achieve articular reduction; screws are passed from lateral into the superior sustentaculum tali, which is quite dense and can be seen on an intraoperative axial view. The articular restoration should be at least 1 mm, and subtalar arthroscopy as well as adequate light has helped in achieving more perfect reductions. The articular fragment is then supported either by appropriate plate configuration to the restored lateral column using screws near the cuboid articulation and near the tuberosity with very few supporting structures in the central part of the calcaneus. During this part of the reduction traction on the calcaneus and achievement of axial alignment and lateral length are critical. The plate utilized should be low profile, and it will not be weight bearing until fracture healing has been achieved. During reduction, use of the arthroscope and intraoperative fluoroscopy with a proper Broden view and axial views are important. Bone graft is only used for very selective cases and is discouraged. The postoperative course concentrates on movement, but not weight bearing until bone union is achieved. If articular reconstruction is impossible, then the goals should be hindfoot realignment and lateral length of the calcaneus, which can be achieved either by closed means using a fixator or by open means. Consideration of a primary fusion can be addressed at that time, although this is not universally accepted. Most surgeons would wait to do a subtalar fusion at a later date after restoration of hindfoot architecture.

We are just beginning to see the first series of results using the technique discussed; the complications of tip necrosis, peroneal tendinitis, sural nerve neuritis, and subtalar stiffness and pain are to be expected. The open approach, if possible, seems to provide the best possible outcome in a difficult situation. Good outcomes require proper equipment, proper timing, an educated operating room staff, and experienced techniques since there is certainly a learning curve for this fracture.

Robert S. Adelaar, M.D.

Complex Foot and Ankle Trauma,
edited by Robert S. Adelaar,
Lippincott–Raven Publishers, Philadelphia © 1999.

11

Long-Term Results of Treatment of Displaced Intraarticular Calcaneal Fractures

Roy Sanders

Although fractures of the calcaneus were described as early as 1843 by Malgaigne, it was not until the 1930s that Böhler (1) classified them and described their mechanism of injury. Despite extensive attempts over the last 50 years to improve on the functional outcome after a displaced intraarticular calcaneus fracture, it has been recognized that the end results following treatment, whether conservative or operative, have been far from optimal. Over the last 10 years, however, great strides have been made regarding the treatment of these fractures. This chapter reviews the pertinent data found in the literature.

HISTORICAL PERSPECTIVE

Until recently the historical precedent has been nonoperative therapy for these fractures, even though Böhler (1,2) advocated open reduction. The principle reason for this shift was the technical problems associated with surgery. Anesthesia was at best mediocre, x-ray and fluoroscopy were in their infancy, antibiotics, flaps, and stainless steel plates were nonexistent, and a sound understanding of the principles of internal fixation

R. Sanders: Department of Surgery, Division of Orthopaedics, University of South Florida, Tampa, Florida 33612; Department of Orthopaedics, Tampa General Hospital, Tampa, Florida 33606.

were lacking. The resulting problems of infection, malunion, nonunion, and amputation led to a sobering realization that surgery was best left to the masters.

In 1948, Palmer (3) published his classic work on calcaneal fractures in the *Journal of Bone and Joint Surgery*. It featured a lateral Kocher approach, reduction of the joint with bone graft to hold up the fragment, and casting. He stated that his patients did well and that many returned to work. Similarly, in 1953, Essex-Lopresti (4) reported on his life's work. He suggested that when the articular surface was displaced, a tongue or joint depression fragment resulted. Although tongue-type fractures were reduced by percutaneous leverage, joint depression fractures required formal open reduction and internal fixation. Again, his results in patients under the age of 40 were reasonable.

About this time I. L. Dick (5) in Canada began advocating primary subtalar fusions for these patients. He cited excellent results with early return to work. This prompted a wave of fusions throughout Canada. Dewar and Lindsay (6) evaluated these patients in long-term follow-up. More than 50% of the patients were lost to follow-up, but because the authors personally found and interviewed the rest, the data were well received. Their findings indicated that fusions were being unnecessarily performed, that operative intervention was fraught with problems, and that the best results were seen in those patients treated nonoperatively. As a result of this article, which was widely read in the United States, operative treatment of calcaneal fractures fell into disfavor.

Fortunately, this approach has changed. Better anesthesia, antibiotics, the AO/ASIF [Arbeitsgemeinschaft für Osteosynthesefragen (Association for the Study of Internal Fixation)] principles of internal fixation, computed tomography (CT) scanning, and fluoroscopy have allowed many authors to report on good outcomes with operative treatment. We now review these findings.

CLASSIFICATION

Perhaps one reason why so much difficulty has been encountered in the treatment of fractures of the os calcis is the lack of understanding of the pathology of these fractures, primarily due to limitations in radiographic technique. Because similar fracture patterns were not analyzed, differing treatment regimens resulted in varying degrees of success. As a result, the author developed a CT scan classification based on the number and location of articular fracture fragments (Fig. 1). It is a natural progression of the classification of Soeur and Remy (7) and has been applied to over 400 fractures.

The classification system is based on coronal and axial CT scan sections (Fig. 1). Using that section with the widest undersurface of the posterior facet of the talus, the talus is divided into three equal columns by two lines, A and B. These two lines separate the posterior facet of the calcaneus into three potential pieces: medial, central, and lateral columns. A third fracture line, C, corresponding to the medial edge of the posterior facet of the talus, separates the posterior facet from the sustentaculum and results in a total of four potential pieces. The lines are named A, B, and C, from lateral to medial because as the fracture line moves medially, intraoperative visualization of the joint becomes more difficult and the ability to obtain an anatomic reduction decreases.

All nondisplaced articular fractures, irrespective of the number of fracture lines, are considered type I fractures; they benefit from early motion without the need for operative intervention unless an extraarticular component exists that is severely displaced. Type II fractures are two-part fractures of the posterior facet, similar in appearance to a split fracture of the tibial plateau. Type III fractures are three-part fractures that feature a centrally depressed fragment similar to a split depressed tibial plateau, die-punch distal radial fracture, or posterior wall acetabular fracture with marginal impaction. Type IV fractures, or four-part articular fractures, feature a highly comminuted posterior facet and are best treated with a primary subtalar fusion. Occasionally more than four articular fragments exist.

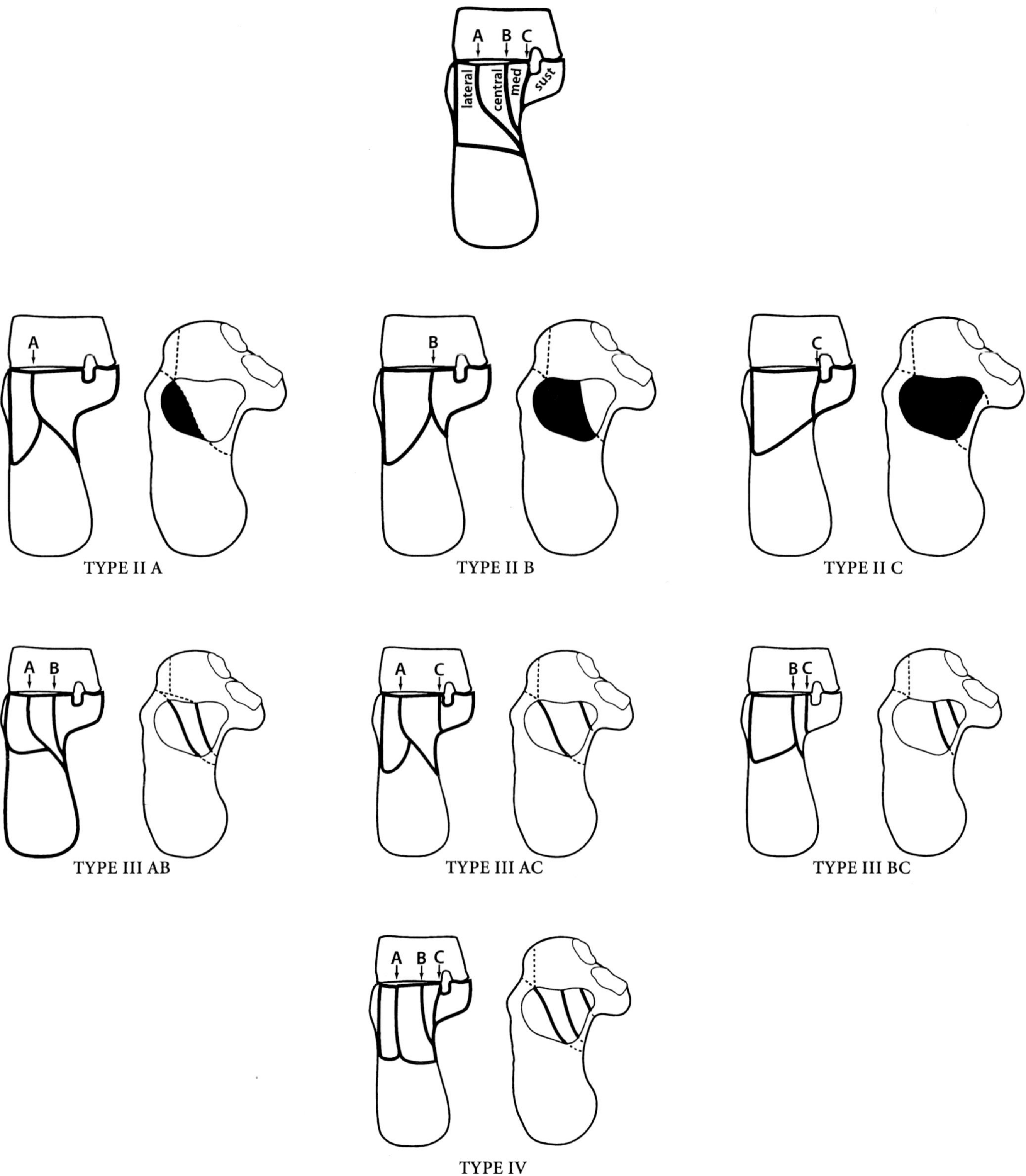

Figure 1. Sanders calcaneal CT classification.

TREATMENT

Three categories of treatment for the acute displaced intraarticular calcaneal fracture exist: (a) nonoperative treatment, (b) open reduction and internal fixation, and (c) primary arthrodesis.

Nonoperative Treatment

Nonoperative treatment of displaced intraarticular fractures of the calcaneus offers the patient little chance of a return to normal function. Of concern is the fact that a reduction of the articular surface is never obtained, the heel remains short and wide, the talus remains dorsiflexed in the ankle mortise, and the lateral wall causes impingement and binding of the peroneal tendons. Nonetheless, there are specific indications for nonoperative treatment: (a) nondisplaced fractures, (b) open fractures, or fractures in patients with life-threatening injuries that preclude early intervention, (c) soft tissue compromise, such as blistering and massive prolonged edema, which prevent surgery, (d) severe peripheral vascular disease or diabetes, and (e) severe infirmity.

Operative Treatment Using a Lateral Approach

Ideally, surgery should be performed within the first 3 weeks of injury to prevent difficulties with reduction secondary to early consolidation of the fracture. Surgery should not be attempted until after swelling in the foot and ankle has significantly decreased. Because this may take 7 to 14 days, immediate elevation and the use of a Jones dressing with a posterior splint are employed. The patient is seen back in the office on a weekly basis, with surgery performed as soon as swelling permits. If this is not accomplished, the window of opportunity for fixation may be lost.

The patient is placed in either the lateral decubitus or prone position on a translucent table or cardiac pacemaker insertion board (pacer board) so that fluoroscopy may be used intraoperatively. After exsanguination, the tourniquet is inflated to 325 to 350 mmHg. The calcaneus is approached through an extensile right-angled lateral incision. This approach minimizes the sequelae of peroneal tendonitis and devascularization of the anterior skin flap by adherence to the peroneal artery angiosome, as well as preserving the sural nerve, which should be entirely within the flap. The peroneal tendon sheath is held anterior to the fibula by the use of three K-wires, one in the fibula, one in the talus, and one in the cuboid.

The lateral wall is gently pried open to expose the articular fracture fragments. After clot removal, the posterior facet is evaluated. The depressed fracture fragment is first rotated out from within the body of the calcaneus. This immediately decompresses the lateral wall. After identification of all remaining articular fracture fragments, preliminary reduction of the facet is obtained using K-wires. Intraoperative fluoroscopic Broden's views (8,9) may be obtained to aid in joint reduction. When the reduction is satisfactory, K-wires are exchanged for 3.5-mm lag screws. Reduction of the tuberosity fragment is then performed through the lateral approach. This can most easily be accomplished by placing an axial spike or transverse traction pin into the tuberosity fragment. Then a calcaneal plate is used to reduce the body and buttress the lateral wall. The patient is kept on a non-weight-bearing protocol for 8 weeks with progressive weight bearing begun after that. Full weight bearing is allowed by 3 months.

Controversy exists about grafting the defect that remains after the superolateral fragment of the posterior facet has been lifted from the body. Originally described by Palmer (3), graft was needed because lag screws were not available. Since the advent of osteosynthesis, many authors feel that grafting is not necessary (10–13).

Primary Fusion

A primary fusion of the subtalar joint is not advisable after a two- or three-part displaced intraarticular calcaneal fracture, because the fusion only addresses subtalar pain. Primary arthrodesis does not solve the problem of a widened heel, peroneal entrapment or dislocation, a dorsiflexed talus, malleolar impingement caused by flattening of the heel, or the overall cosmetic problem, which is especially distressing to women. When the patient presents with a four or more part displaced intraarticular calcaneal fracture, however, the articular surface may be so disrupted that the surgeon's technical skill will still not permit an anatomic reconstruction of the articular surface. It is in these fractures that the author has combined an anatomic restoration of the calcaneus using internal fixation with a primary fusion (14). In this way, all problems associated with these fractures may be addressed simultaneously. Early experience in 32 type IV fractures treated in this manner and followed for 2 years has been surprisingly encouraging, with 28 of 32 patients returning to work within 6 months of injury.

COMPLICATIONS

Wound Dehiscence/Calcaneal Osteomyelitis

Should the wound be impossible to close at surgery, a delayed primary closure may be attempted. Skin grafting alone in this region has been unsuccessful, and in this situation a free tissue transfer will be required (15). Postoperatively, the wound may dehisce as late as 4 weeks, usually at the angle of the incision. Daily whirlpools with wet to dry dressing changes should be employed; if these are unsuccessful, a free flap will be needed as soon as possible to avoid osteomyelitis. Once an infection has occurred, repeat debridements must be performed. If the infection is superficial, the plate and screws may be retained. After the wound bed is deemed clean, a free tissue transfer combined with 6 weeks of intravenous antibiotics is used. If osteomyelitis exists, the hardware must be removed together with all necrotic and infected bone. After repeated debridements and 6 weeks of culture-specific antibiotics, salvage, fusion, or amputation based on the amount of remaining calcaneus is performed.

Subtalar Arthritis

Most commonly the result of a poorly reduced joint, subtalar arthritis may occur even in the presence of a normal x-ray and arthrogram, secondary to cartilage necrosis at the time of injury. In either case, the patient should initially be treated with conservative means. Activity change, shoe modifications, and antiinflammatory medications may often be successfully employed. If these modalities are unsuccessful, a subtalar injection should verify the location of the pain. If the injection is successful, subtalar or triple arthrodesis should be contemplated.

Sural Neuritis

Sural neuritis often occurs after a lateral approach. Because the nerve travels with the peroneal tendons, it is often stretched, contused, or cut during surgery using the standard lateral Kocher incision. The most consistent solution to this problem is to use the extensile approach, centered well away from the fibula, as previously described. Should a symptomatic neuroma develop, proximal resection is advised. Since employing this incision we have had no instances of sural neuritis or neuromas.

RESULTS

Literature Review

The literature is filled with accounts expounding the merits of various modalities in the treatment of intraarticular calcaneal fractures. Simpson et al. (16) reviewed the 62 largest series up to 1983. The reader is cautioned against making conclusions based on this information. Simple nondisplaced fractures will do well; conversely, highly comminuted fractures will do poorly, regardless of the treatment employed. Clearly, if nonoperative methods are used in highly displaced fractures and operative methods are reserved for minimally displaced fractures, the results would favor operative reduction. Finally, because classification schemes and postoperative assessment were not consistent, difficulty arises in understanding what these series represented. Thus, the entire body of literature before CT scanning was available is ambiguous at best. Since 1983, several series using more modern methods have been published (10,11,13,17–22). Stephenson (11) reported on 22 displaced intraarticular calcaneal fractures using medial and lateral approaches with 77% good to excellent results and return to work within 6 months in all but one patient. Leung et al. (19) had similar findings with 64 displaced intraarticular calcaneal fractures. Although follow-up was only 10.6 months, over 80% of the patients returned to work within 6 months.

Prognostic Classifications

Müller et al. (23), in his classification of fractures, addressed the question of prognosis after an articular fracture. The more comminuted an articular fracture was, the worse was the outcome expected. Until the advent of CT scanning, however, evaluation of the subtalar joint and hence a prognostic classification for intraarticular calcaneal fractures was not possible. CT scan classifications of intraarticular fractures of the calcaneus must be prognostic and must aid the surgeon in determining both treatment and outcome.

Closed Treatment

Crosby and Fitzgibbons (24) evaluated the results of closed treatment using a CT scan classification based on the fracture pattern involving the posterior facet. They classified small or nondisplaced fractures as type I, displaced fractures as type II, and comminuted fractures as type III. Their series included 13 type I, 10 type II, and 7 type III fractures. Fractures were treated with a variety of closed methods, depending on the individual surgeon's preference. Based on this classification they were able to predict which fractures did well, and which did poorly using closed treatment. They concluded that all type I and some type II fractures did well, but all type III fractures did poorly with closed treatment.

Unfortunately, as Sangeorzan et al. (25) and others (26) have pointed out, numerous questions were raised concerning treatment methods, positioning of the foot during CT scanning, and analysis of results using a new and unproven rating scale. In general, however, this classification does appear to anticipate the expected outcome using closed techniques.

Operative Treatment

Buckley and Meek (27) reported on a series of 34 calcaneal fractures; half were treated operatively and half were treated nonoperatively. Additionally, these patients were matched cohorts with respect to age, sex, work type, and time to follow-up. The authors concluded that unless a perfect, anatomic reduction of the joint surface was possible, there was no difference in the two treatment plans. Unfortunately, there were significant problems with the study. No CT scan classification was performed, so that fractures were not consistently classified. More importantly, 12 different surgeons operated on 17 fractures and all used different techniques. It is doubtful whether these patients were truly matched cohorts because the very issues in question (i.e., which fractures one operates on and how you perform a reproducible procedure) were never addressed.

More recently, four large series of operatively treated displaced intraarticular calcaneal fractures [Bezes et al. (17), 83 patients; LeTournel (12), 126 patients; Zwipp et al. (18), 123 patients; and Sanders et al. (10), 120 patients] reported data indicating that a good result is possible with operative treatment. All cases within each series were treated by the same surgeon, using the same surgical technique, and all fractures were classified by a consistent method. The last series is described in detail below.

Sanders et al. (10) reported on 132 displaced, intraarticular calcaneal fractures (types II to IV) using their CT scan classification with follow-up in 120 cases (range 12 to 56 months; average 29.3 months). All fractures were treated using a lateral approach, lag screw fixation of the joint, H-plate fixation of the body, and no bone grafting. All patients had preoperative, postoperative, and 1-year follow-up CT scans. Clinical outcome was based on the Maryland Foot Score. Reductions in heel height, length, and width were 98%, 100%, and 110% of normal, respectively, regardless of fracture type. Böhler's and Gissane's angle were reduced within 5 degrees of normal in all but three cases. In type II fractures, 68 of 79 fractures (86%) had a radiographic anatomic reduction of the articular surface as verified by follow-up CT scan. There were ten near-anatomic articular reductions and one approximate reduction. The clinical outcome in 58 (73%) fractures was graded as good or excellent. Eight (10%) fractures had a fair result, and 13 (17%) were failures, with 10 of 21 requiring subtalar fusion. In these cases, arthrogram, CT scan, and inspection of the joint at time of isolated subtalar fusion verified an anatomically reduced articular surface with damaged cartilage.

In type III fractures, there were 18 of 30 (60%) radiographically verified anatomic reductions, 8 near-anatomic, and 4 approximate reductions. Clinically, there were 21 (70%) excellent to good results, three (10%) fair results, and six (20%) failures. Seven fractures ultimately required a subtalar fusion: four of these were in fractures that had been anatomically reduced. In the type IV fractures, there were no (0%) anatomic, three (27%) near-anatomic reductions, two (18%) approximate reductions, and six (54%) complete failures of reduction. Clinically, there was one (9%) excellent to good result, two fair (18%) results, and eight (73%) complete failures. The one good and two fair results were in patients with near anatomic reductions.

When results were compared by year, a distinct learning curve appeared. Worse results occurred at the start of the series whereas the number of good to excellent results improved each successive year. When these data were analyzed further, with respect to fracture type and year, it appeared that type II fractures were easier to fix than type III fractures. With time even type III results improved. Despite a better outcome for type II and III fractures over time, however, the results of operative intervention in type IV fractures were not improved on even after 4 years of experience.

DISCUSSION

Previously, many authors have noted the type of fracture and the number of fragments present, the scheme of Essex-Lopresti (4) being the most widely used. None of these authors focused on the joint reduction itself, being more concerned with restoration of overall shape and correction of Böhler's angle to prevent disability. As a result, McReynolds (28,29) and others (30–33) stressed the importance of a medial approach to reconstruct the shape of the extraarticular calcaneal body. Unfortunately, this approach results in an indirect and incomplete reduction of the joint surface. As a result, Stephenson (11,34,35) employed a medial approach for body reduction, and a lateral approach for joint reduction.

The most recent series all use a lateral approach (10,13,18,19,25). Reduction of the body with reconstitution of height, width, and length is consistently reproducible, irrespective of the amount of comminution. Joint reduction, when technically possible, is easy through the lateral approach as well. It appears, therefore, that a medial approach is only rarely needed.

In our series (10), most of the II and III part fractures had an anatomically reduced posterior facet. Even so, 14 anatomically reduced fractures ultimately required a subtalar fusion. It appears, therefore, that although an anatomic articular reduction is necessary for a good outcome, it cannot guarantee it, probably due to cartilage necrosis from the original injury.

The use of bone graft is still controversial. Palmer (3) was unhappy with contemporary internal fixation techniques and therefore suggested bone graft to hold up the articular surface. LeTournel (12,13), using internal fixation, suggested that bone graft was unnecessary because lag screws were able to hold the articular surface together, Stephenson (11) used no bone graft and only had one late collapse, whereas Leung et al. (19) used bone graft in all cases and felt it was needed. In our series (10), bone grafting was not employed and in no case was there a subsequent loss of articular reduction. Consequently, the author believes there is little need for bone graft, and in fact the graft can block articular reduction.

Our protocol eliminated as many variables as possible to determine if the articular fracture classification was prognostic. Interestingly, an unforeseen variable appeared, a surgeon-dependent learning curve. The curve appears to require between 35 and 50 cases, or roughly 2 years, before results can become fairly predictable for type II and III fractures. Type IV fractures are so severe that even the most experienced surgeon may find it difficult to piece these fractures together. Knowing this in advance will allow the surgeon and patient to prepare for the possibility of a primary fusion.

CONCLUSIONS

Displaced intraarticular fractures of the calcaneus require anatomic reduction with stable internal fixation to maximize the chances for good joint function. The recent literature indicates that open reduction and internal fixation within 10 days of injury yields the most satisfactory results. Treatment should be tailored to the personality of the fracture. This is best evaluated using a prognostic fracture classification. CT scanning is the only accurate method of analyzing this complex fracture and therefore only a CT scan classification can be prognostic. Using such a classification, the following conclusions can be reached.

Most intraarticular calcaneal fractures are type II fractures and are amenable to operative intervention. Good results and return to work can be expected. Type III fractures are less frequent and have a worse prognosis. Patients should be counseled that disability, and the possible need for a late subtalar fusion, may occur. Type IV fractures are rare injuries. Operative intervention is suggested in these fractures, if only to restore calcaneal shape; if the joint cannot be restored, primary arthrodesis should be considered. With operative intervention a learning curve exists, and the surgeon should expect significant improvement after approximately 35 cases or 2 years.

REFERENCES

1. Böhler L. Diagnosis, pathology and treatment of fractures of the os calcis. *J Bone Joint Surg* 1931;13:75–89.
2. Böhler L. *The treatment of fractures.* New York: Grune & Stratton, 1958.
3. Palmer I. The mechanism and treatment of fractures of the calcaneus. *J Bone Joint Surg [Am]* 1948;30A:2–8.
4. Essex-Lopresti P. The mechanism, reduction technique, and results in fractures of the os calcis. *Br J Surg* 1952;39:395–419.
5. Dick IL. Primary fusion of the posterior subtalar joint in the treatment of fractures of the calcaneum. *J Bone Joint Surg [Br]* 1953;35:375.
6. Lindsay WRN, Dewar FP. Fractures of the os calcis. *Am J Surg* 1958;95:555–576.
7. Soeur R, Remy R. Fractures of the calcaneus with displacement of the thalamic portion. *J Bone Joint Surg [Br]* 1975;57:413–421.
8. Broden B. Roentgen examination of the subtaloid joint in fractures of the calcaneus. *Acta Radiol* 1949;31:85–91.
9. Sanders R, Dipasquale T. Intra-operative Broden's views in the operative treatment of calcaneal fractures. *Orthop Trans* 1989;13.
10. Sanders R, Fortin P, Dipasquale T, and Walling A. Operative treatment in 120 displaced intraarticular calcaneal fractures. Results using a prognostic computed tomography scan classification. *Clin Orthop* 1993;290:87–95.
11. Stephenson JR. Surgical treatment of displaced intraarticular fractures of the calcaneus. A combined lateral and medial approach. *Clin Orthop* 1993;68–75.
12. Letournel E. Open reduction and internal fixation of calcaneal fractures. In: Spiegel P, ed. *Topics in orthopedic surgery.* Baltimore: Aspen Publishers, 1984:173–192.

13. Letournel E. Open treatment of acute calcaneal fractures. *Clin Orthop* 1993;290:60–67.
14. Stephens HM, Sanders R. Calcaneal malunions: results of a prognostic computed tomography classification system. *Foot Ankle Int* 1996;17:395–401.
15. Levin LS, Nunley JA. The management of soft-tissue problems associated with calcaneal fractures. *Clin Orthop* 1993;290:151–156.
16. Simpson LA, Shulak DA, Spiegel PG. Intraarticular fractures of the calcaneus: a review. *Contemp Orthop* 1983;6:19–28.
17. Bezes H, Massart P, Delvaux D, Fourquet JP, Tazi F. The operative treatment of intraarticular calcaneal fractures. Indications, technique, and results in 257 cases. *Clin Orthop* 1993;290:55–59.
18. Zwipp H, Tscherne H, Thermann H, Weber T. Osteosynthesis of displaced intraarticular fractures of the calcaneus. Results in 123 cases. *Clin Orthop* 1993;290:76–86.
19. Leung KS, Yuen KM, Chan WS. Operative treatment of displaced intraarticular fractures of the calcaneum. Medium-term results. *J Bone Joint Surg [Br]* 1993;75:196–201.
20. Laughlin RT, Carson JG, Calhoun JH. Displaced intra-articular calcaneus fractures treated with the Galveston plate. *Foot Ankle Int* 1996;17:71–78.
21. Thordarson DB, Krieger LE. Operative vs. nonoperative treatment of intraarticular fractures of the calcaneus: a prospective randomized trial. *Foot Ankle Int* 1996;17:2–9.
22. Crosby LA, Fitzgibbons TC. Open reduction and internal fixation of type II intra-articular calcaneus fractures. *Foot Ankle Int* 1996;17:253–258.
23. Muller ME, Nazarian S, Koch P. *Classification AO des fractures.* Berlin: Springer–Verlag, 1987.
24. Crosby LA, Fitzgibbons T. Computerized tomography scanning of acute intra-articular fractures of the calcaneus. *J Bone Joint Surg [Am]* 1990;72A:852–859.
25. Sangeorzan BJ, Benirschke SK, Carr JB. Surgical management of fractures of the os calcis. *Instr Course Lect* 1995;44:359–370.
26. Ebraheim NA, Biyani A, Padanilam T, Paley K. A pitfall of coronal computed tomographic imaging in evaluation of calcaneal fractures. *Foot Ankle Int* 1996;17:503–505.
27. Buckley RE, Meek RN. Comparison of open versus closed reduction of intraarticular calcaneal fractures: a matched cohort in workmen. *J Orthop Trauma* 1992;6:216–222.
28. McReynolds IS. The case for operative treatment of fractures of the os calcis. In: Leach RE, Hoaglund FT, Riseborough EJ, eds. *Controversies in Orthopedic Surgery.* Philadelphia: WB Saunders, 1982:232–254.
29. McReynolds IS. Trauma to the os calcis and heel cord. In: Jahss M, ed. *Disorders of the foot and ankle.* Philadelphia: WB Saunders, 1984:1497–1538.
30. Burdeaux BD Jr. Fractures of the Calcaneus. In: Chapman M, Madison M, eds. *Operative orthopedics. Vol. 3.* Philadelphia: JB Lippincott, 1989:1723–1736.
31. Burdeaux BD Jr. Fractures of the calcaneus: open reduction and internal fixation from the medial side—a 21 year prospective study. *Foot Ankle Int* 1997;18:685–692.
32. Burdeaux BD Jr. Reduction of calcaneal fractures by the McReynolds medial approach technique and its experimental basis. *Clin Orthop* 1983;177:87–103.
33. Burdeaux BD Jr. The medical approach for calcaneal fractures. *Clin Orthop* 1993;290:96–107.
34. Stephenson JR. Displaced fractures of the os calcis involving the subtalar joint: the key role of the superomedial fragment. *Foot Ankle* 1983;4:91–101.
35. Stephenson JR. Treatment of displaced intra-articular fractures of the calcaneus using medial and lateral approaches, internal fixation, and early motion. *J Bone Joint Surg [Am]* 1987;69:115–130.

EDITORIAL COMMENTS

Long-Term Results of Displaced Intraarticular Calcaneal Fractures

Roy Sanders

Dr. Sanders has been a modern pioneer in the treatment of calcaneal fractures; he has advocated the extensile-type approach to fractures in the Sanders II and III category (i.e., "fixable"). A CT scan is the only way to evaluate these fractures appropriately with routine x-ray views. Many challenges still exist to the surgical treatment of these calcaneal fractures in the literature, but these series do not adequately classify the fractures that undergo open reduction and internal fixation, nor do they evaluate those fractures compared with conservative care. The type IV fractures described in this chapter defy open reduction, but the goal is somehow to maintain hindfoot architecture so that future reconstructive surgery can focus on the articular destruction rather than a three-dimensional misshapen bone. The goal with the severely comminuted fracture is to restore the calcaneal architecture (by either closed means, external fixation, or open reduction) so that in the future one can directly concentrate on the articular fusion or the posterior hindfoot distraction arthrodesis to elevate the talus. One should be able to decrease the amount of lateral wall extrusion and axial malalignment by either closed or open means with the severe fractures. We also feel, as does Dr. Sanders, that grafting is not necessary in calcaneal fractures since a portion of the calcaneus is devoid of bone and even grafting is not going to help obtain better fixation. The key factor in evaluating whether you can improve a situation by open reduction and internal fixation is to look at the number of articular pieces and also the areas where screw purchase is good near the articular surface, tuberosity, and calcaneocuboid joint. If those areas are severely comminuted, plating is probably not advantageous. I would agree that a primary fusion should be considered in severely comminuted fractures, but we do not do it at the time of injury; we try to restore the hindfoot architecture and then allow the bone to heal. Later we do a fusion. With our attempts at primary fusion, we have still had loss of the talo–calcaneal angle. We agree with Dr. Sanders that, if indicated, an open reduction and internal fixation is best, performed by the technique described here and using a Sanders-type plate to support the articular surface along with the rest of the body.

Robert S. Adelaar, M.D.

Complex Foot and Ankle Trauma,
edited by Robert S. Adelaar,
Lippincott–Raven Publishers, Philadelphia © 1999.

12

Calcaneal Malunions and Their Treatment

Roy Sanders

Although the recent literature advocates operative treatment of displaced intraarticular calcaneal fractures, many surgeons continue to treat these injuries nonoperatively because of the fear of operative complications (1–3). Unfortunately, complications of nonoperative treatment of calcaneal fractures may be equally significant and include (a) peroneal tendon impingement, subluxation or dislocation, which results in pain and/or instability; (b) post-traumatic subtalar and/or calcaneocuboid arthritis; (c) hindfoot malalignment resulting in altered shoe wear and/or gait patterns; and (d) posterior tibial or sural neuritis (4). These problems are all due to the development of a calcaneal malunion; they result in pain and functional disability in a surprisingly large number of patients (5–9). In an effort to improve the outcome in this group of patients, treatment must be centered around correction of the specific anatomic problems encountered. Preoperative evaluation must include a careful clinical examination, footprints, plain films, and computed tomography (CT). Surgery is then offered, based on these findings.

CLINICAL EXAMINATION

A detailed history is obtained, specifically asking the patient for difficulty with uneven ground (subtalar joint arthrosis), buckling, or giving way (peroneal tendon dislocation), leg length discrepancy (calcaneal shortening), difficulty with shoe size (lat-

R. Sanders: Department of Surgery, Division of Orthopaedics, University of South Florida, Tampa, Florida 33612; Department of Orthopaedics, Tampa General Hospital, Tampa, Florida 33606.

eral wall enlargement), abnormal lateral shoe wear (varus/valgus hindfoot), and/or numbness or paresthesias (nerve impairment). Physical examination should begin with the patient standing, facing away from the examiner, with the legs together. In this way, hindfoot shortening and varus or valgus is noted. At this time footprints are made and the patient's shoes are observed, to see if the lateral counter is misshapen, or there is abnormal wear. The patient is then seated and an evaluation of the skin, noting any previous surgical wounds or scars, is performed. Neurologic damage, such as injury to the sural or posterior tibial nerve, is also documented. Acquired deformities such as equinus, cavus, varus, or a combination, are noted. Ankle and subtalar motion is tested next. The best way to test subtalar motion is to dorsiflex the ankle, lock the anterior portion of the dome of the talus in the mortise with the thumb and index finger of the left hand, and then forcibly invert and evert the calcaneus with the right hand. Pain, limitation of motion, and peroneal spasm are noted.

Standard radiographs are then reviewed; these will show a calcaneal malunion with shortening of the heel and dorsiflexion of the talus, both of which can best be seen on the lateral view. Aside from these findings, plain radiographs do not offer much information other than an indication that subtalar and/or calcaneal–cuboid joint arthritis exists. Once the malunion is diagnosed, however, a CT scan should be obtained in both the coronal and transverse planes. These images will allow the surgeon to diagnose peroneal tendon dislocations, hindfoot varus, lateral wall exostoses, calcaneocuboid and subtalar arthritis, and any associated talar or ankle pathology. A reproducible treatment algorithm based on a CT scan classification of calcaneal malunions developed by the author can then be used to plan operative intervention (5).

Type I malunions include a large lateral exostosis, with or without extremely lateral subtalar arthrosis (Fig. 1). Type II malunions include a lateral wall exostosis combined with significant subtalar arthrosis across the width of the joint (Fig. 2). Type III malunions include a lateral exostosis, severe subtalar arthrosis, and a calcaneal body malunited in hindfoot varus or valgus (Fig. 3). In addition to these findings, the calcaneocuboid and ankle joints can be clearly seen, as well as any peroneal pathology. Treatment is then based on malunion type.

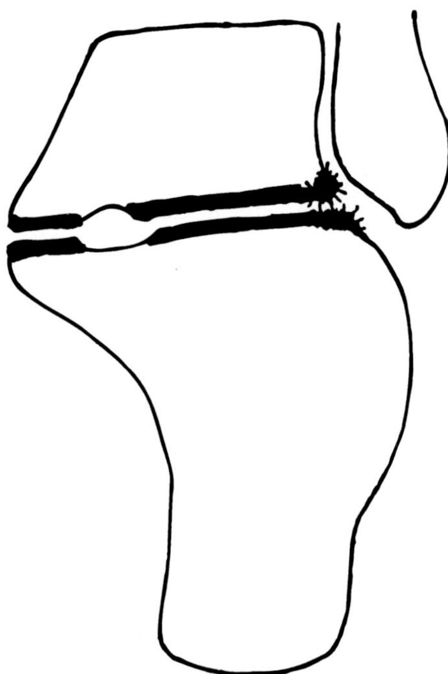

Figure 1. Type I malunions include a large lateral exostosis, with or without extremely lateral subtalar arthrosis.

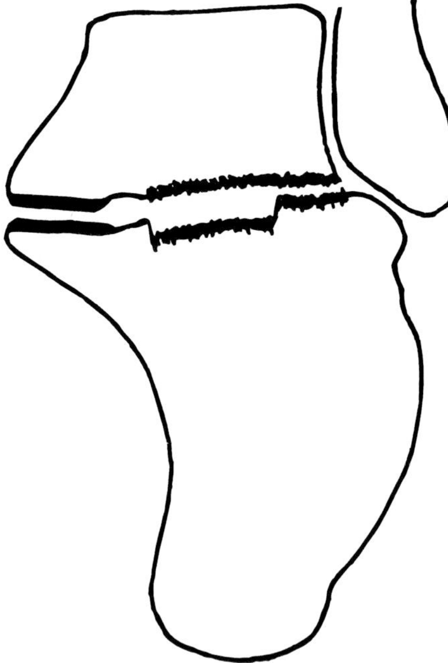

Figure 2. Type II malunions include a lateral wall exostosis combined with significant subtalar arthrosis across the width of the joint.

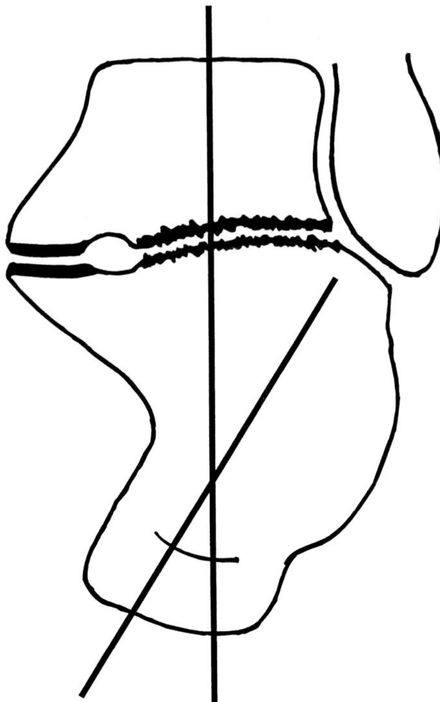

Figure 3. Type III malunions include a lateral exostosis, severe subtalar arthrosis, and a calcaneal body malalignment in varus.

SURGICAL TREATMENT

Incisions

Many surgical approaches have been advocated to address these complex problems. Specifically, Romash (10) has championed the Ollier incision for both a subtalar fusion and a calcaneal osteotomy. Similarly, Carr et al. (11) have suggested using the longitudinal posterior incision of Picot, avoiding the lateral extension because of wound problems. In this author's experience, only an extensile approach (12,13) can appropriately address all the possible pathology to be encountered. Furthermore, because this is not an acute injury, the flap is not at risk. The only limitation of this approach is an inability to close the wound when *significant* lengthening has occurred. In these cases, the Ilizarov method should be used (14).

Surgical treatment should therefore begin with the same modified Kocher extensile approach used for acute fractures, with the patient in a lateral decubitus position. This approach spares the sural nerve, permits a formal peroneal tenolysis, and allows ample room for a calcaneal exostectomy. The ankle ligament complex, calcaneocuboid joint, and calcaneal tuber (for Dwyer osteotomy) can all be approached as well. Once this is performed, the subtalar joint can be visualized with ease. In cases of fracture–dislocation, in which the lateral wall and joint are one piece and subluxed over the lateral talus, care must be taken not to enter the ankle joint. When in doubt, fluoroscopy is an invaluable aid in identifying these joints. When medial pathology needs to be addressed, the patient should be placed in a prone position. In this position, a medial incision, as well as a lateral incision, can be performed with ease.

Treatment Options

Type I Malunions

Cotton and Henderson (15) wrote in 1916 that "the man who breaks his heel bone is 'done,' so far as his industrial future is concerned." Formerly treated conservatively, the salvage of calcaneal malunions has proved to be a complex and demanding undertaking. Cotton (7) described the lateral exostectomy procedure commonly used for treatment of calcaneal malunions either as an isolated or combined procedure. He stated that "the key to this whole question is the doing of enough surgery . . . often leaving what seems not half the joint" (7). Therefore, in our experience, a peroneal tenolysis and lateral wall exostectomy, coupled with a very lateral joint resection and early motion is all that is required for type I malunions (16).

Type II Malunions

In the past, triple arthrodesis was advocated for these patients (17). More recently, however, most authors have agreed that a fusion of the transverse tarsal joints seems unwarranted because of the additional loss of motion, especially with respect to pronation and suppination (9,18–20). An isolated subtalar fusion with specific attention to the restoration of a plantigrade hindfoot is now considered the treatment of choice. The type of subtalar fusion performed for a calcaneal malunion has also been the subject of some interest in recent years. The bone block technique described by Carr et al. (11) is felt to restore heel height and improve talar inclination. Results from Seattle were very good, with six of eight having a satisfactory result. Unfortunately, other series using this technique have been associated with a high number of patients who developed a varus malunion. Myerson and Quill-Ge (21) reported only 7 of 14 patients with a good result using this technique; 2 patients had varus malunions requiring reoperation. Sanders et al. (22) reported on series of 15 patients treated with this technique with four varus malunions two of which required reoperation. Therefore, type II malunions without significant loss of height undergo a peroneal tenolysis, a lateral wall exostectomy, and an in situ subtalar fusion, using the local bone as graft (5,23). It is important to take the lateral wall as one large piece. If significant loss of height is present and associated with collapse of Bohler's angle such that the talus is dorsiflexed, a tricortical iliac crest bone block (as described by Carr et al.), should be used to correct the deformity. Care must be taken not to overdistract the subtalar joint, however, or the hindfoot will fall into varus. Although Carr et al. (11) suggested the use of a medial femoral distractor to prevent this from occurring, the deltoid ligament can only be stretched a fixed amount before the hindfoot is shifted into varus by the oversized graft. If additional length is needed, a calcaneal osteotomy and slide, coupled with an Achilles tendon lengthening should be employed instead.

The fusion should be secured using two cannulated 6.5- to 8.0-mm lag screws. Carr et al. (11) suggest the use of fully threaded position screws (nonlag), to prevent shortening created by the lag effect. It has been the author's experience that with a bone graft in place, this theoretical shortening is not a concern. Conversely, if position screws are used, nonunion of the fusion with screw breakage may occur because no compression exists at the fusion site.

Type III Malunions

Type III malunions are treated with a peroneal tenolysis, a lateral calcaneal exostectomy, a subtalar fusion, and a calcaneal osteotomy to correct hindfoot malalignment or shortening. Although this osteotomy can be performed through the original fracture line, as described by Romash (24), not only is this difficult, but lengthening may not allow for wound closure. As a result, if complete restoration of length is required, an osteotomy through the fracture line is performed, and an Ilizarov frame is applied. In all other cases, the principle problem is varus or valgus, and a Dwyer osteotomy addresses this pathology. If shortening is still a concern, as mentioned above, an Achilles tendon lengthening coupled with an inferior slide of the osteotomy, may be required. The osteotomy can be held with the same cannulated lag screws used for the fusion, or it can be stabilized with supplemental fixation. Type II and III malunions require 10 to 12 weeks of non-weight-bearing immobilization in a cast to allow the fusion and/or osteotomy to unite.

Associated Problems

All other problems should be addressed at this time as well. Often the peroneal tendons are subluxed, but removal of the lateral wall exostectomy corrects this problem. If the tendons are dislocated, stapling of the sheath, a small fibula bone block, or deepening of the fibula groove will solve the problem. If the patient has calcaneocuboid arthritis, a fusion should be done at this time. Finally, if the lateral ankle ligament complex is damaged, a Brostrom repair will address this.

RESULTS

Using our protocol we analyzed 26 patients with 26 malunions at an average of 32 months (range 12 to 57 months) after treatment (5). There were seven type I malunions, 15 type II malunions, and four type III malunions. There were six excellent and one good result in the type I patients. These patients had restoration of approximately 50% of their subtalar motion postoperatively. Lateral impingement pain was eliminated in all but one patient, who continued to complain of persistent sinus tarsi pain.

There were 11 excellent, 3 good, and 1 fair results in the type II subgroup. All had limitations in their ability to walk on uneven surfaces secondary to the subtalar fusions. None, however, required assistive devices. Twenty percent (three of 15) had mild pain that altered certain activities of daily living. Women's shoewear was limited to a less than 1-in. heel. Most patients preferred a lace-up walking shoe, with one patient requiring orthotics. There were no problems with the heel counter impinging on the malleoli or symptomatic limitation of ankle dorsiflexion in the type II patients.

Type III malunion patients presented with two excellent, one good, and one poor result. Type III patients had similar shoewear requirements as the type II patients. All patients had pain that caused changes in certain activities of daily living. One patient walked with a moderate limp and required an orthosis.

There were no wound complications or infections in this series. All arthrodeses went on to successful union. None of the type II patients developed varus malunions requiring revision. There was one superficial wound infection that resolved with a course of oral antibiotics and a case of peroneal instability that was corrected at the time of surgery. Finally, triple arthrodesis has been advocated for salvage when the subtalar joint is incongruent and arthritic. It was interesting to note that in our series, although calcaneocuboid involvement was present in a number of the original fractures, only one patient was symptomatic enough to warrant fusion of this joint. No patient in our series required a triple arthrodesis.

CONCLUSIONS

Patients with nonoperative treatment of calcaneal fractures may develop a disabling calcaneal malunion causing impingement of the peroneal tendons, arthritis of the subtalar joint, and a varus hindfoot. CT scanning has permitted us to analyze these malunions and develop a three-part classification that defines both the injury and the treatment outcome. If these principles are employed, most patients will see a significant improvement in their function.

REFERENCES

1. Sanders R, Fortin P, Dipasquale T, Walling A. Operative treatment in 120 displaced intraarticular calcaneal fractures. Results using a prognostic computed tomography scan classification. *Clin Orthop* 1993;290:87–95.
2. Sanders R. Intra-articular fractures of the calcaneus: present state of the art. *J Orthop Trauma* 1992;6:252–265.
3. Buckley RE, Meek RN. Comparison of open versus closed reduction of intraarticular calcaneal fractures: a matched cohort in workmen. *J Orthop Trauma* 1992;6:216–222.
4. Paley D, Hall H. Intra-articular fractures of the calcaneus. A critical analysis of results and prognostic factors. *J Bone Joint Surg [Am]* 1993;75:342–354.
5. Stephens HM, Sanders R. Calcaneal malunions: results of a prognostic computed tomography classification system. *Foot Ankle Int* 1996;17:395–401.
6. St C Ibister JF. Calcaneo-fibular abutment following crush fracture of the calcaneus. *J Bone Joint Surg [Br]* 1974;56:274–278.
7. Cotton FJ. Old os calcis fractures. *Ann Surg* 1921;74:294–303.
8. Pennal GF, Yadov MP. Operative treatment of comminuted fractures of the os calcis. *Clin Orthop* 1973;4:197–211.
9. Dick IL. Primary fusion of the posterior subtalar joint in the treatment of fractures of the calcaneum. *J Bone Joint Surg [Br]* 1953;35:375.
10. Romash MM. Reconstructive osteotomy of the calcaneus with subtalar arthrodesis for malunited calcaneal fractures. *Clin Orthop* 1993;290:157–167.
11. Carr JB, Hansen ST, Benirske SK. Subtalar distraction bone block fusion for late complications of os calcis fractures. *Foot Ankle* 1988;9:81–86.
12. Gould N. Lateral approach to the os calcis. *Foot Ankle* 1984;4:218–220.
13. Zwipp H, Tscherne H, Thermann H, Weber T. Osteosynthesis of displaced intraarticular fractures of the calcaneus. Results in 123 cases. *Clin Orthop* 1993;290:76–86.
14. Paley D, Fischgrund J. Open reduction and circular external fixation of intraarticular calcaneal fractures. *Clin Orthop* 1993;290:125–131.
15. Cotton FJ, Henderson FF. Results of fractures of the os calcis. *Am J Orthop Surg* 1916;14:290.
16. Braly WG, Bishop JO, Tullos HS. Lateral decompression for malunited os calcis fractures. *Foot Ankle* 1985;6:90–96.
17. Conn HR. The treatment of fractures of the os calcis. *J Bone Joint Surg* 1935;17:392–405.
18. Gallie WE. Subastragalar arthrodesis in fractures of the os calcis. *J Bone Joint Surg* 1943;XXV:731–736.
19. Hall MC, Pennal GF. Primary subtalar arthrodesis in the treatment of severe fractures of the calcaneum. *J Bone Joint Surg [Br]* 1960;42:336–343.
20. Harris RI. Fractures of the os calcis: treatment by early subtalar arthrodesis. *Clin Orthop* 1963;30:100.
21. Myerson M, Quill-Ge J. Late complications of fractures of the calcaneus. *J Bone Joint Surg [Am]* 1993;75:331–341.
22. Sanders R, Fortin P, Walling A. Subtalar arthrodesis following calcaneal fracture. *Orthop Trans* 1991;15:656.

23. Kalamchi A, Evans J. Posterior subtalar fusion. *J Bone Joint Surg [Br]* 1977;59:287–289.
24. Romash MM. Fracture of the calcaneus: an unusual fracture pattern with subtalar joint interposition of the flexor hallucis longus. A report of two cases. *Foot Ankle* 1992;13:32–41.

EDITORIAL COMMENTS

Calcaneal Malunions and Their Treatment

Roy Sanders

In previous chapters, we have stressed that the primary treatment of calcaneal fractures would be to avoid significant malunion problems at a later date since they are so difficult to treat. Therefore, with judicious use of x-ray film including axial and Broden's views and surgical open reduction for type II and III Sanders fractures, the severe problems with calcaneal malunion (other than the subtalar arthritis) should be eliminated. The subtalar arthritis can occur just from the damage of the articular surface even after excellent articular reduction. Pain after calcaneal fractures does not necessarily mean that problems exist with lateral wall impingement, calcaneocuboid arthritis, or hindfoot malalignment, but these areas must be investigated. We use axial views and CT scans to evaluate these problems in the post-calcaneal-fracture pain patient. We also use judicious injections in the subtalar joint as well as along the lateral wall of the fibula to try to distinguish arthritic from impingement problems. If the problem is demonstrated to be secondary to an impingement from malunion, a decompression or calcaneal osteotomy may be indicated. If the problem is with subtalar arthrosis, a subtalar fusion needs to be done, making sure that the calcaneocuboid joint does not need to be included within the fusion site.

When one does a subtalar fusion, it is important to align the talus with the first metatarsal axis on a weight-bearing lateral view because calcaneal fractures, if there is a malunion, are usually accompanied by a horizontal flattening of the talus. If such flattening is present, a hindfoot posterior arthrodesis with distraction through the subtalar joint elevating the talus is required. Very rarely is a triple arthrodesis needed except for very old calcaneal malunions that have developed talonavicular arthrosis in addition to the subtalar arthrosis or are associated with forefoot deformities. We personally like to use autogenous iliac crest strut grafts when needed for malunion patients for the posterior distraction arthrodesis.

Robert S. Adelaar, M.D

Complex Foot and Ankle Trauma,
edited by Robert S. Adelaar,
Lippincott–Raven Publishers, Philadelphia © 1999.

13

Fractures of the Navicular and Cuboid

Michael M. Romash

ANATOMY

Osseous Anatomy

The navicular and cuboid occupy unique positions in the foot. The navicular is the keystone of the longitudinal arch of the foot (Fig. 1). It is wider dorsally than plantarly when viewed laterally. It is wider medially than laterally when viewed anteroposteriorly (AP), lengthening the foot's medial column. It is the proximal bone of the midfoot, initiating the bridge from the larger bones (talus and calcaneus) to the individual rays. Proximally it makes up half of the transverse tarsal articulation. Distally it articulates with the three cuneiforms. The distal surface is relatively flat. The proximal surface is curved concavely to articulate with the talus. Its proximal joint enjoys a significant arc of motion intimately related to inversion and eversion; the distal joints move very little. Force transmitted from the medial metatarsals is consolidated and passed on to the talus. This establishes complex internal strain and stress within the navicular by compression and shear applied through the ligamentous anatomy. The cuboid articulates with the anterior calcaneus proximally and the fourth and fifth metatarsals distally, thus accepting and consolidating the stress of two rays. It is a connecting link, and its length constitutes a portion of the lateral column of the foot. The calcaneocuboid articulation is the lateral portion of the transverse tarsal articulation.

The navicular cuneiform joints are supported by dorsal and plantar cuneonavicular ligaments. Medially and plantarly, the navicular is supported by the spring (plantar calcaneonavicular) ligament and the insertions of the posterior tibial tendon. Talonavicular ligaments reinforce the support both dorsally and plantarly, along with some fibers of the anterior deltoid ligament. Laterally there is an inconstant articulation with the cuboid and enveloping cuboidonavicular ligaments (1).

M. Romash: Department of Surgery, Uniformed Services, University of the Health Sciences, Bethesda, Maryland 20814; Department of Surgery, Chesapeake General Hospital, Chesapeake, Virginia 23320.

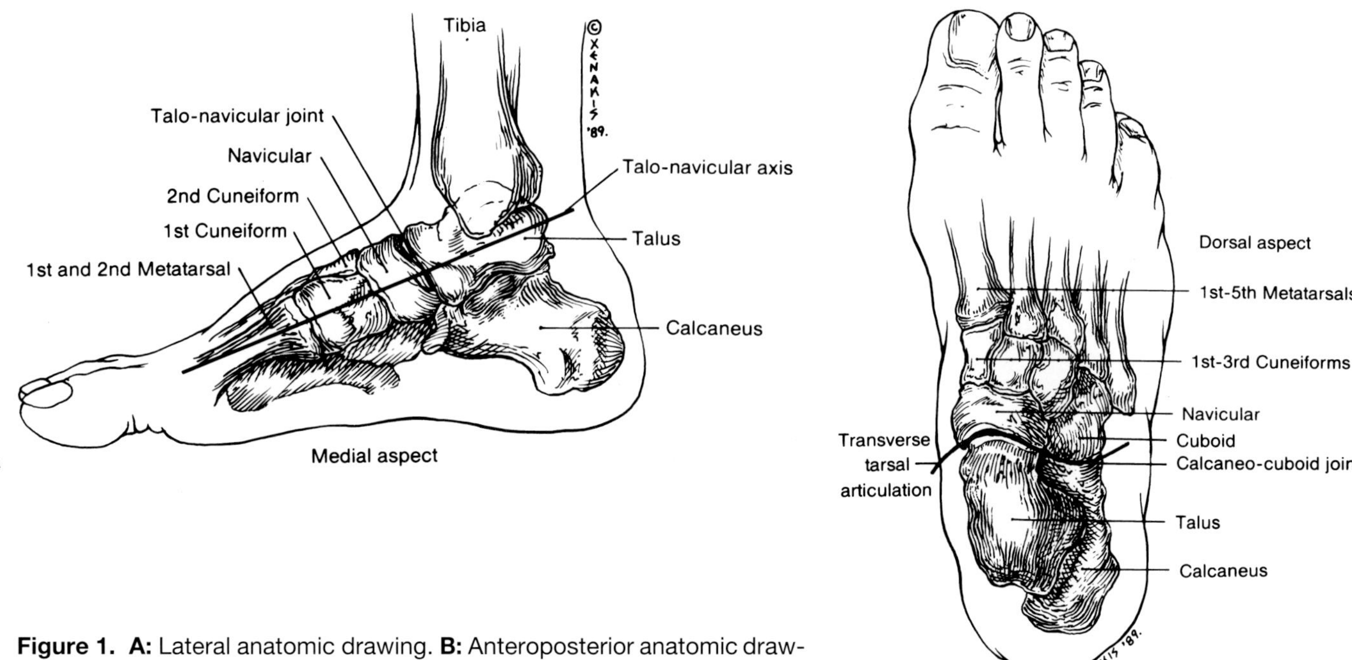

Figure 1. A: Lateral anatomic drawing. **B:** Anteroposterior anatomic drawing.

Lehman and Eskeles (2) postulated that the cuneiform navicular ligaments are weaker than the talonavicular connections. They believe that this results in failure of the naviculocuneiform ligaments with forced plantar flexion. This permits subluxation and their further compression, causing compression fracture of the navicular.

Vascular Anatomy

Torg et al. (3) have shown that the navicular is well vascularized at its periphery but is relatively avascular centrally (Fig. 2). The vessels originate dorsally from the dorsalis pedis and plantarly from the medial plantar artery, through the tuberosity from an anastomosis of these two. The relatively avascular central area may predispose this portion of the navicular to stress fractures.

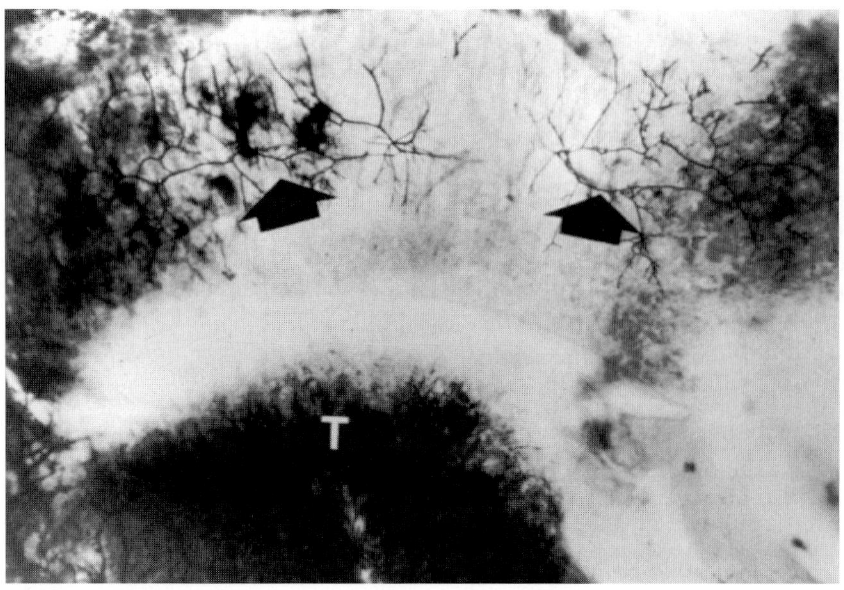

Figure 2. Vascular anatomy the navicular. The *arrows* point to the relatively avascular central portion of the navicular. *T*, talus. (From ref. 3, with permission.)

Anatomic Variants

The os tibiale externum or accessory scaphoid lies in the insertion of the posterior tibial tendon to the navicular (Fig. 3). There is a synchondritic joint between it and the navicular, represented by a smooth and regular line. It is present in 15% to 25% of the population (4) and is bilateral 90% of the time. It is possible for a synchondritic fracture to occur in adults (5) (Figs. 4 and 5).

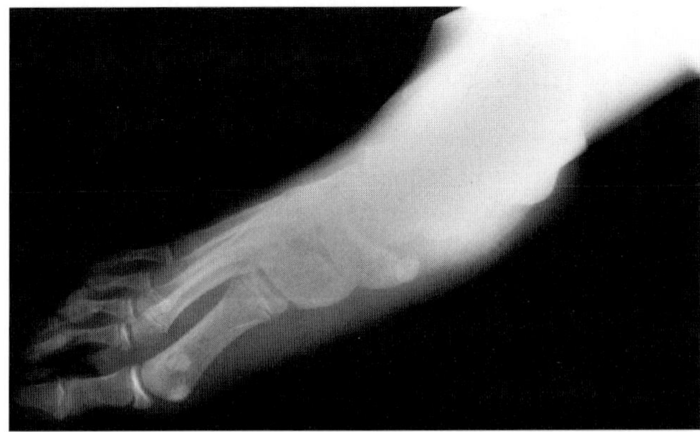

Figure 3. Os tibiale externum.

A

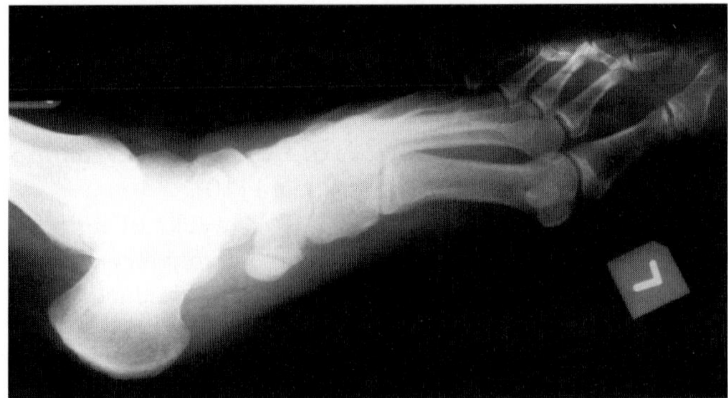

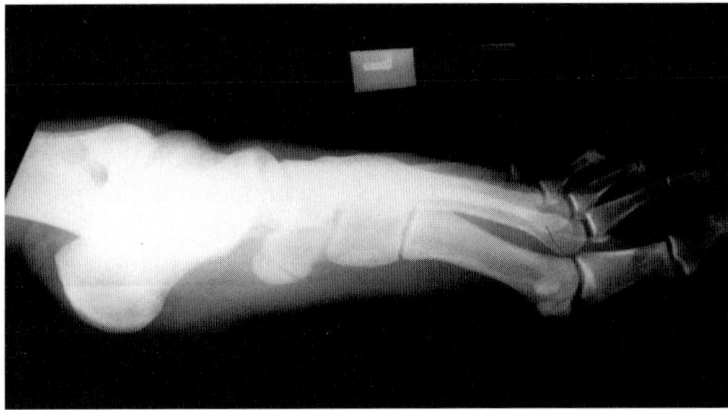

B

Figure 4. A,B: Reverse or medial oblique view of the foot demonstrating synchondrosis.

A

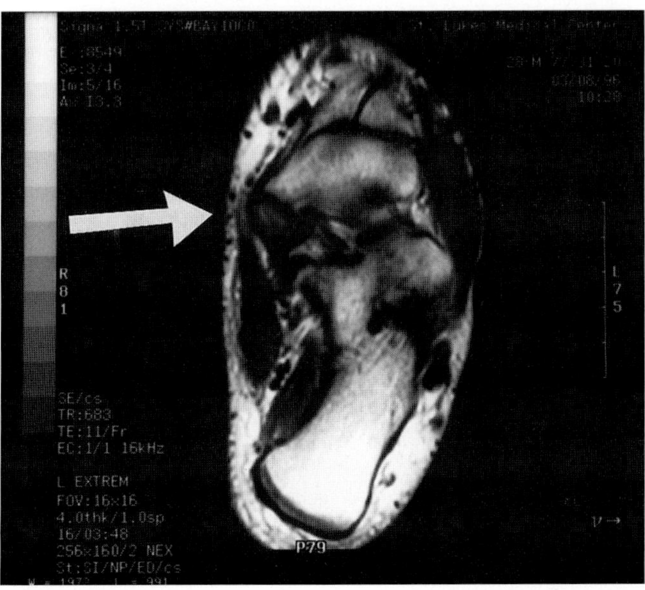

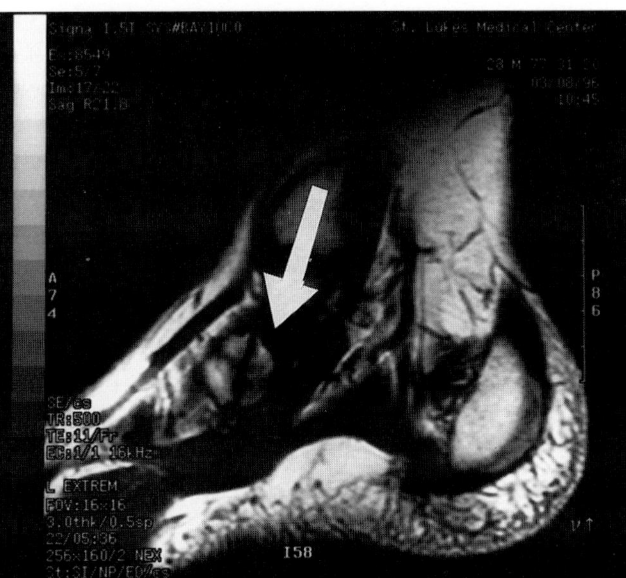

B

Figure 5. A,B: MRI of synchondritic fracture (*arrows*) of the navicular.

MECHANISMS OF INJURY

The navicular and cuboid are routinely involved in pronation and supination in normal gait. Forced motion beyond the normal limits of this motion can cause failure through fracture. Forced dorsiflexion or plantarflexion will also cause fracture. Combinations of the above may occur. Pure axial loading may occur and may also be combined with other stresses causing fracture.

Severe axial loads that injure the forefoot, splitting the rays (often between the first and second ray) can continue the injury pattern through the cuneiforms and then through the navicular (6).

NAVICULAR FRACTURES

DeLee (7) and Sangeorzan et al. (8) have provided a classification system of navicular fractures, expanding classifications by Watson Jones (9). These are tuberosity fractures, dorsal lip fractures, fractures of the body, and stress fractures. The fractures of the body have been subdivided into nondisplaced and displaced and the displaced fractures then subdivided into type I (coronal plane fracture line with a large dorsal fragment), type II (oblique dorsal plantar fracture with a large medial fragment), and type III (central comminution with naviculocuneiform disruption). An additional fracture of the body occurs in conjunction with forefoot disruption.

Dorsal Lip Fracture

A severe plantarflexion force will cause tension on the dorsal talonavicular ligament. The ligament then avulses a portion of the navicular (Fig. 6). An associated midfoot subtalar or ankle sprain may be present and should be considered (10).

Treatment here is symptomatic initially. Short periods of 3 to 4 weeks of immobilization or support are recommended (10,11). If the dorsal fragment contains a significant portion of the articular surface, 20% to 25% or greater, then open reduction and internal fixation should be considered (6). (This fracture pattern is to be differentiated from the type I body fracture.)

Symptomatic fragments, causing discomfort by their prominence, may be excised.

A
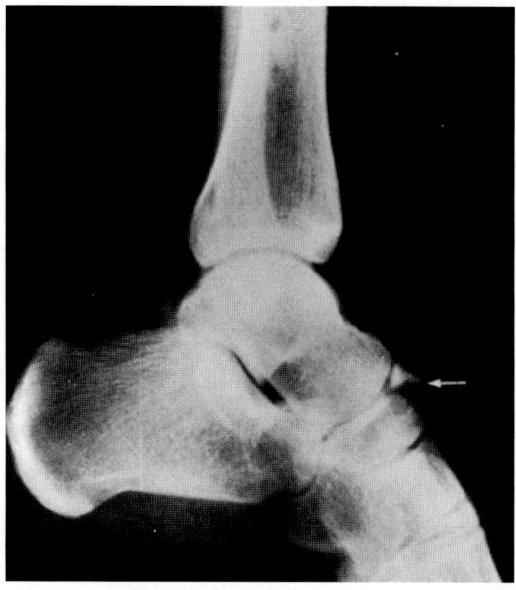
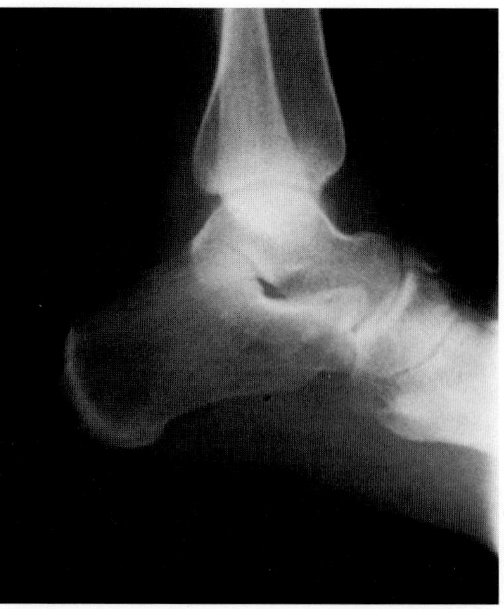
B

Figure 6. A,B: Dorsal lip fracture.

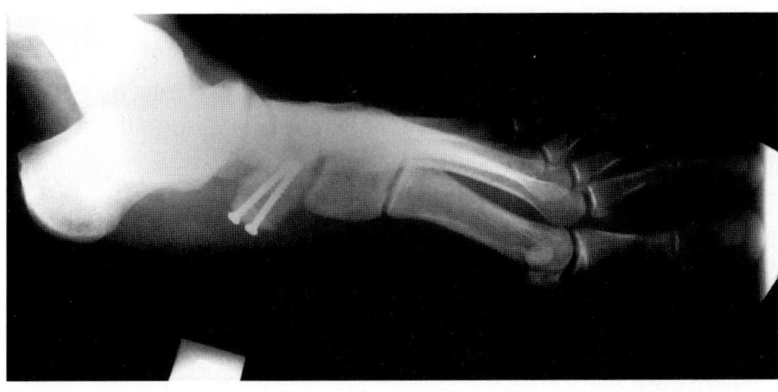

Figure 7. Internal fixation of synchondritic tuberosity fracture.

Tuberosity Fracture

The posterior tibial tendon inserts on the tuberosity of the navicular. An acute eversion of the foot can lead to fracture of the tuberosity, which fails under tension due to the resistance of the posterior tibial and associated medial ligaments. The continuation of the posterior tibial insertion plantarly, distally, and laterally (on the plantar aspect) often prevents significant displacement. As the foot everts, the lateral column is compressed, and cuboid fractures caused by this compression may occur.

It is important to differentiate an acute fracture from the synchondritic joint of an accessory navicular. The accessory navicular is often present bilaterally. The junction of the accessory navicular with the body may be injured by eversion of the foot and should be considered (4,5).

Displacement of the minor fragment (carried by the posterior tibial tendon) can be demonstrated on oblique x-ray film of the foot.

These fractures are treated by 4 to 6 weeks of support by casts or compressive dressings. The foot may be placed in an inversion (12) or neutral position in this period.

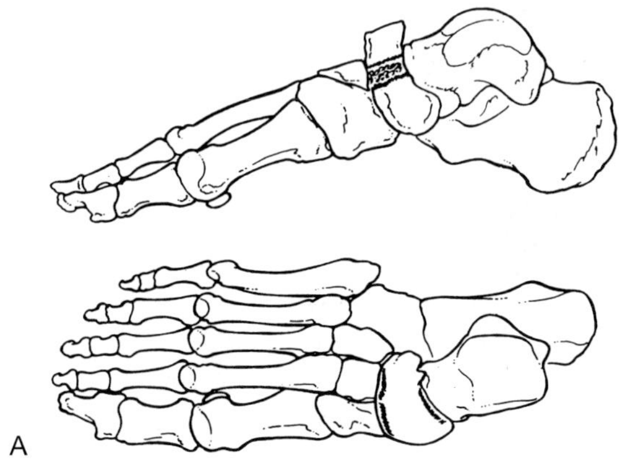

A

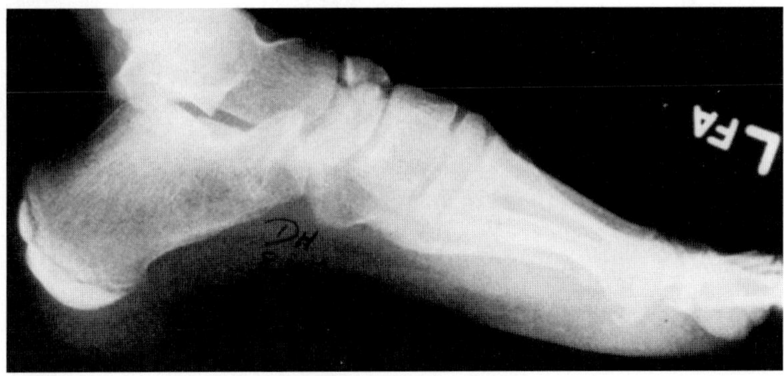

B

C

Figure 8. A (from ref. 8, with permission), **B:** Sangeorzan type I fracture. **C:** Internal fixation of Sangeorzan type I fracture.

Asymptomatic fibrous unions occasionally occur. If the tuberosity fragment is large enough, internal fixation may be performed (Fig. 7).

Continued symptoms are treated by excision of the tuberosity fragment accompanied by advancement and reimplantation of the posterior tibial tendon, similar to the Kidner procedure (13).

Body Fractures

Fractures of the body of the navicular can be isolated fractures or combined with other midfoot disruptions. Direct blows to the navicular may be the cause, or the force

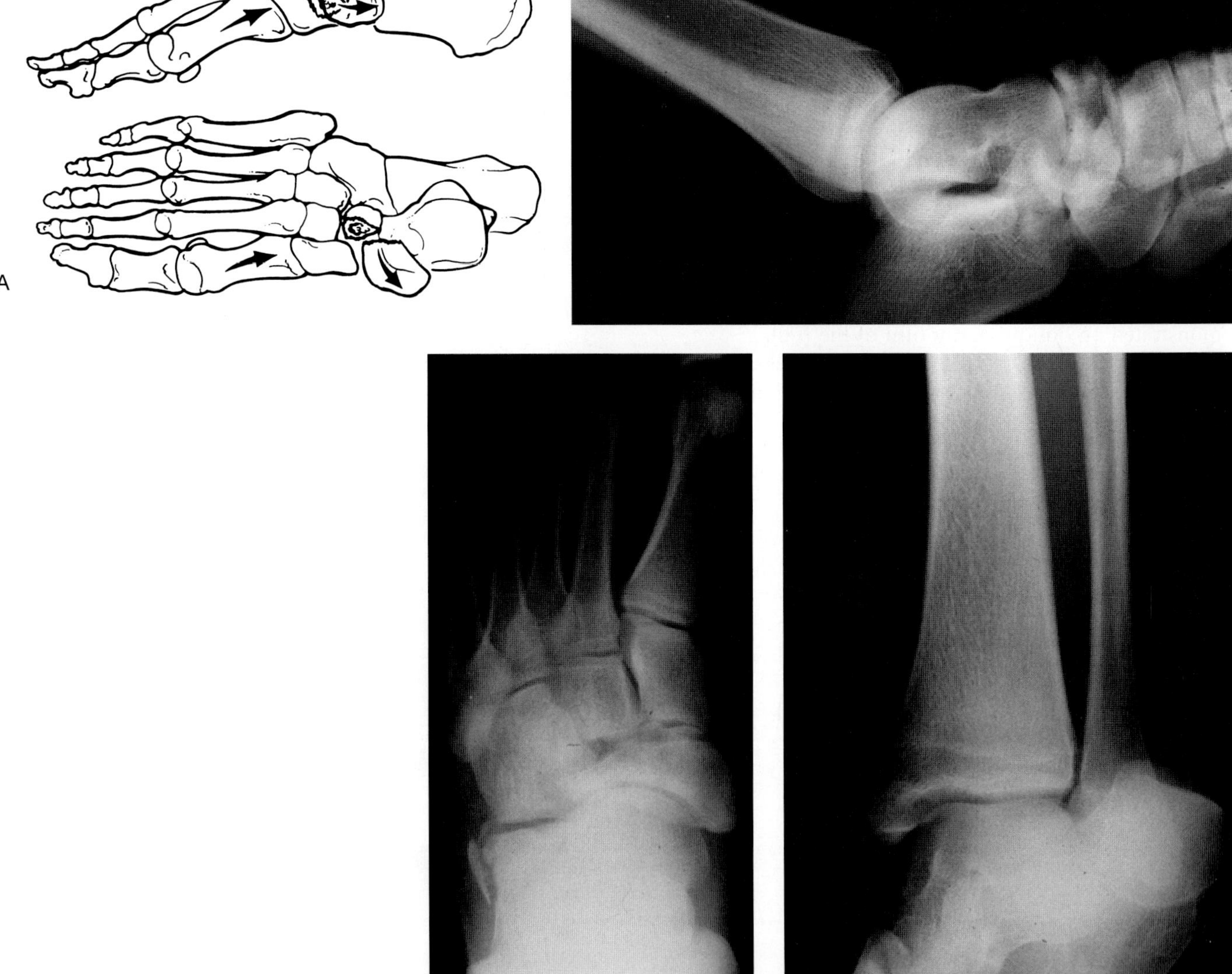

Figure 9. Diagram (**A,** from ref. 8, with permission) and x-ray films of anteroposterior **(B),** lateral **(C),** and oblique **(D)** views of Sangeorzan type II fracture. The lateral side of the calcaneous fracture is noted in **C.** *Arrows* in **A** indicate the axial load applied to the medial column of the foot with resultant displacement of the navicular fracture.

may be transmitted from the metatarsals to the cuneiforms to the navicular and talus as the plantarflexed foot is loaded in a fall. The latter mechanism is more likely to cause other midfoot disruptions. In the latter case, as the injury progresses, dorsal subluxation of the navicular at the talonavicular *or* navicular cuneiform joints can concentrate pressure on the plantar aspect of the navicular. Abduction or adduction occurring during the injury also influences the fracture pattern. Fracture lines also tend to occur along the longitudinally oriented extensions of the intercuneiform joints.

Vaishya and Patrick (14) feel that the strong spring ligament plantarly holds the inferior portion, while bone fails in tension. Inferior comminution may occur. This may be considered a variant of the dorsal lip fracture. The injury can lead to shortening of the medial column of the foot. Restoring the length of the medial column seems to be key in management of the fracture, combined with reconstruction of the articular surfaces. Sequelae are posttraumatic arthritis, deformity, and avascular necrosis, all of which should be considered in planning treatment.

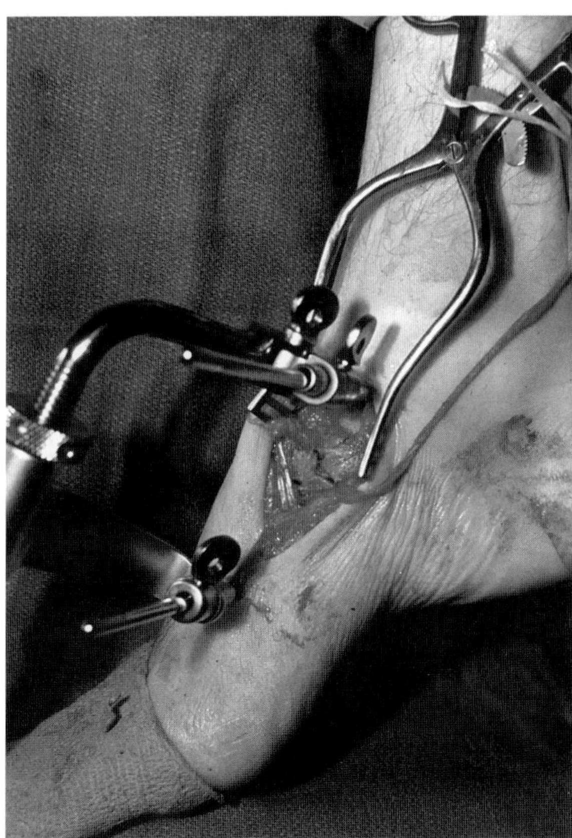

E

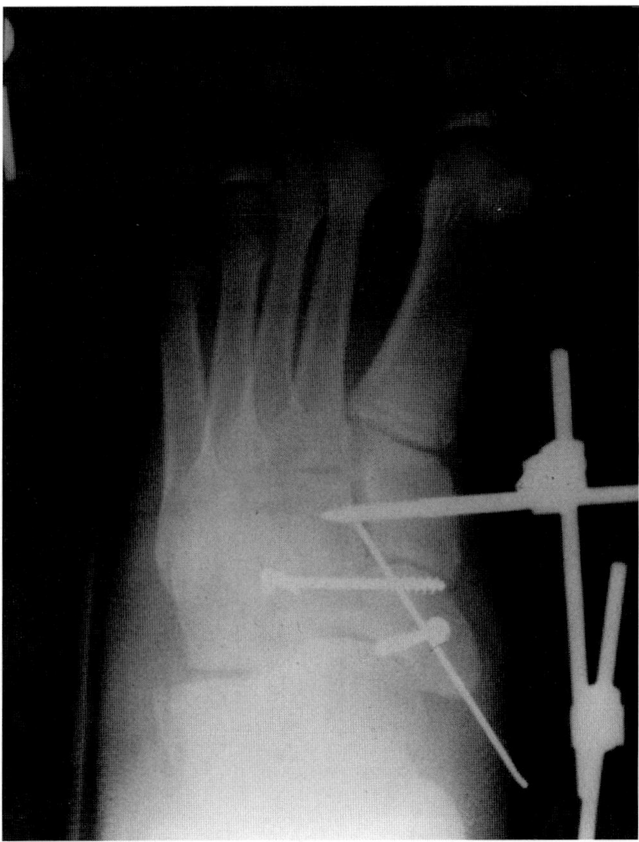

F

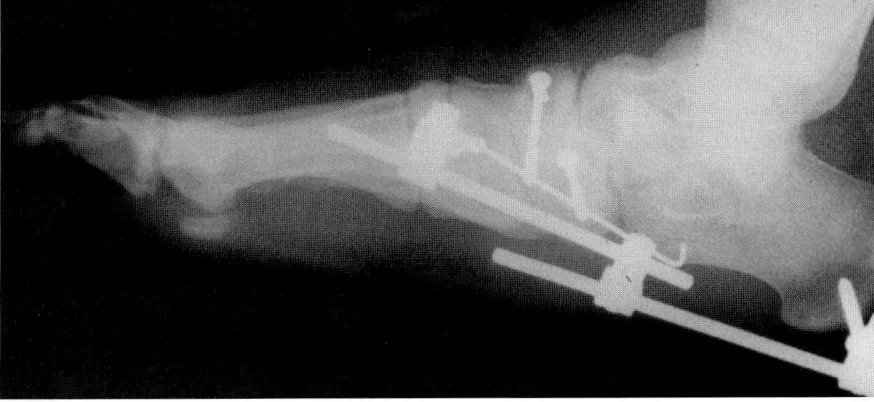

G

Figure 9. *(Continued.)* **E:** External fixator applied to medial column of foot to restore its length during open reduction and internal fixation of navicular fracture. **F,G:** Fixation of type II fracture.

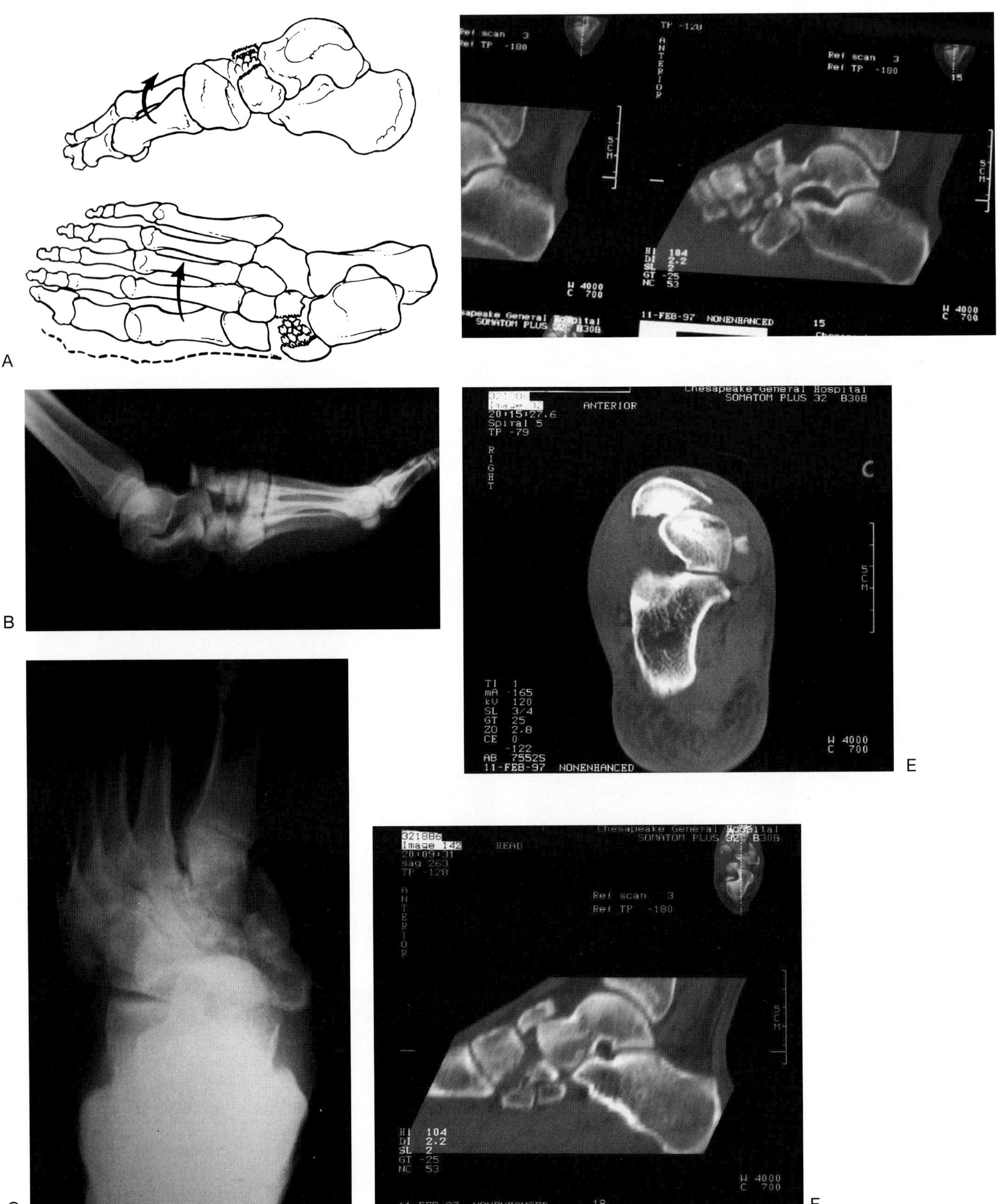

Figure 10. Diagram [**A** (from ref. 8, with permission)], x-ray film **(B** and **C)**, and CT scans **(D–F)** of type III fracture.

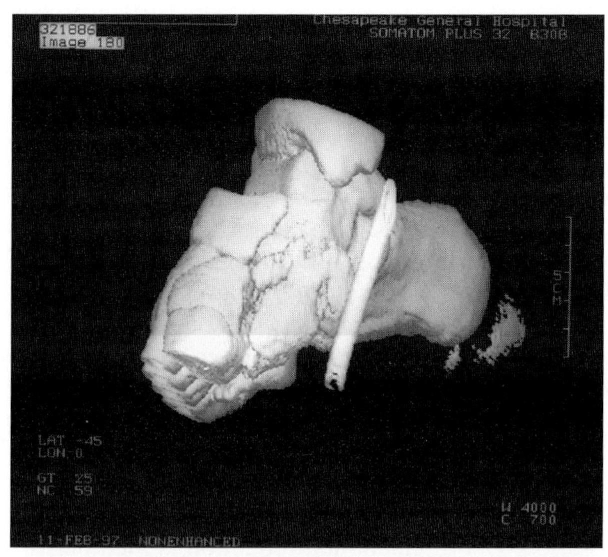

G

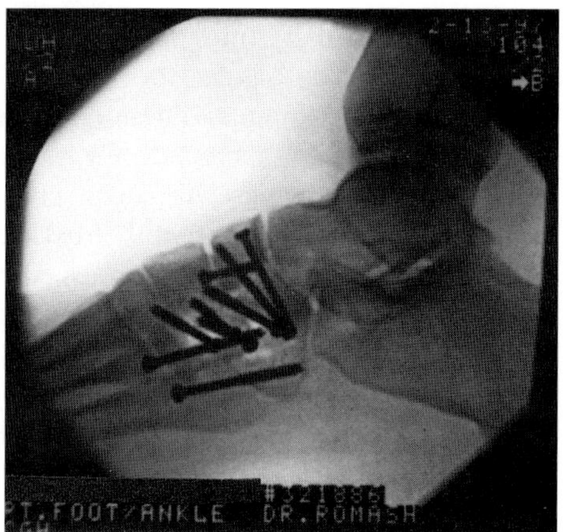

J

H

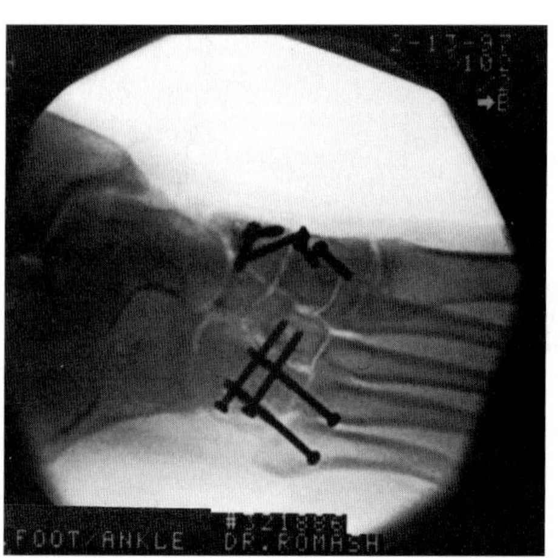

K

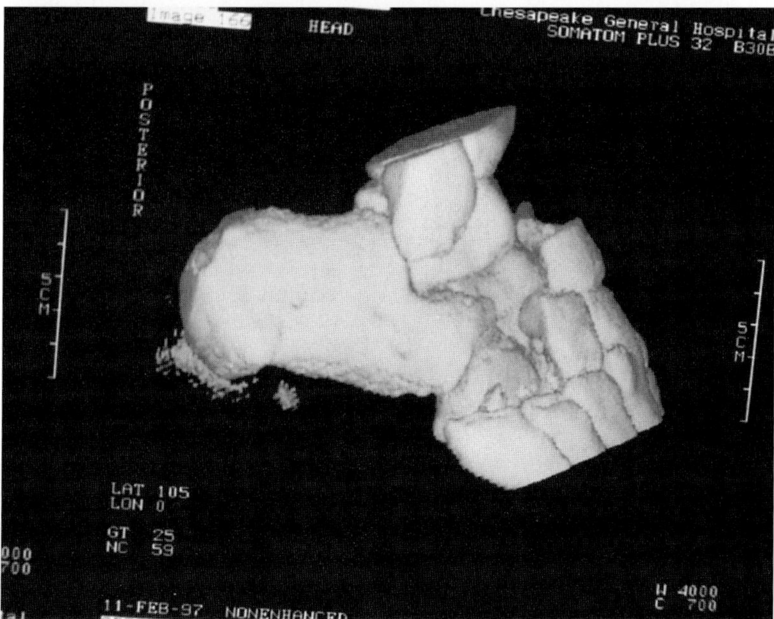

I

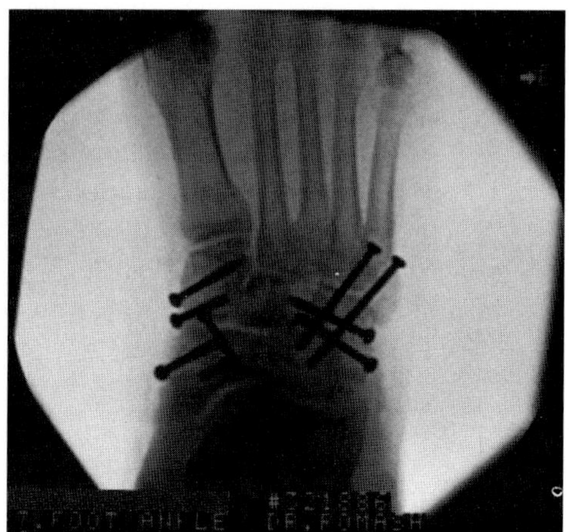

L

Figure 10. Three-dimensional volumetric construction **(G–I)** and reduction and internal fixation **(J–L)** of type III fracture.

Nondisplaced body fractures may be treated by 6 to 8 weeks of immobilization followed by an orthotic device to support the arch. Sangeorzan et al.'s (8) classification of body fractures I, II, and III describe the position and displacement of the fragments as well as the foot.

Attempts to treat displaced fractures by closed reduction have been made. Reduction can be achieved, but maintenance of the reduction is difficult. This is especially true when there has been comminution. When the medial column is shortened, as in a Sangeorzan type II fracture, an adduction deformity of the foot may become manifest. When the foot has moved laterally, as in a Sangeorzan type III fracture, a flattened foot with medial prominence may result. Because closed treatment of these fractures is unreliable, open reduction and internal fixation through an anteromedial approach is recommended.

Sangeorzan et al. (8) described the subtleties of the problem and recommended solutions. The type I fracture may be addressed directly and fixation accomplished by lag screws within the navicular (Fig. 8). The type II fractures pose more of a problem (Fig. 9 A–D). The medial column has shortened and the medial navicular moved proximally. To reduce the fracture, the length of the medial column must be restored. A miniexternal fixator/distraction device placed from the talus to the first metatarsal provides this restoration. Debridement and reduction is then performed (Fig. 9E). Direct lag screw fixation into the lateral navicular is done, if possible. If the lateral fragment is too small to accept fixation, the medial fragment is fixed to the second and third cuneiforms by screws, removed after union has been accomplished (Fig. 9F,G). The fixation scheme for type III fractures follows type II method (Fig. 10). The fixation devices are removed before weight bearing and motion is begun, usually at 8 weeks after operation. Custom arch supports are then used, with 70% good results.

When destruction of the articular cartilage is severe, primary arthrodesis should be considered. The medial column length must be restored and maintained by the arthrodesis. A defect will predictably occur due to the comminution and debridement of bony fragments. This should be addressed by bone grafting. Controversy exists over the magnitude of the arthrodesis effort. Authors have advocated isolated talonavicular arthrodesis, talonavicular cuneiform arthrodesis, or triple arthrodesis. (The triple arthrodesis permits some shortening of the lateral column, which may help in ''balancing'' the foot.) In light of the controversy, decisions as to the magnitude of the arthrodesis may be made after assessment of the degree of damage to the joints.

Sangeorzan et al.'s (8) work helps to predict the outcome. Axiomatically, the most severe injuries had the poorest outcome. Satisfactory reduction was accomplished in 100% of type I (four fractures), 67% of type II (12 fractures), and 50% of type III (four fractures). (Satisfactory reduction was defined as restoration of 60% of the articular surface.) When satisfactory reduction was achieved, ''good'' results (i.e., no pain or occasional pain during vigorous activities but no restriction in activities of daily living) could be anticipated. The foot is not considered normal by the patient, and although Sangeorzan et al. (8) do not comment on range of motion, some stiffness of the foot is to be anticipated.

The sequela of avascular necrosis can be anticipated, but it does *not* always lead to osseous collapse of the entire bone.

Stress Fractures

The navicular is a locus of stress fractures, and this diagnosis is now recognized more frequently (3,15). The vascular anatomy may contribute to this process. The symptom of poorly defined pain along the medial arch makes diagnoses difficult but should also raise a red flag. This fracture has been recognized in high-performance (professional) athletes. It should be diagnosed before displacement can occur. Abnor-

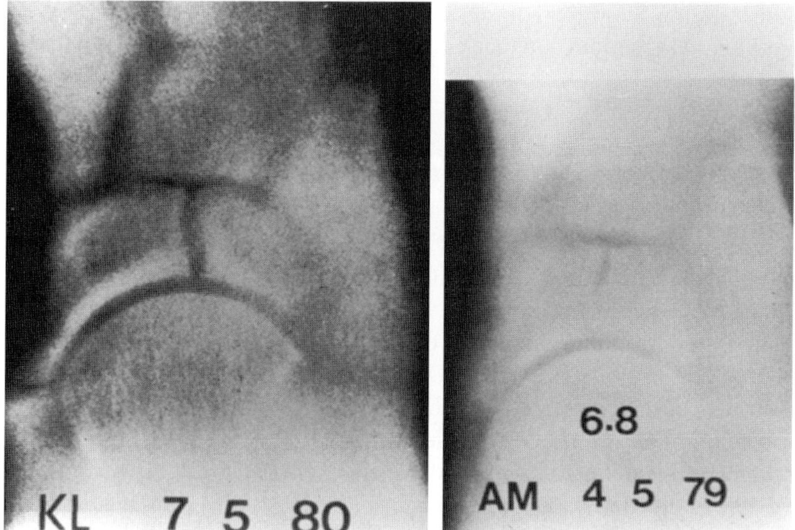

Figure 11. Stress fracture.

mal architecture of the foot can contribute to the cause. Adduction of the forefoot or limited ankle and subtalar motion may increase or change the distribution of stress on the navicular.

The fracture is vertically oriented and occurs in the midportion of the navicular. It is not oriented along the intercuneiform lines. Torg et al. (3) note that a coned down *true* AP view of the navicular is needed (Fig. 11). The fracture may be incomplete, involving only the dorsal portion of the bone. Bone scans will be positive before

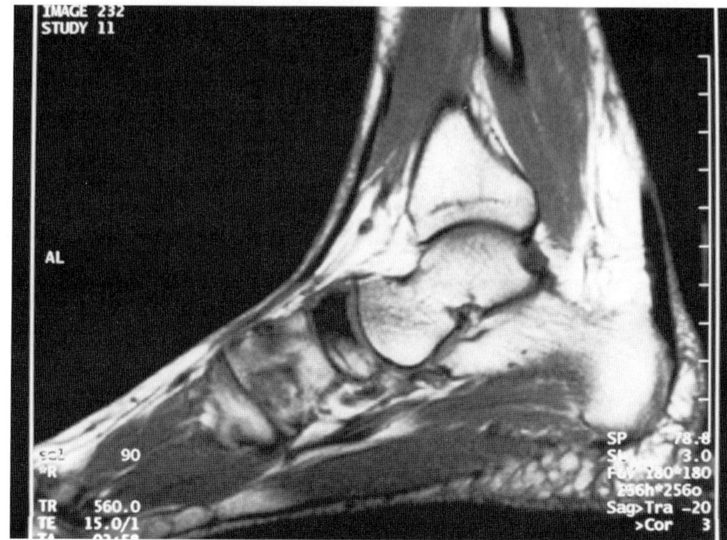

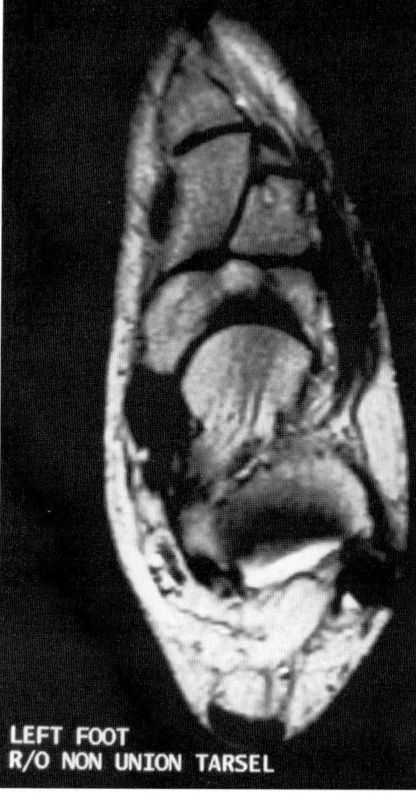

Figure 12. A,B: MRI of stress fracture.

radiographs demonstrate the fracture. Tomograms and/or computed tomography (CT) scans are effective later. Magnetic resonance imaging (MRI) is also sensitive and will demonstrate the fracture (Fig. 12).

Treatment

If the fracture is diagnosed early by means of bone scan, MRI, or radiograph before displacement has occurred, the initial treatment is immobilization in a non-weight-bearing short leg cast for 8 weeks.

If union is not achieved by immobilization or if displacement has occurred, then operative intervention is indicated. The fracture should be bridged by a bone graft and secure internal fixation accomplished by means of a lag screw. This should be followed by 8 weeks of non-weight-bearing immobilization.

Ancillary treatment by means of external pulsed electromagnetic fields or internal bone stimulators may be considered, but there are no scientific studies showing efficacy of these treatments in this specific situation. The principle involved in this application is sound.

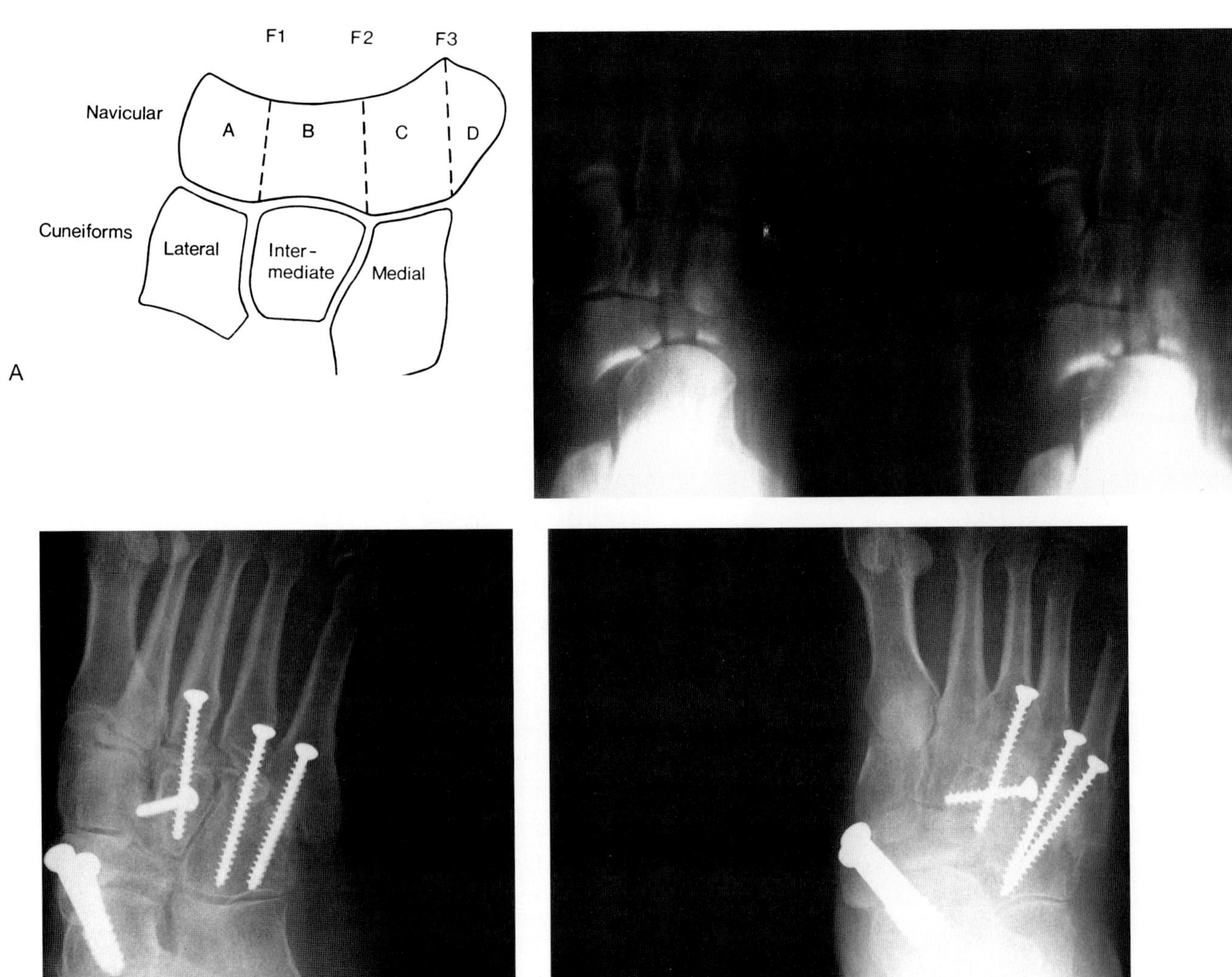

Figure 13. A,B: Navicular fracture with midfoot disruption. **C:** Final salvage of fracture with talonavicular and midfoot arthrodesis.

Fractures of the Navicular with Forefoot Disruption

The axial load along the shafts of the metatarsal that produces the Lisfranc fracture (dislocation at the metatarsal cuneiform junction) can be transmitted proximally (15a), causing failure in the intercuneiform joints and fracture of the navicular (6) (Fig. 13A). The navicular fracture occurs along the lines of fracture previously noted and displaces in a similar fashion (Fig. 13B). Management is complicated by the need to stabilize the intercuneiform joints and the metatarsal–cuneiform/cuboid junction.

Shortening of the medial column due to proximal displacement of the medial fragment of the navicular, cuneiform, and great toe metatarsal must be corrected. The previously noted techniques are applicable to this situation. Stabilization of the medial fragment of the navicular to the lateral fragment of the navicular is then accomplished. Reduction and stabilization of the intercuneiform joints is also performed, in conjunction with reduction and stabilization of the metatarsal cuneiform joints. The magnitude of this injury is greater than that of the isolated navicular fracture. The postinjury recuperative time is prolonged, and later salvage by arthrodesis of the involved joints may be necessary (Fig. 13C).

FRACTURES OF THE CUBOID

To review the anatomy, the cuboid articulates with the fourth and fifth metatarsals, the lateral cuneiform, and the anterior calcaneus. Little motion occurs at the metatarsal cuneiform junction or cuneiform articulation. There is motion at the calcaneocuboid joint, as this joint moves during inversion and eversion of the foot. The length of the cuboid contributes to the length of the lateral column of the foot. The peroneal tendons course by the cuboid laterally, the peroneus longus turning plantarly under the cuboid. The inconsistent os peroneum is found in the peroneus longus adjacent to the cuboid.

Mechanism of Injury

Severe abduction of the forefoot or axial loading of the fourth and fifth metatarsals produces a compressive force on the lateral column. The cuboid is caught in a ''vise'' or ''nutcracker'' between the metatarsal bases and the calcaneus. The cuboid then fails in compression.

Fracture Patterns

The fracture patterns produced may occur along lines of internal shear produced by the compression, in an ''explosive'' type pattern as the cuboid shortens and *widens* as it is crushed, or in a pure compressive mode as one or the other of the articular surfaces is driven into the body of the cuboid. Fractures of the cuboid are often associated with tarsometatarsal or midtarsal fracture dislocations. Avulsion fractures of the navicular may also occur, due to the violent abduction force opposed by the posterior tibial tendon's insertion on the navicular.

Radiographs

The oblique view demonstrates the cuboid on plane film. CT scans of the foot in axial, coronal, and sagittal cuts or reconstructions give detailed information of the fracture (Fig. 14).

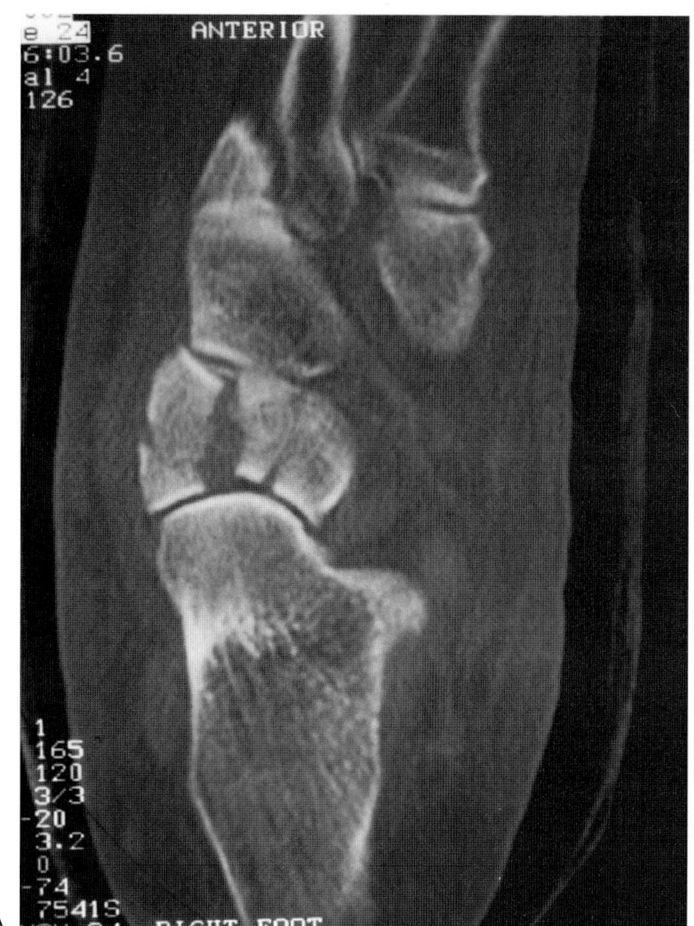

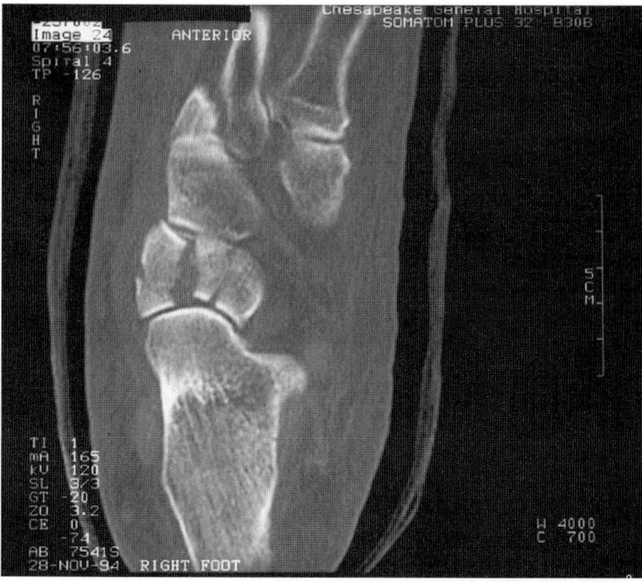

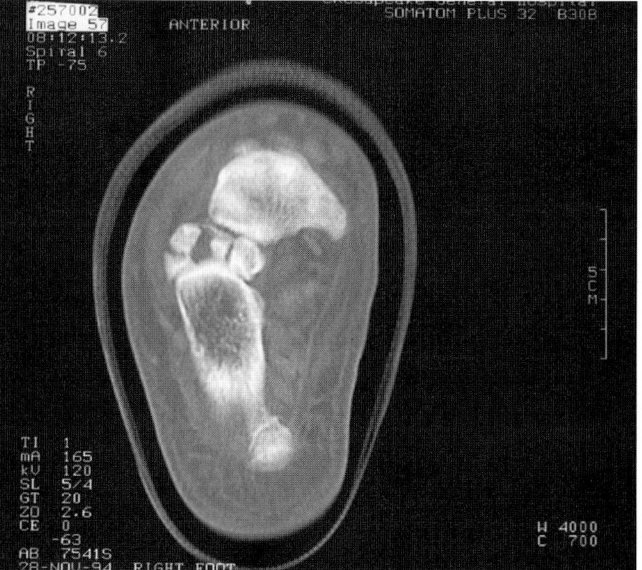

Figure 14. A–C: CT scan of cuboid fracture.

Treatment

The older literature (16–18) may reflect poor results with conservative management, as Hermel and Gerson-Cohen (19) recommend primary midtarsal fusion when the fracture is comminuted. Their premise is that the lateral column of the foot is relatively immobile, hence arthrodesis may be performed with few sequelae.

More recent literature (6,20) reflects more enthusiasm for anatomic reconstruction. The principles applied are (a) reestablishing the length of the lateral column and (b) reduction of the articular surfaces with (c) adequate fixation. CT imaging allows preparation for the procedure.

When fractures occur along internal shear lines, reduction and fixation is satisfactory. When the cancellous bone of the cuboid has been crushed, the length of the cuboid must be reestablished. This may be done with cancellous bone grafts or cortical–cancellous grafts. Fixation may be secured with screws and may be buttressed with a plate and screws (Fig. 15). Sangeorzan and Swiontkowski (20) reported satisfactory results in a group of four patients so treated.

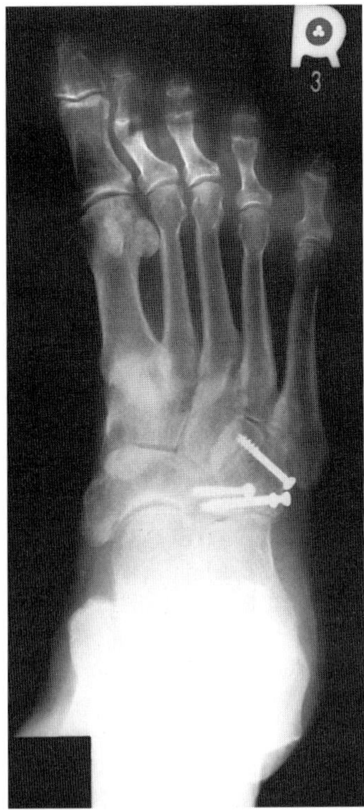
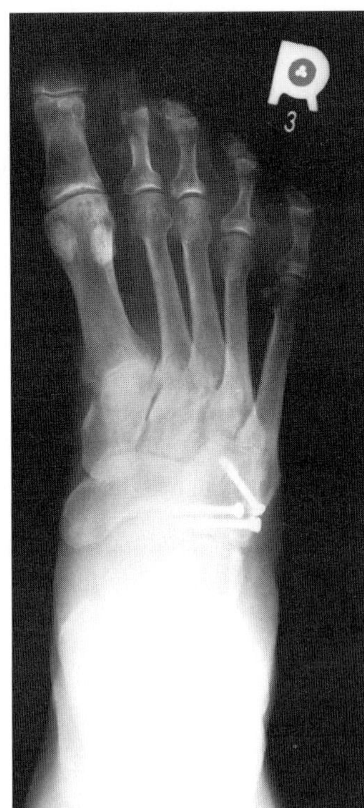
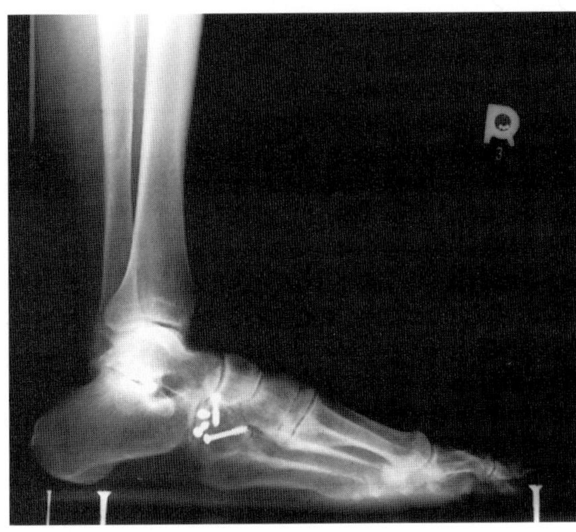

A–C

Figure 15. A–C: Postoperative open reduction and internal fixation of cuboid fracture.

Salvage may be accomplished by arthrodesis. At this time there is again some enthusiasm for isolated calcaneocuboid arthrodesis with lengthening of the lateral column for painful flat feet with forefoot abduction (21). This principle may be applied in the treatment of malunions or posttraumatic arthritis at the calcaneocuboid joint. Hindfoot motion appears to diminish slightly when the calcaneocuboid joint is arthrodesed.

REFERENCES

1. Sarrafian SK. *Anatomy of the foot and ankle.* Philadelphia: JB Lippincott, 1983.
2. Lehman EP, Eskeles IH. Fracture of the tarsal scaphoid. With notes on the Mechanism. *J Bone Joint Surg* 1928;10:108–113.
3. Torg JS, Pavlov H, Cooley LH, et al. Stress fracture of the tarsal navicular. *J Bone Joint Surg [Am]* 1982;64:700–712.
4. McKeever FM. Fractures of the tarsal and metatarsal bones. *Surg Gynecol Obstet* 1950;90:735–745.
5. Mygind HB. The accessory tarsal scaphoid. *Acta Orthop Scand* 1954;23:142–151.
6. Heckman JD. Fractures and dislocations of the foot. In: Rockwood CA, Green DP, eds. *Fractures in adults,* 2nd ed, vol 2. Philadelphia: JB Lippincott, 1984:1789–1796.
7. DeLee JC. Fractures and dislocations of the foot. In: Mann RA, Coughlin MJ, eds. *Surgery of the foot,* 6th ed. St. Louis: CV Mosby, 1993:1600–1617.
8. Sangeorzan BJ, Benirschke SK, Mosca V, Mayo KA, Hansen ST. Displaced intra-articular fractures of the tarsal navicular. *J Bone Joint Surg [Am]* 1989;71:1504–1510.
9. Watson-Jones R. *Fractures and joint injuries,* 4th ed, vol 2. Baltimore: Williams & Wilkins, 1955.
10. Giannestras NJ, Sammarco GJ. Fractures and dislocations in the foot. In: Rockwood CA Jr, Green DP, eds. *Fractures,* vol 2. Philadelphia: JB Lippincott, 1975.
11. Chapman MW. Fractures and fracture dislocations of the ankle and foot. In: Mann RA, ed. *DuVreis' surgery of the foot,* 4th ed. St. Louis: CV Mosby, 1978:1601–1613.
12. Coker TP Jr, Arnold JA. Sports injuries to the foot and ankle. In: Jahss MH, ed. *Disorders of the foot,* vol 2. Philadelphia: WB Saunders, 1982:1573–1606.
13. Kidner FC. The prehalux (accessory scaphoid) in its relationship to flatfoot. *J Bone Joint Surg* 1929;11:831.
14. Vaishya R, Patrick JH. Isolated dorsal fracture-dislocation of the tarsal navicular. *Injury* 1991;22:47–48.
15. Hunter LY. Stress fractures of the tarsal navicular. *Am J Sports Med* 1981;9:217–219.

15a. Eichenholtz SN, Levine DB. Fractures of the tarsal navicular bone. *Clin Orthop* 1964;34:142–157.

16. Bohler L. *The treatment of fractures,* 5th ed, vol 3. New York: Grune & Stratton, 1958.
17. Conwell HE, Reynolds FC. *Key and Conwell's management of fractures, dislocations, and sprains,* 7th ed. St. Louis: CV Mosby, 1961.
18. Heck CV. Fractures of the bones of the foot (except for the talus). *Surg Clin North Am* 1965;45:103–117.

19. Hermel MB, Gershon-Cohen J. The nutcracker fracture of the cuboid by indirect violence. *Radiology* 1953;60:850.
20. Sangeorzan BJ, Swiontkowski MF. Displaced fractures of the cuboid. *J Bone Joint Surg [Br]* 1990;72B:376–378.
21. Sangeorzan BJ, Mosca V, Hansen ST. Effect of calcaneal lengthening on relationships among the hindfoot, midfoot, and forefoot. *Foot Ankle* 1993;14:136–141.
22. Hillegass RC. Injuries to the midfoot: a major cause of industrial morbidity. In: Bateman JE, ed. *Foot science*. Philadelphia: WB Saunders, 1976.
23. Main BJ, Jowett RL. Injuries of the midtarsal joint. *J Bone Joint Surg [Br]* 1975;57:91.

EDITORIAL COMMENTS

Fractures of the Navicular and Cuboid

Michael M. Romash

The navicular and cuboid occupy an important position at the pinnacle of the longitudinal arch and the midfoot. Injuries to both these bones can affect the forefoot rotation, abduction, and adduction. Small deformities of these structures may result in significant alteration of the normal plantar surface stress relationship of the forefoot. The key principle in dealing with these injuries is recognition and suspicion of injury. Injury to these structures should be suspected if there is axial force significant enough to create a tarsometatarsal injury and when injuries have a great deal of rotation, with a fixed portion of the foot. These injuries are often missed, particularly if they appear as crush injuries of the cuboid on initial screening; they depend on clinical tenderness and alteration of the normal architecture of the foot. I have found that the CT scan is very valuable in both navicular and cuboid injuries in determining the degree of articular involvement and amount of loss of substance of the bone when one is determining whether an open reduction is necessary. We also advocate, as does Dr. Michael Romash, the use of external fixation devices, both medial and lateral, for restoration of length. These fixators may need to stay on for 6 to 8 weeks; then a reconstruction should be planned to support the midfoot, which has collapsed, since the use of the fixator alone without restoration of anatomy will not be appropriate. On the lateral side, the length of the lateral column can be restored by fusion of the calcaneocuboid joint, which does not seem to affect the hindfoot motion significantly. One can also add length to the anterior portion of the calcaneus, but the foot must be fairly supple for this to occur. Iliac crest grafts are utilized in my practice by taking full-thickness central segments about 1 cm long. Restoration of the navicular by fusion is more difficult because the blood supply is not as good as on the lateral side due to poor interosseous circulation; it is difficult to use internal fixation by means of plates on that side for absolute rigidity. Therefore, one is utilizing screws that do not provide absolute rigid fixation. A final word on this fracture is recognition and absolute anatomic restoration to maintain the normal architectural relationships. As noted in this chapter, even if treatment is perfect, patients can still have symptomatic problems in this region of the foot that require orthotic support for long periods.

Robert S. Adelaar, M.D.

Complex Foot and Ankle Trauma,
edited by Robert S. Adelaar,
Lippincott–Raven Publishers, Philadelphia © 1999.

14

Treatment of Tarsometatarsal Injuries

Robert S. Adelaar

Severe injuries of the forefoot were frequently reported in the equestrian age of Lisfranc (Fig. 1). The Royal Infirmary in Edinburgh in the mid-twentieth century reported a 0.2% incidence of tarsometatarsal injuries (1,2). These low-velocity injuries were usually a result of longitudinal compression and twisting of the forefoot. They have been reported by Lisfranc in 1840, Gissane in 1951, Watson-Jones in 1955, and Jeffreys in 1963 (1–4).

The modern incidence of high-velocity tarsometatarsal injuries has been reported at the Hannover Germany Medical School to be approximately 120 cases in a series of 1,580 complex foot and ankle problems (5).

ANATOMY

The anatomy of the area is critical in understanding the mechanism of injury and the rationale for appropriate treatment. The second metatarsal is the keystone of the metatarsal arch, which has been found to be similar to a roman arch. The width of the bones on the dorsal surface is greater than the width of those on the plantar surface, providing architectural stability (Fig. 2). The second metatarsal is usually the longest and most rigid and is felt to be the keystone of the foot with its articulation with the first, second, and third cuneiform. The key to reduction of the complex tarsometatarsal dislocation is the second metatarsal. The fourth and fifth metatarsals are mobile and articulate with the cuboid. The cuboid third cuneiform articulation is also important

R. S. Adelaar: Department of Orthopaedics of Virginia Commonwealth University, Medical College of Virginia, Richmond, Virginia 23298.

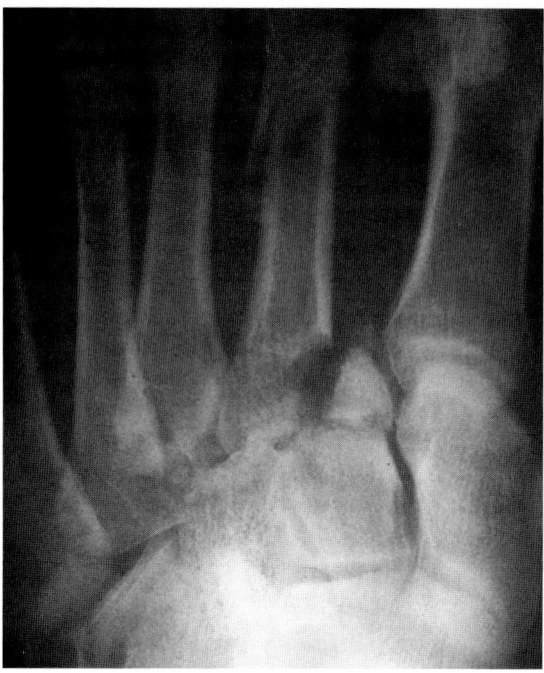

Figure 1. X-ray film of a tarsometatarsal dislocation demonstrating a lateral dislocation of the second through fifth metatarsals and an avulsion fracture of the Lisfranc ligament.

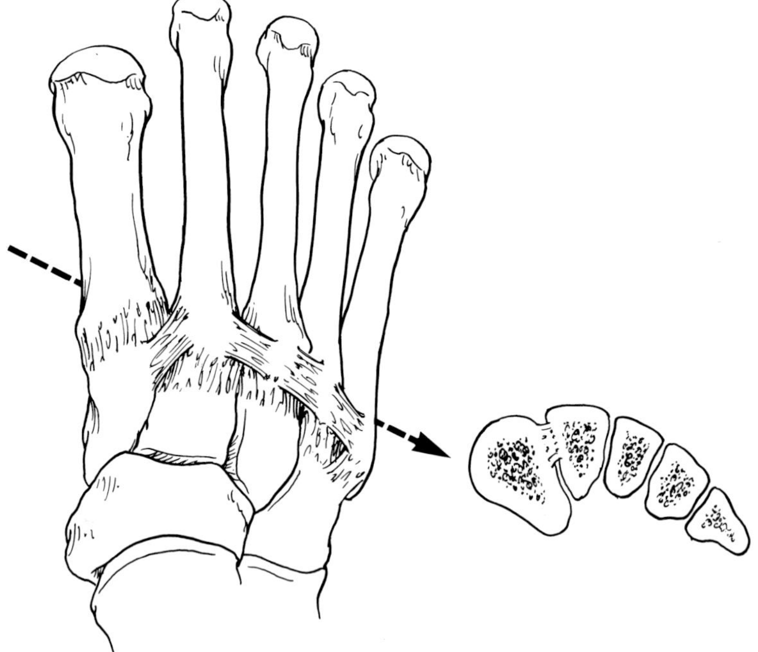

Figure 2. Anatomy of tarsometatarsal region.

for mobility of the lateral complex. The base of the first metatarsal is stabilized by the capsule and the anterior tibialis and peroneus longus tendons. There is no interosseous ligament between the base of the first and second metatarsal bones, but there are strong plantar and dorsal ligaments (Fig. 2).

The dorsal and central interosseous ligament between the medial cuneiform and the second metatarsal is well developed and is known as Lisfranc's ligament. In this injury it is often noted that an avulsion of the second metatarsal will remain with the Lisfranc ligament, and its anatomic reduction is critical in analyzing the reduction (Fig. 1). Most of the dislocations occur in a dorsal direction (Fig. 3) due to the basic intrinsic stability of the bone architecture and the fact that the plantar ligaments and supporting structures are stronger than the dorsal, consisting of the plantar fascia, intrinsic musculature, and peroneus longus.

The arterial anatomy is critical since the anterior tibialis artery has an intermetatarsal branch which anastomoses with the plantar circulation (Fig. 4). The anterior tibialis creates the first dorsal metacarpal artery and first plantar metacarpal artery, which are critical to circulation of the medial portions of the foot. In injuries to this area, as reported by Gissane, the arterial anastomosis can be disrupted, causing significant hemorrhage and increased compartment pressure (2). The close relationship between the first and second metatarsal and cuneiform is critical to establish the reduction and reduce the stress on the vascular system. It is interesting that the plantar branches from

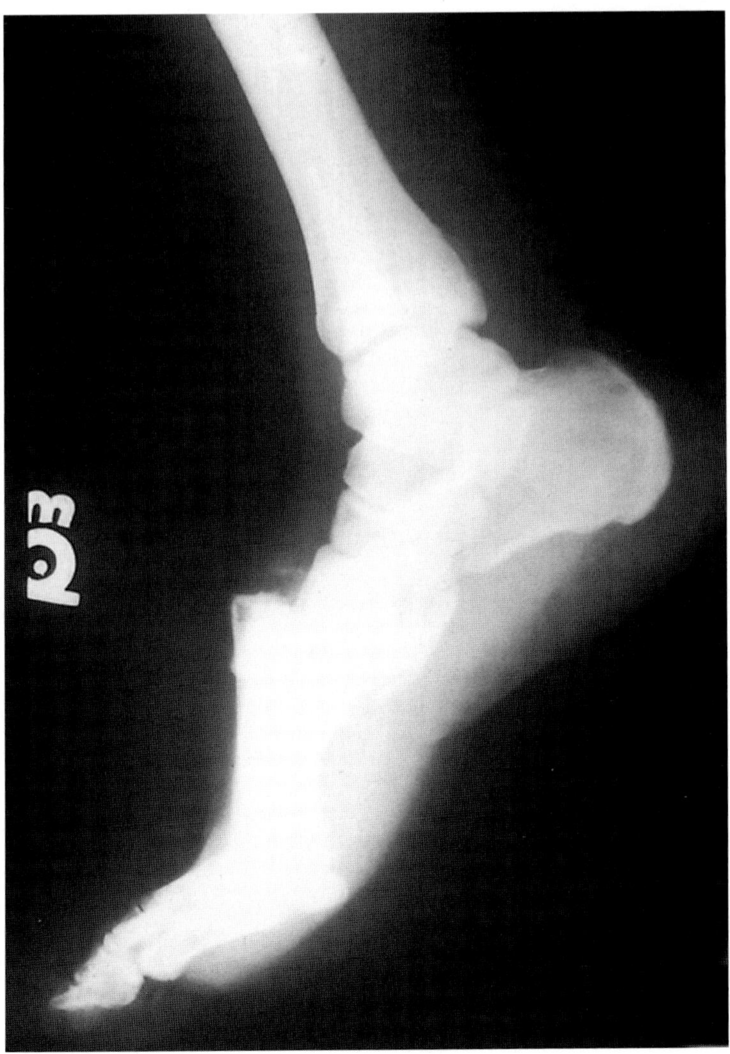

Figure 3. Typical dorsal dislocation of the tarsometatarsal joint.

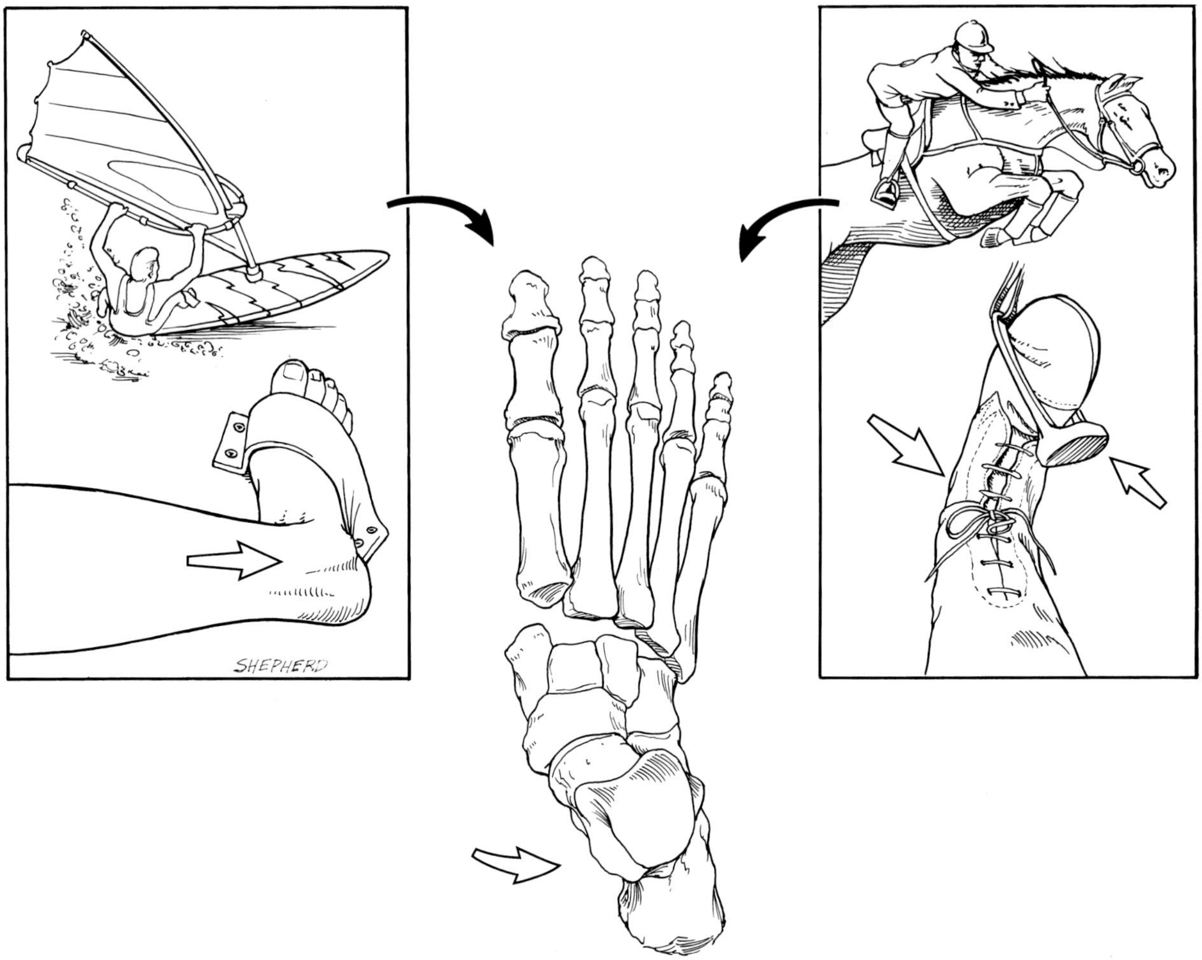

SHEPHERD

A

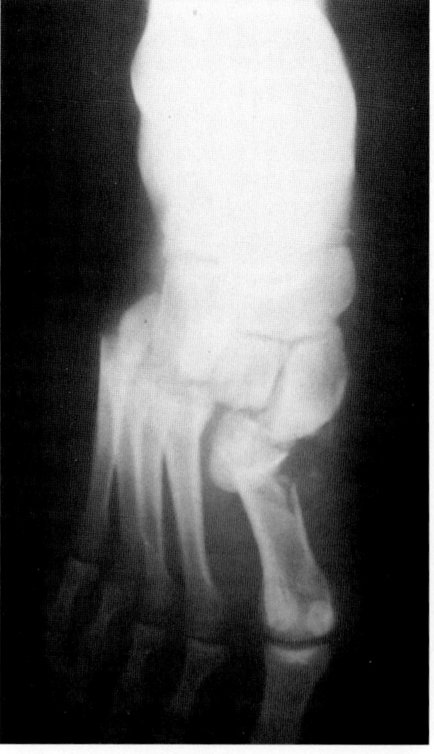

B

Figure 4. A: Tarsometatarsal dislocation mechanism with the forefoot caught and the hindfoot rotated around the fixed axis. **B:** Typical x-ray film of the result of the mechanism shown in A.

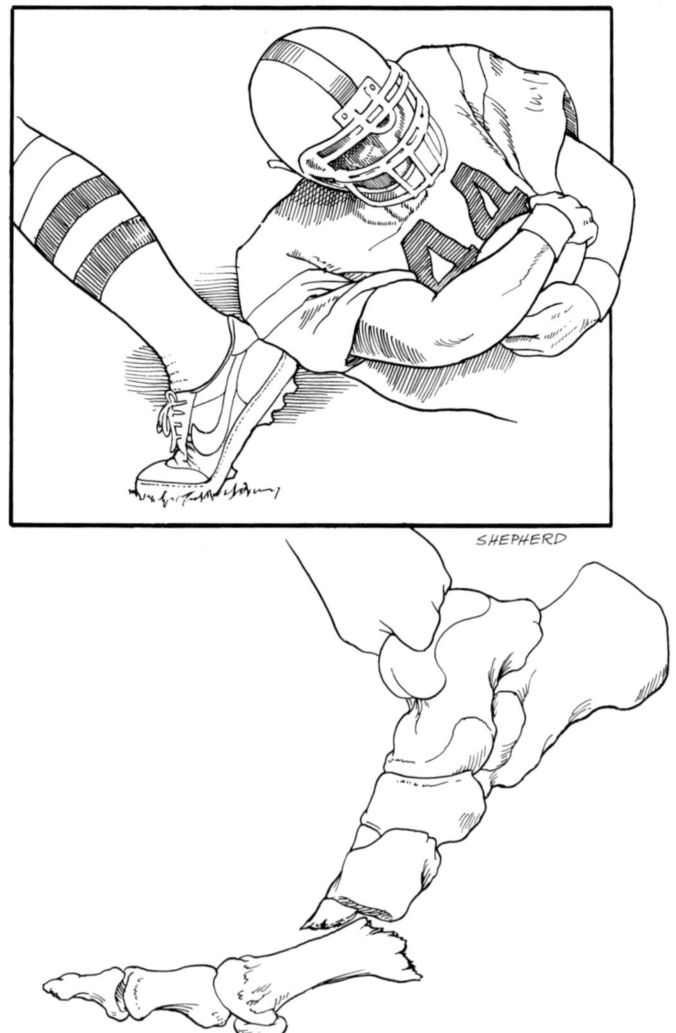

C

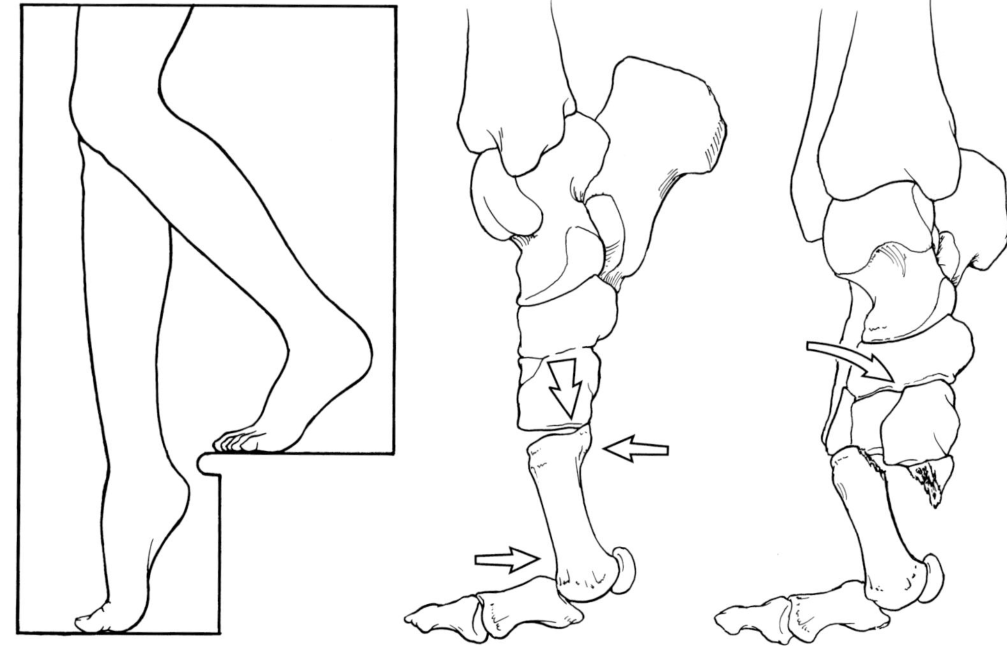

D

Figure 4. *Continued.* **C:** Mechanism of injury at the tarsometatarsal joint with the hindfoot loaded and the forefoot fixed. **D:** Mechanism of tarsometatarsal injuries in dancers.

the anterior tibiales artery are used for microsurgical tissue transplantation of the great toe.

MECHANISM OF INJURY

The mechanism of injury can occur from three different actions. In the equestrian age of Lisfranc, a twisting injury to a fixed forefoot pulled into abduction was critical to these injuries. This injury occurred when a soldier was thrown from his horse with his foot remaining in the stirrup (1,6–8) (Fig. 4A,B). These injuries are characterized by fractures of the base of the second metatarsal, the cuboid, and the metatarsal necks. The second type of injury, which is more common today particularly in athletic competition, is that of an extrinsic heel loaded with the foot in fixed plantar flexion (9). This occurs in football when the planted plantarflexed heel is loaded by an opposing lineman (Fig. 4C). Another mechanism that often causes occult injury is a twisting injury to a dancer with the collapse in the extreme point position (Fig. 4D) or to a large lineman on his toes pass blocking. Crushing injuries cause the rarer plantar dislocations.

CLASSIFICATION

At the Medical College of Virginia we use the basic classification developed by Hardcastle (7,8,10) (Fig. 5A). In type I, there is total incongruity; this has also been called homolateral, with the entire tarsometatarsal group traveling in one direction (Fig. 5B). Type II, which is more common, is partially incongruent or isolated; the first metatarsal or the lateral four tarsometatarsals are involved only (Fig. 5C). These can be either medial or lateral, with the force on the metacarpal determining whether the injury is at the base or the metacarpal necks. In type III, which is most common, the

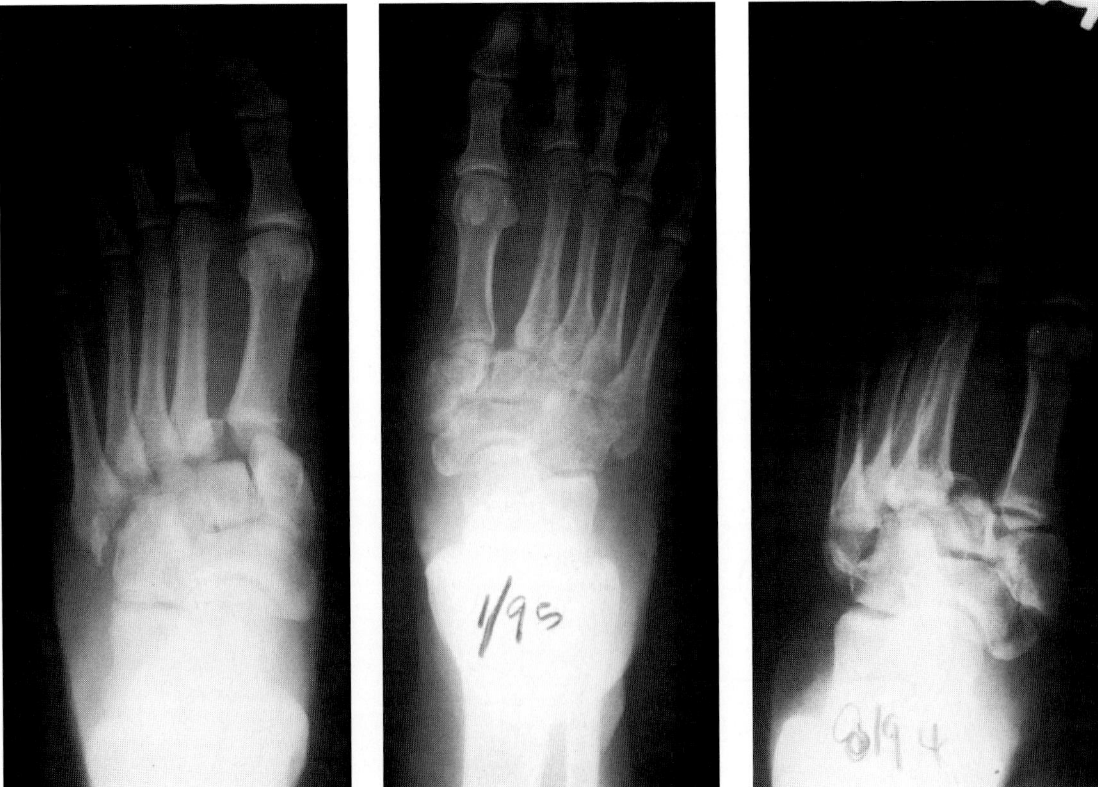

Figure 5. The Hardcastle mechanism of tarsometatarsal injuries. **A:** Typical homolateral dislocation. **B:** Isolated type of tarsometatarsal dislocation. **C:** Divergent type of tarsometatarsal dislocation.

first metatarsal and lateral four metatarsals diverge into opposite directions (Fig. 5D). There can be fractures at the metacarpal bases or necks. Myerson (9) has grouped injury segments into columns, with the medial column consisting of a medial cuneiform and first metatarsal, the middle column consisting of a second and third cuneiform and second and third metatarsals, and the lateral column consisting of a fourth and fifth metatarsal and cuboid (7,9). These columns are useful in describing reduction fixation techniques.

RADIOLOGIC CRITERIA

The normal radiographic anatomy is important in the diagnosis of tarsometatarsal injuries. The characteristic views taken are anteroposterior AP, lateral, and 30-degree oblique. The normal anatomic findings are the following: the medial fourth metatarsal aligns with the medial cuboid; the lateral third metatarsal aligns with the lateral third cuneiform; the medial second metatarsal aligns with the medial second cuneiform; and the first metatarsal aligns with the first cuneiform (9,11) (Fig. 6).

Some characteristic danger signs to look for on x-ray film are the avulsion fracture of the Lisfranc ligament with a small piece of the second metatarsal attached (Fig. 1). Cuboid fractures also represent significant abduction-type injuries with stress to the fourth and fifth metatarsal. A decrease in varus of the first metatarsal indicates an injury to the base of the articulation, with loss of support. The injury pattern usually includes the navicular cuneiform complex; therefore, look for widening or an avulsion of the medial portion of the navicular, which indicates a possible injury to the medial complex.

Jeffreys (6) has done an experimental study on tarsal metatarsal dislocations in which he fixed the forefoot and attempted to reproduce the dislocation patterns. He found that

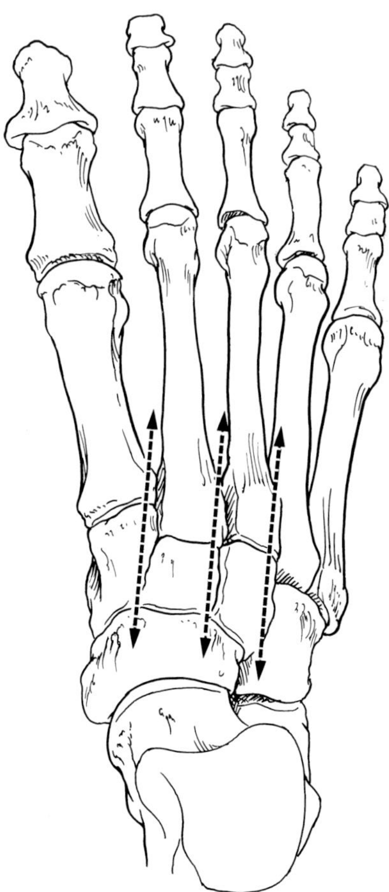

Figure 6. Normal anteroposterior view of the foot with alignment criteria of tarsometatarsal joints.

pronation of the hindfoot produced lateral dislocations of all metatarsal bases, with all five metatarsals being displaced together. Supination of the hindfoot with the forefoot fixed caused displacement of the first metatarsal cuneiform joint. Further supination did not increase the displacement as long as the second metatarsal remained intact. When the second metatarsal fractured, the medial and dorsal displacement in the bases of the lateral four metatarsals occurred. Therefore the two main patterns of injury are lateral dislocation produced by pronation of the hindfoot and medial dislocation of the first metatarsal cuneiform complex produced by supination of the hindfoot, followed by complete dislocation after disruptions of the second metatarsal base (6).

TREATMENT

Treatment should be dictated by the nature of the injury mechanism or wound or the amount of swelling present. Care should be taken to rule out significant arterial injury between the dorsal and plantar circulation (Fig. 2) and injury to the deep peroneal nerve. The treatment principles are that an anatomic reduction will give you the best possible chance for a good to excellent result in the future. Anesthesia by foot and ankle block, regional or general, and traction would be appropriate for closed and possible open reduction. X-ray film is provided by image intensification in the operating room, but a regular radiograph would need to be done to look for reduction parameters if any doubt existed. Stress x-ray film should also be taken to define the extent of injury, particularly the first metatarsal, navicular–cuneiform, and lateral complex. Usually one would want to try an anatomic reduction by closed or open means within at least the first 2 weeks, but reduction can be tried for up to 6 weeks, at which time it is more difficult. The goal is an absolutely perfect radiologic reduction as close to the time of injury as possible.

Compartment syndrome can occur with a crushing type or vascular injury. Measurements of the forefoot compartments may be indicated. Most of the tarsometatarsal injuries are closed. An attempt is made to treat these injuries as early as possible due to the multiple disruptions that require reduction. Our goal is to treat all injuries closed or open to obtain anatomic reduction within the first 6 weeks. After the first 3 weeks it is much more difficult to obtain a closed reduction and the procedure must be open. In our experience, some of the injuries can be treated by closed pinning or percutaneous screw methods if approached early enough, but we do not hesitate to open if reduction is not adequate.

All injuries are initially treated closed in the operating room unless they are open to start with. Closed treatment depends on placing traction on the second and third metatarsals under adequate anesthesia (Fig. 7). Up to 20 pounds of traction should be used initially to obtain a reduction of the second metatarsal complex. After reduction of the second metatarsal complex, the first metatarsal, followed by the lateral three, is reduced. The metatarsal head fractures will usually not require fixation unless the periosteal cuff is ruptured, and then pinning is required. The metatarsal heads can be pinned by the plantar percutaneous approach or by using bioabsorbable pins. The plantar pins need to be discontinued by 3 to 4 weeks since they are difficult to handle in that area and can lead to extension contractures of the metatarsal phalangeal joint. Percutaneous pins or cannulated screws (4.5 or 5.0 mm) are used from the first metatarsal to the first and second cuneiforms; at least two pins or screws are required (Fig. 8). Screws should also be passed from the second metatarsal to the second cuneiform or first cuneiform to second metatarsal. When fixing from distal to proximal, an inset screw technique should be used. The lateral complex requires two to three 0.062 pins. An image intensifier is utilized to obtain reduction, and 0.062 K-wires or 4- to 5-mm cannulated screws are used for percutaneous methods. Final AP, lateral, and oblique x-ray film are mandatory to check the final reduction. Percutaneous pin or screw fixation is recommended, at least for any displaced tarsometatarsal injury after reduction. Cast containment of displaced fractures does not preserve anatomic reduction.

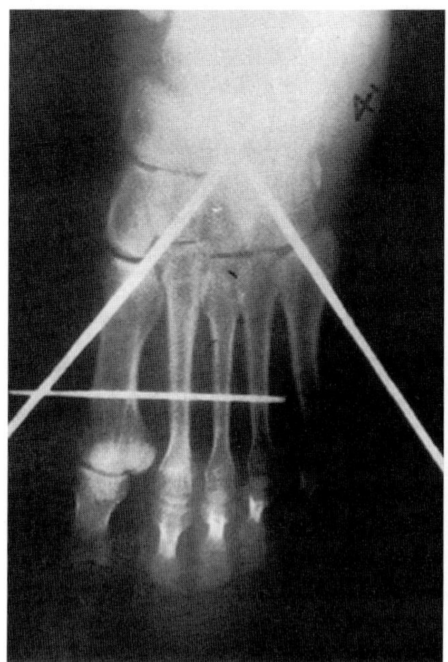

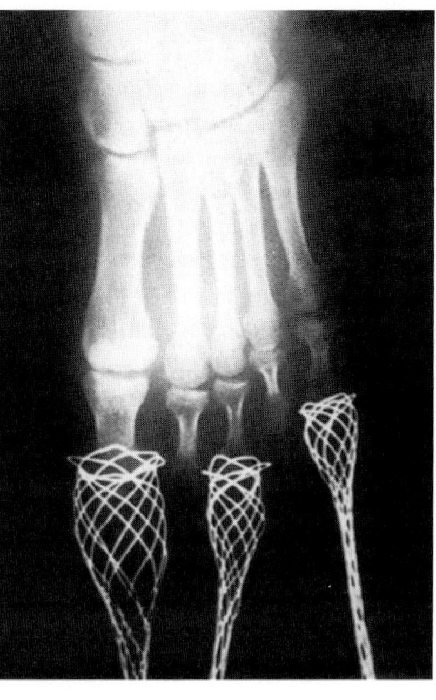

Figure 7. Traction is applied and fixation achieved with cannulated screws or K-wires.

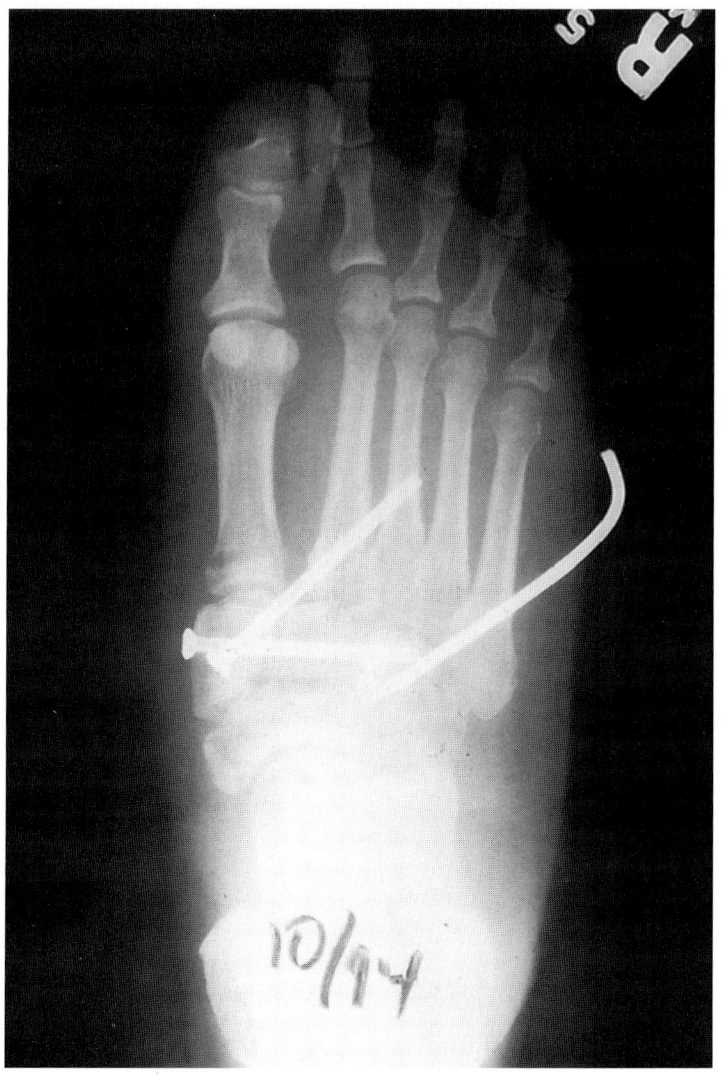

Figure 8. Adequate fixation would be with screws and pins.

Open treatment is usually necessary if anatomic reduction cannot be obtained closed. The incision will be dorsal between the first and second metatarsals, and additional incisions between the fourth and fifth or medial cuneiform–navicular may be required. Care is taken to preserve the arterial anastomosis between the dorsal and plantar circulations or to look for an arterial injury in that area (Fig. 9). A significant hematoma on approach to the base of the first and second metatarsals indicates injury to a portion of the anterior tibialis circulation. The anatomic reduction criteria used are as follows: less than 3 to 4 mm of space between the first and second metatarsal; less than a 15-degree angle between the lateral talar metatarsal axis; lateral shifting of the third, fourth, and fifth metatarsals; and reasonable reduction of the metatarsal head fractures (7,8,9,12). It should be noted that the second metatarsal is treated first since the lateral three metatarsals will not locate if the second metatarsal complex is not anatomic. A recent cadaver study has shown that up to 3 mm of dorsolateral subluxation between the second metatarsal and cuneiform would decrease the contact area and increase the peak pressure by one-third (13).

The type of fixation utilized depends on the judgment of the surgeon. There has been a movement toward screw fixation of at least the medial and middle columns injuries and continued pin fixation of the lateral columns (Fig. 10). The pin fixation usually can not last more than 6 to 8 weeks due to pin track problems, and it usually takes a long-term containment to maintain an anatomic reduction. When using (Fig. 11) screw fixation from distal to proximal, we make a cortical recessed area in the metatarsal base with a bur to facilitate placement of the screw and avoid cracking the cortex. We prefer percutaneous or open self-tapping cannulated systems. The jury is out as to whether to remove these screws or not. I would recommend removal after 1 year and leaving the joint with a fibrous union. A formal fusion should be done when there is severe irre-

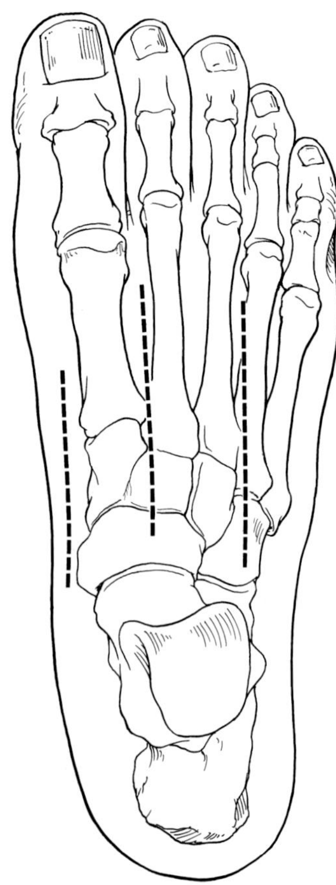

Figure 9. Placement of incisions for open reduction and internal fixation. The *dotted lines* represent the recommended incisions.

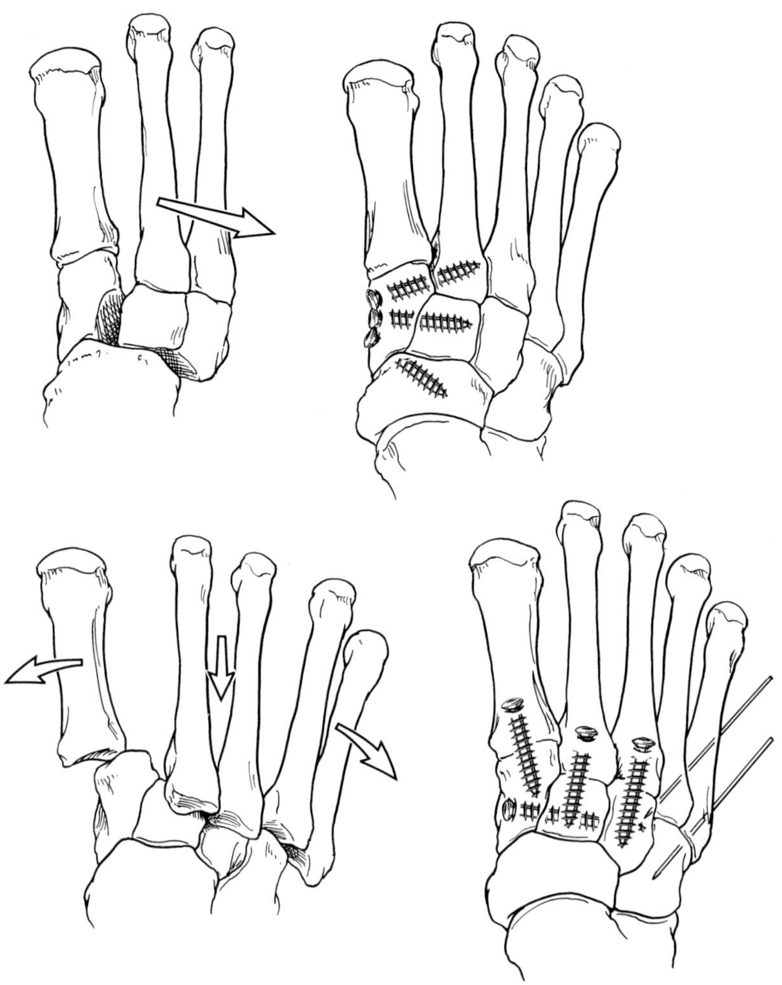

Figure 10. Recommendation would be for fixation with open reduction and internal fixation or the percutaneous method.

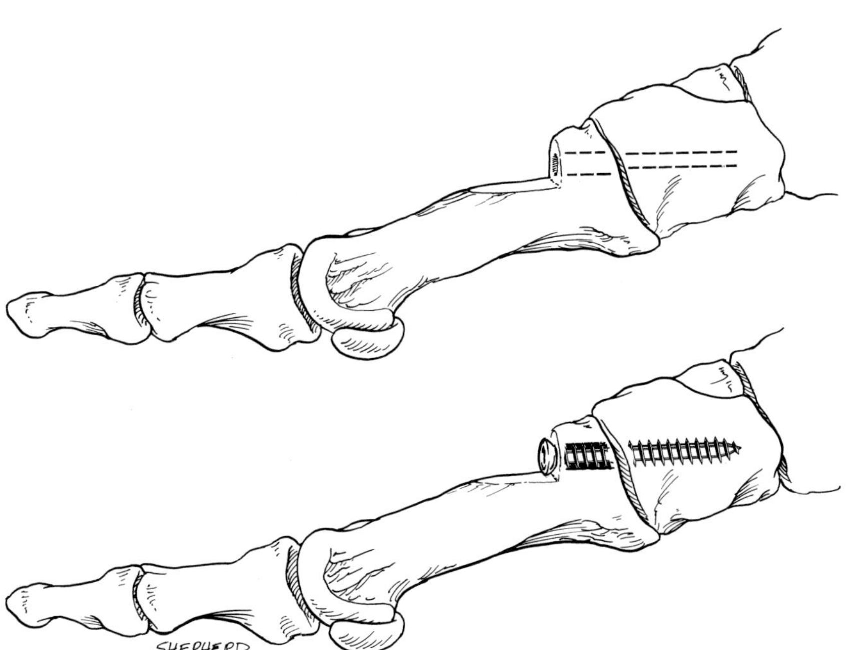

Figure 11. Method of distal to proximal screw fixation.

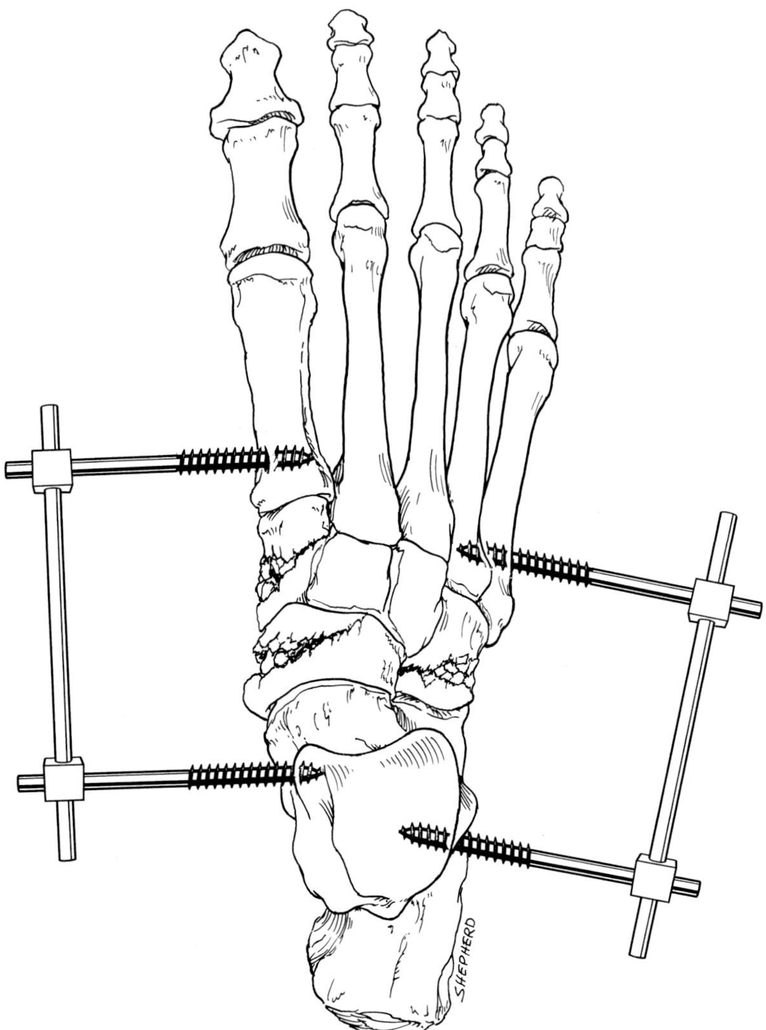

Figure 12. An external fixator can also be used for severe midtarsal collapse.

constructable articular damage or in a chronic injury of longer than 6 months. In the fusion method the dimensions of the bones should be maintained. An external fixator can also be used to maintain correction of severe midtarsal injuries (Fig. 12).

Our postoperative care has been a non-weight-bearing cast for 3 months. Then a plastizote semirigid full-length orthotic with metatarsal and longitudinal support is utilized for at least 1 year. Physical therapy has been helpful for mobilization of the forefoot, midtarsal, and gastroc soleus complex.

An unusual condition has been reported when the first metatarsal will not reduce. The anterior tibialis tendon or portion of the tendon can be entrapped between the first and second metatarsal; this will require an open reduction.

RESULTS

The results of tarsal metatarsal dislocations are scarce in the literature. Wilson (14) and Wilppula (15) stated that a closed anatomic reduction gives the best long-term results. They accepted only a slight initial separation between the first and second metatarsals and a reduction of the lateral three metatarsal dislocations. Treatment after 6 weeks did not yield good results in their reports. The most recent report on long-term follow-up of tarsal metatarsal injuries is that of the University of Maryland Shock Trauma group, with a 4.2-year follow-up (16). They reported that an anatomic reduction was the key to decreasing long-term morbidity. Eighty-one percent of patients with a good anatomic reduction by the criteria given had good to excellent results. Only 20% of those who did not have a good anatomic reduction had good to excellent results. They also found that degenerative changes on x-ray film did not necessarily correlate with pain at the tarsometatarsal joints. Other centers have not found as good a result with open anatomic fixation. A recent cadaver study demonstrates that computed tomography (CT) scans would be more accurate to determine reduction. Dorsolateral subluxation of up to 3 mm caused significant reduction in articular surface, which would increase peak pressure (16). Therefore, a routine x-ray series may not be enough to ensure accurate reduction.

Our results have been that an anatomic reduction gave the best result for pain. Forefoot stiffness, loss of metatarsal arch, and intrinsic contractures have been a problem. We have had an occasional sympathetic dystrophy in crush injuries.

OCCULT INJURIES

Tarsometatarsal occult injuries usually occur during athletic activities with rotation of the hindfoot on the fixed forefoot or activity on the standing forefoot. Usually the patient feels a pop and has pain in the tarsometatarsal area fairly well localized to the site of injury. The x-ray film can be characteristically normal, and stress x-ray or weight-bearing films are recommended to determine whether any separation is present. A bone scan is also quite helpful in determining the site of an occult injury. A CT scan would be needed for diagnosis of subtle subluxations. A history of tenderness in the tarsometatarsal area usually implies some type of Lisfranc ligament or interosseous ligament injury. Treatment of these disorders is long-term containment with a cast and orthotic as long as the reduction is acceptable. If the reduction is not acceptable on a stress test, then the same criteria would be followed for open reduction or closed pinning. A high index of suspicion on clinical examination would lead to this diagnosis. These injuries are often morbid, with loss of participation for the season in athletes. When using a surgical technique, percutaneous screws to the medial and middle column are preferred.

CONCLUSIONS

At the Medical College of Virginia we have treated the tarsometatarsal fracture dislocation complex in a classical fashion. Our main goal is to obtain an anatomic reduction with 3 to 5 mm of space between the first and second metatarsals and accurate AP, oblique, and sagittal reduction of the lateral complex. A CT scan may be needed to check for accurate reduction. Attention should be focused on metatarsal head reduction, particularly if it is directed in a plantar direction. We have not had difficulty utilizing traction and percutaneous screw or wire methods to obtain and maintain reduction if surgery is performed within the first 2 weeks. We do not hesitate to use open techniques. Our results, like those of others, show that an anatomic reduction will give the best long-term results; forefoot stiffness, loss of metatarsal arch, and inequality of metatarsal head plantar pressure are always problems. We use a long-term cast to hold our reduction and long-term orthotics for support of the longitudinal and metatarsal arch complexes. Compartment syndromes and vascular injuries can occur in these injuries, and compartment pressure techniques should be used if there is any question of this problem. If open treatment is necessary, delay for up to 2 weeks may be appropriate until the swelling can go down, unless there is no severe crush component. With the crush injuries, dystrophy and causalgia can be complicating factors.

REFERENCES

1. Aitken AP, Poulson D. Dislocations of the tarsometatarsal joint. *J Bone Joint Surg [Br]* 1963;45:546–551.
2. Gissane W. A dangerous type of fracture of the foot. *J Bone Joint Surg [Br]* 1951;33B:535–538.
3. Watson-Jones R. *Fractures and joint injuries,* 4th ed, vol 2. Baltimore: Williams & Wilkins, 1955: 902.

4. English TA. Dislocations of the metatarsal bone and adjacent toe. *J Bone Joint Surg [Br]* 1964;46:700–704.
5. Zwipp H. Severe foot trauma in combination with talar injuries. In: Tscherne H, Schatzker J, eds. *Major fractures of the pilon, the talus, and the calcaneus.* New York: Springer–Verlag, 1993:123–135.
6. Jeffreys TE. Lisfranc's fracture-dislocations. A clinical and experimental study of tarso-metatarsal dislocations and fracture-dislocations. *J Bone Joint Surg [Br]* 1963;45:546–551.
7. Heckman JD. Fractures and dislocations of the foot: injuries of the tarsometatarsal (Lisfranc's) joints. In: Rockwood CA Jr, Green DP, eds. *Fractures in adults,* 2nd ed, vol 2. Philadelphia: JB Lippincott, 1984:1796–1806.
8. DeLee JC. Fractures and dislocations of the foot. In Mann RA, ed. *Surgery of the foot,* 5th ed. St. Louis: CV Mosby, 1986:783–798.
9. Myerson MS. Injuries to the forefoot and toes. In Jahs JMH, ed. *Disorders of the foot and ankle; medical and surgical management,* 2nd ed, vol 3. Philadelphia: WB Saunders, 1991:2233–2273.
10. Hardcastle PH, Reschauer R, Kutscha-Lissberg E, et al. Injuries to the tarsometatarsal joint: incidence, classification, and treatment. *J Bone Joint Surg [Br]* 1987;64:349–356.
11. Stein RE. Radiological aspects of the tarsometatarsal joints. *Foot Ankle* 1983;3:286–289.
12. Myerson MS. Tarsometatarsal joint injuries. *Phys Sports Med* 1993;21:97–107.
13. Febraheim NA, Yang H, Lu J, Biyania A. Computer evaluation of second tarsometatarsal joint dislocation. *Foot Ankle Int* 1996;17:685–689.
14. Wilson DW. Injuries of the tarsometatarsal joints: etiology, classification and results of treatment. *J Bone Joint Surg [Br]* 1972; 54:677–686.
15. Wilpulla E. Tarsometatarsal fracture–dislocation: late results in 26 patients. *Acta Orthop Scand* 1973;44:335–345.
16. Myerson MS, Fisher RT, Burgess AR, Kenzora JE. Fracture dislocations of tarsometatarsal: end results. *Foot Ankle Int* 1986;6:225–242.

Complex Foot and Ankle Trauma,
edited by Robert S. Adelaar,
Lippincott–Raven Publishers, Philadelphia © 1999.

15

Management of Crush and Soft Tissue Injuries of the Foot

Mark S. Myerson

The management of crush and mangling injuries of the foot is challenging. An understanding of the pathogenesis of the injury is often useful in planning treatment, although not necessarily predictive of the final outcome of treatment. These complex injuries invariably involve both the soft tissues and skeletal structures. Although some will require the input of a microvascular surgeon, it is important that the orthopaedist fully comprehend the treatment plan and coverage options.

MECHANISM OF INJURY

The mechanism of crushing is an important factor in treating these injuries. By definition, a crushing type of injury occurs from an extrinsic compressive or shear force applied to the foot over a variable period. These injuries can be further defined by the magnitude of trauma to the soft tissues and bone.

Three types of crush injuries of the foot are usually seen; although there is a continuum of soft tissue damage with each, they are sufficiently different that they require separate approaches. The first type occurs when the foot comes into contact with a crushing object that is broad and heavy. A typical example would be a tractor

M. S. Myerson: Department of Orthopaedic Surgery, The Union Memorial Hospital, Baltimore, Maryland 21218.

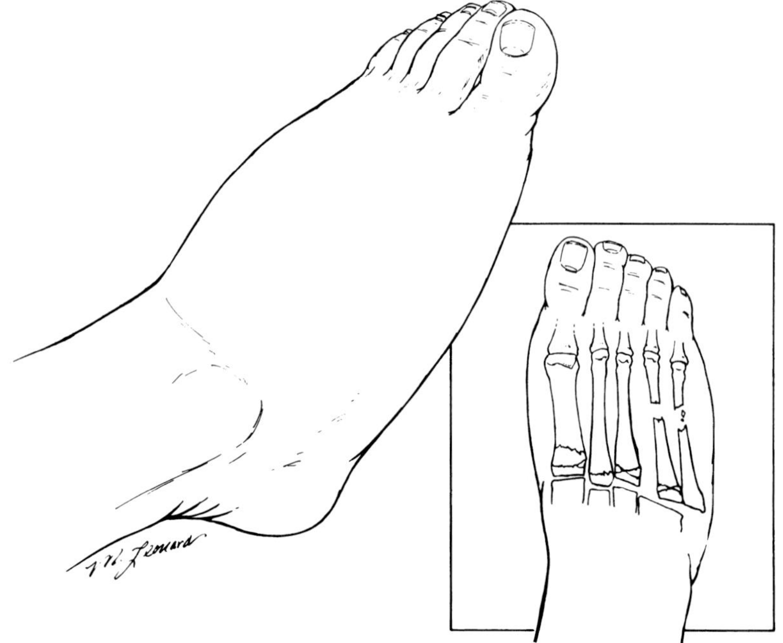

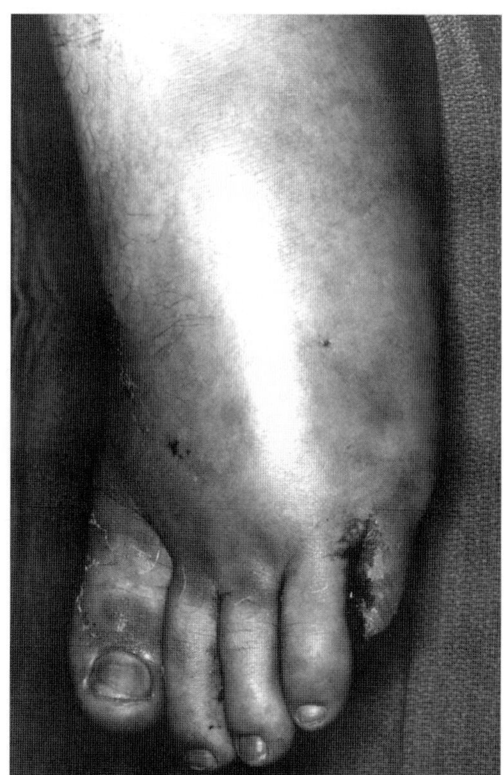

A

B

Figure 1. A: Crush injury of the foot presents with swelling and fractures, typically of the metatarsals. This patient sustained a crush injury when a forklift ran over his foot. **B:** Note marked swelling and ecchymosis with probable midfoot dislocation.

or forklift injury, in which the weight of the object comes into contact with the foot over an extended period. My colleagues and I have termed this a *compressive* type of injury (1,2) (Fig. 1). This type is the one I treat most often, and it is also typically associated with compartment syndromes (see Chapter 16 for details). A variant occurs when the deforming object comes into contact with the foot over a more prolonged period. Under these circumstances, the foot is gradually squeezed and crushed, and *bursting* of tissues then occurs, usually on the plantar aspect of the foot (Fig. 2). This bursting type of injury is similar to the wringer forearm injury (3). Although the concept of a compressive injury embraces that associated with severe crushing and soft tissue loss, more minor compressive injuries may involve the skin and subcutaneous tissues predominantly without fracture or dislocation. This soft-tissue variant may not initially appear serious and is not typically associated with difficult wounds, yet it may be associated with marked morbidity, particularly if nerve injury occurs. My colleagues and I have experienced some difficulty with these more minor injuries, particularly if any underlying neuritis is not recognized early and treated.

A second type of injury occurs when, in addition to crushing, elements of laceration are present, causing severe *mangling* of tissues. These injuries are often associated with industrial or railway accidents, are all open, and are often contaminated, with marked skeletal and soft tissue disruption (Fig. 3). Although mangling occurs in agricultural and lawnmower injuries, the latter are not typically associated with tissue crushing and are not discussed here.

The third type of crushing injury is associated with *shear, degloving,* or avulsion of tissue, as when a tangential force is applied to the surface of the foot (Fig. 4). Cleavage of the skin from its deeper attachments occurs, with soft tissue flaps based both proximally and distally (Fig. 5). Shear degloving injuries are amenable to immediate coverage employing the technique of split-thickness skin excision (STSE; see below).

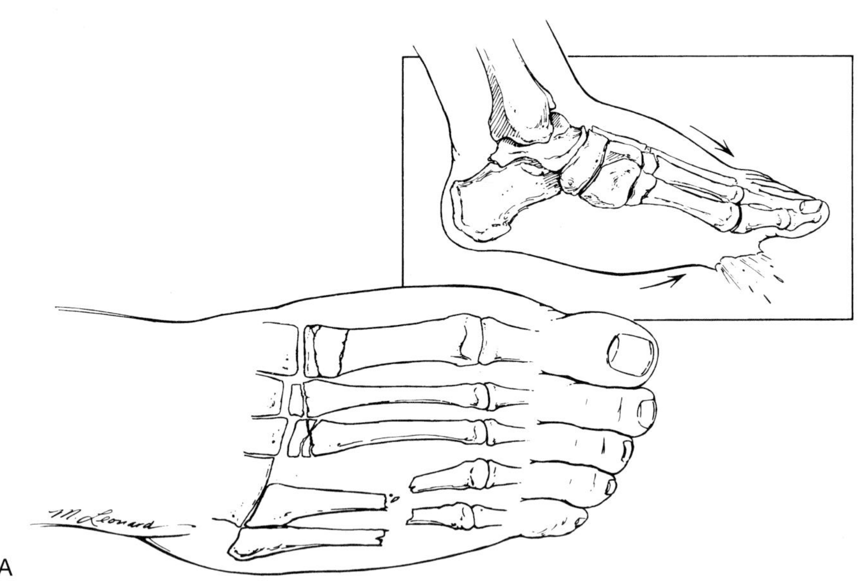

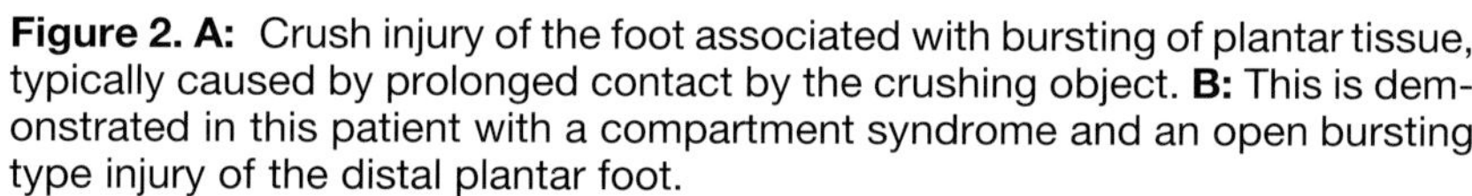

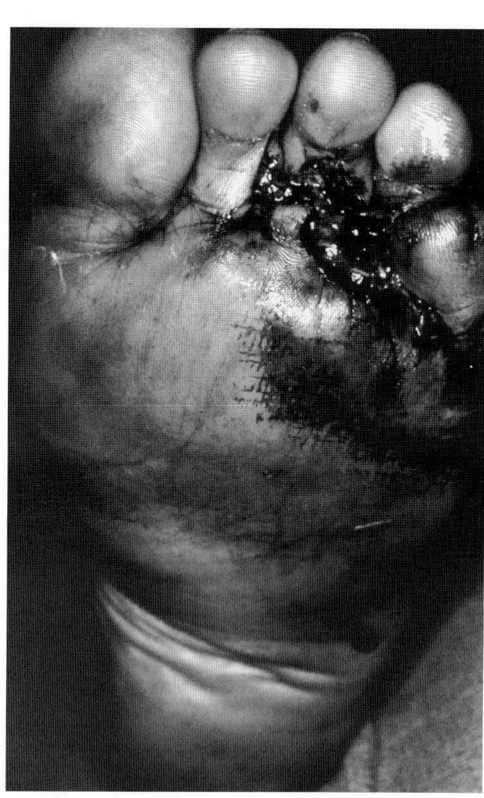

Figure 2. A: Crush injury of the foot associated with bursting of plantar tissue, typically caused by prolonged contact by the crushing object. **B:** This is demonstrated in this patient with a compartment syndrome and an open bursting type injury of the distal plantar foot.

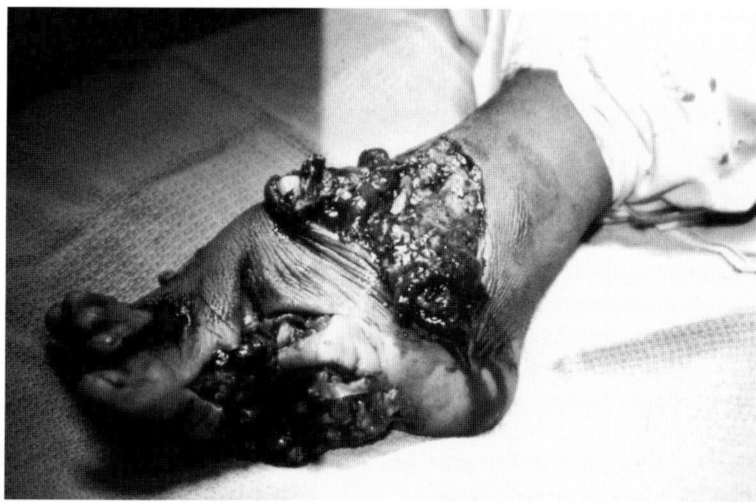

Figure 3. Severe mangling occurs with certain crush injuries, demonstrated in this patient who sustained marked disruption of the skeleton and soft tissues when run over by a train.

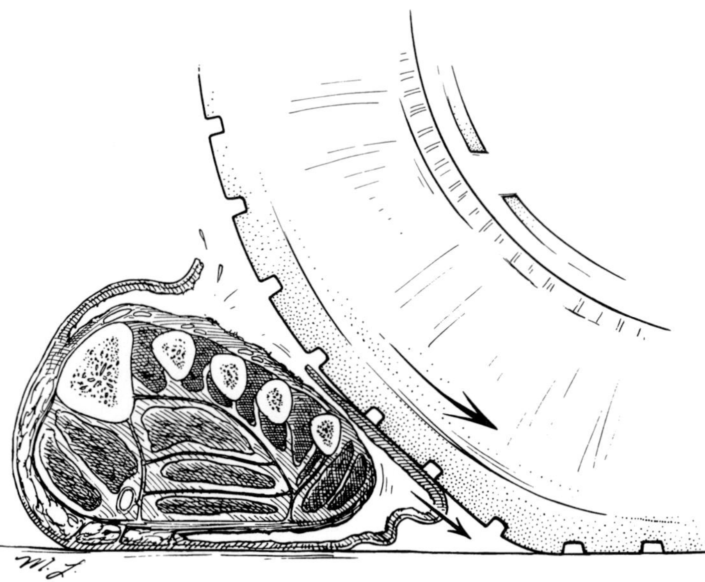

Figure 4. Shear type of crush injury occurs when a force tangential to the surface of the foot is present, as when the foot is run over by a car.

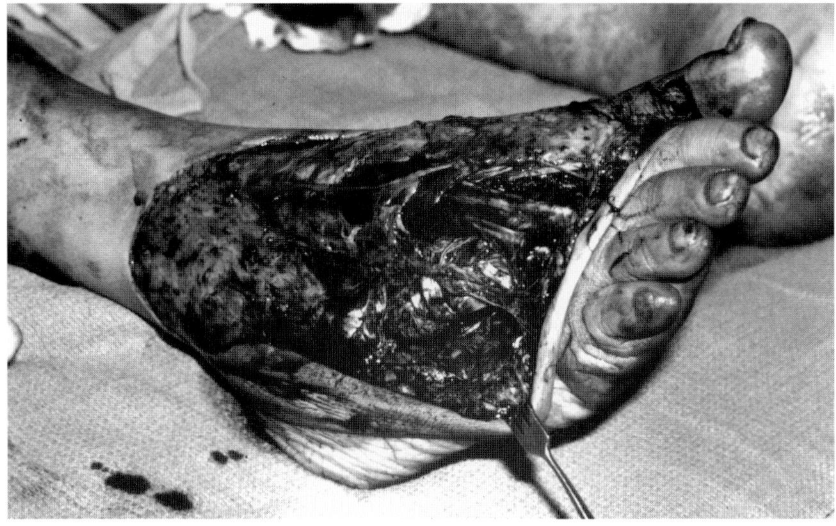

Figure 5. This is a good example of a shear injury of the foot. Note the large skin flap, which has separated from the deeper fascial structures and bone.

INITIAL EVALUATION AND PRINCIPLES OF TREATMENT

A routine history is obtained, including details of the mechanism of injury and the events surrounding the accident, i.e., information about the injury mechanism and the application force, such as a quick blow versus extended contact. The physical examination includes attention to neurovascular status, notation of abrasions and penetrations of the skin, and measurement of pressure in all patients suspected of having compartment syndrome (4).

After the initial examination, my colleagues and I routinely administer a regional ankle block regardless of the type or magnitude of injury. This significantly alleviates discomfort and does not alter decision-making regarding treatment, even in the presence of a compartment syndrome. The ankle block is performed in a standard manner using 20 ml of 0.5% bupivacaine without epinephrine, as described previously (5). For minor open wounds, a first-generation cephalosporin is used, and gentamicin and clindamycin are added if substantial visible dirt or debris is present. Anteroposterior, oblique, and lateral radiographs of the foot and an anteroposterior view of the ankle are obtained.

If closed treatment is planned or surgery is delayed for any reason, a bulky dressing is applied and the extremity is elevated to minimize swelling. My colleagues and I have found that simple elevation of the limb is quite insufficient for reducing the swelling associated with these types of crush injuries of the foot. We now routinely use a pneumatic intermittent compression foot pump (AV Impulse System, Kendall, Mansfield, MA) to reduce swelling (6). This pump effectively reduces both acute and chronic posttraumatic swelling. The "foot pump" consists of a controller and a bladder (Fig. 6). The controller delivers an air impulse of up to 200 mmHg to the bladder, which is placed over the plantar arch of the foot; this pressure is maintained for 3 seconds before venting. The rapid delivery of inflation impulses (every 20 sec) to the plantar region of the foot generates a venous pulse having a stroke volume of around 20 ml, which not only improves venous return, but also seems to enhance arterial inflow. These flow increases result in a higher percentage of the capillary network being open, allowing increased osmotic reabsorption of interstitial fluid. Whereas osmotic reabsorption accounts for 90% of the fluid removed from the interstitial space, increased lymph flow becomes progressively more important as interstitial fluid pressure increases. When bedridden, a patient loses the beneficial effect of the physiologic venous foot pump that intermittently empties the lower veins when bearing weight. Treatment with elevation of the foot and leg works only passively to decrease venous pressure, and exercises that involve the calf muscles have been shown to be less effective in reducing venous pressure than is the physiologic venous foot pump. By its cyclic effect on the capillary bed, which promotes the reabsorption of interstitial fluid, the AV Impulse System may function to mimic ambulatory physiology of the lower extremities of non-weight-bearing patients.

My colleagues and I apply the pump as soon as the patient is admitted to the hospital. The pressure from the pump is occasionally painful at first; however, over the ensuing hour, the patients invariably get used to the intermittent compression. If pain is intolerable, intermittent or continuous patient-controlled anesthesia may be used. In many of these patients, a regional ankle block is used to control pain. After any crush injury

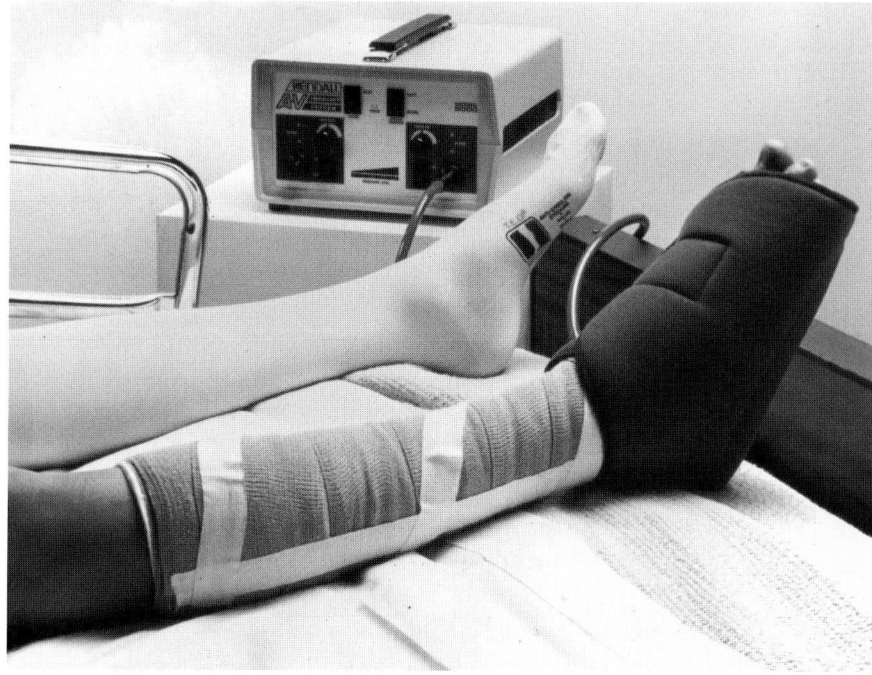

Figure 6. The AV Impulse foot pump (Kendall Co., Mansfield, MA) consists of a controller and a bladder delivering an impulse of compressed air to the foot.

to the foot, the potential for compartment syndrome exists. By using an ankle block to control pain, is there added risk of masking the pain from elevated compartment pressures? This has not been a clinical problem, and we use the foot pump in conjunction with the ankle block to control pain and simultaneously decrease swelling. My colleagues and I, as well as others, have identified a beneficial effect of intermittent compression on elevated compartment pressures, and we have encountered no problem with its use in this setting (6,7).

ZONE OF INJURY AND TIMING OF SOFT TISSUE COVERAGE

The injury to the foot is often far worse than immediately and grossly apparent. There is always an extended area of pathologic involvement of the soft tissue and bone beyond the point of impact on the foot. This ''zone of injury'' concept has significant implications for treatment, because the true extent of the injury is often underestimated (Fig. 7). Although this extended area at risk is a common problem associated with crushing, it is present with almost all injuries to the soft tissue envelope as well as those to the bone, regardless of the mechanism of injury (1,8,9).

Because we are accustomed to debriding only what is obviously nonviable, there is a tendency to underestimate and possibly treat these injuries inadequately. The absolute extent of this extended zone of injury is never apparent macroscopically and therefore forms the basis for serial debridement of soft tissue and bone. This is integral to the successful management of the wound, because all nonviable tissue has to be removed before definitive wound closure or coverage. It is frequently recommended that one should let the wound ''settle down'' over a few days until the true extent of the injury becomes apparent. In this manner, the nonviable areas demarcate, and final debridement

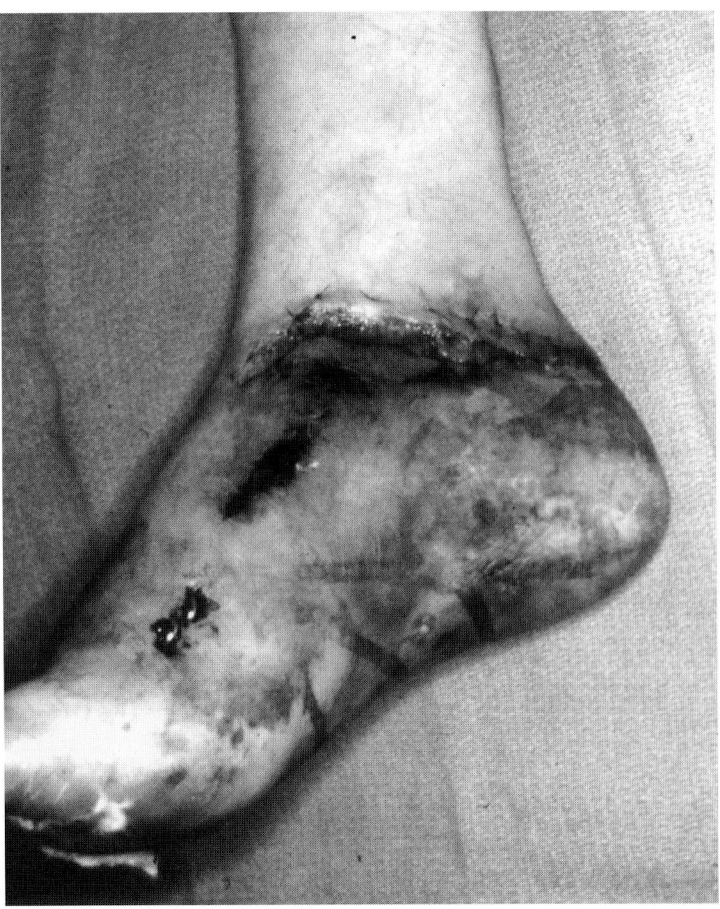

Figure 7. This patient sustained a crush injury when his foot was caught between the couplings of a train. Shown here is the appearance of the foot 10 days after injury. The extended area of skin discoloration represents full-thickness skin loss, which could have been diagnosed immediately on evaluation after injury. This is the zone of injury.

is more easily accomplished. This approach is not ideal; under most circumstances, the earlier definitive coverage is obtained, the less is the likelihood of wound compromise, infection, and failure. One should not, of course, remove potentially viable tissue, particularly if these are vital structures or integral to the function of the foot. However, the result of inadequate debridement is an ever-expanding area of cellular necrosis associated with edema and, finally, increased focal fibrosis and stiffness.

Certain tissues, such as cortical bone, articular cartilage, and tendon devoid of peritenon, do not survive if exposed. One is therefore faced with the dilemma of covering these wounds as soon as possible to protect these underlying structures, while recognizing the increased potential for infection where the recipient bed is marginal (Fig. 8). The risk of infection is less after immediate coverage. As an alternative to early coverage, one can attempt to keep these vital structures viable with moist or wet dressing changes performed every 6 to 8 hours. The goal of this type of treatment is the formation of granulation tissue that would support a simpler form of coverage, such as a split-thickness skin graft. Unfortunately, my colleagues and I have found that these tissues invariably desiccate despite wet dressings, and one is faced with an extending margin of necrosis. In such patients, the results may be the sacrifice of tissue—and perhaps vital structures—that may have been preserved by earlier coverage.

There are clearly significant advantages to a more aggressive approach to debridement and definitive earlier coverage. It has been my experience, and that of others, that the longer the wait before final coverage, the greater is the incidence of wound contamination, bacterial colonization, and infection (10–13). These results are attributed to increased fibrosis, which can extend up to 10 cm from the wound into all tissues, including tendons, muscles, and neurovascular structures. On occasion, delay is determined by the condition of the wound, but it may also be due to patient problems and physician decision making. It is now accepted that far better results occur if coverage is performed expeditiously (14). Early coverage provides an overall lower failure rate,

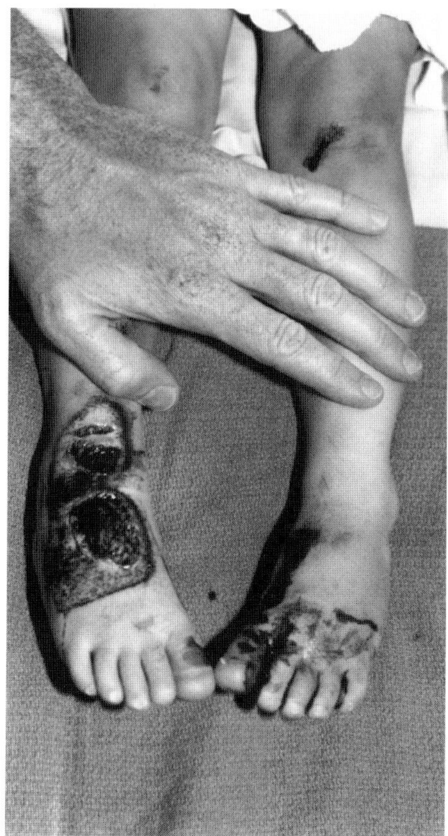

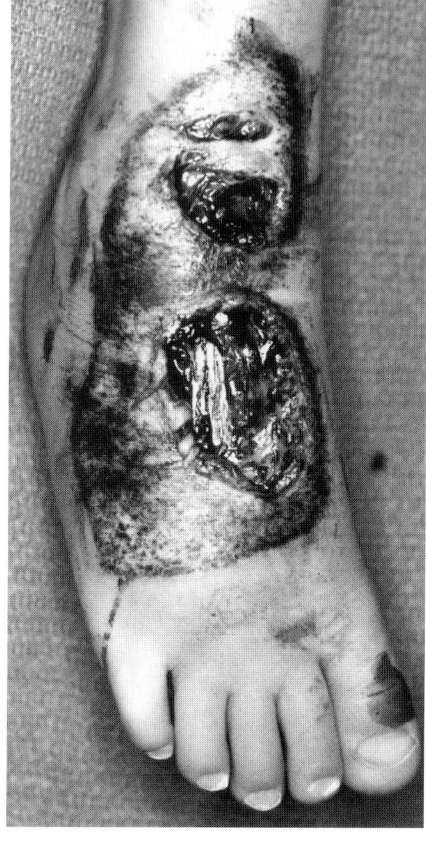

A,B

Figure 8. This child sustained this injury when her foot was run over by a car. Note the bilateral injuries (**A**) and the exposed deeper tissues, including extensor tendon and bone (**B**).

decreased infection rate, fewer overall surgical procedures, increased rate of bone union, and decreased hospital stay (14).

Whatever the choice and form of soft-tissue coverage, I have found that a more aggressive approach to obtaining earlier coverage has led to the most optimal results. Delay in coverage is associated with an increasing zone of injury and a progression of the level of unusable recipient vessels. These wounds have marked contamination and tissue devitalization, and it is tempting to return the patient to the operating room every 48 hr for serial debridement. However, this remaining necrotic tissue is the source of infection and also an extended zone of tissue loss and fibrosis (Fig. 9). There is no substitute for meticulous debridement and pulsatile lavage, which is laboriously continued and repeated until the wound is completely clean.

This is particularly true for crush injuries that involve high-energy forces, crushing, and contamination. Soil and other debris are often embedded in multiple tissue planes and are difficult to remove even with lavage. It is important, therefore, to look carefully in between muscle and soft tissue planes for more debris that can be removed only manually.

A similar problem is encountered in the ''road burn'' injury: the dirt and gravel are extremely difficult to remove without mechanical abrasion. In addition to vigorous cleansing of the skin and exposed subcutaneous tissue with a sterile scrubbing brush, these tissues have to be sharply excised, often leaving large exposed areas that require skin grafting. In performing this debridement, it is important to identify the branches of the superficial peroneal and sural nerves. It is preferable to preserve these nerves unless they are avulsed or crushed, in which case they should be sharply divided and buried in the nearest available muscle. On the dorsal surface of the foot, the nerve is usually buried in the extensor brevis muscle by imbricating the muscle over the nerve with a buried absorbable 4-0 or 5-0 suture. With these avulsion shear-type injuries, one should also try to preserve any peritenon over exposed tendons. The peritenon is often lacerated or avulsed and can be gently reapproximated and sutured with an absorbable 5-0 or 6-0 suture. A split-thickness skin graft will ''take'' over peritenon, but not exposed tendon, and it is important to identify and preserve the peritenon. Although this may not be significant for the intrinsic extensors, it is particularly relevant if the anterior or posterior tibial or peroneal tendons are involved.

Another difficult wound to cleanse and debride is that contaminated with oil or grease. Degreasing agents can be purchased at the hardware or grocery store and are more effective than some of the more abrasive solvents commercially available. Frequent applications, followed by pulsatile lavage, are required.

It is important to recognize the zone of injury as early as possible and to identify contused, crushed, and devitalized tissue in a reproducible, easy, and reliable manner. The conventional parameters used to determine tissue viability include color, bleeding, contractility, and consistency of muscle. These are unfortunately often inconclusive and do not allow clear differentiation of viable from nonviable tissue. The differentiation of viable from nonviable tissue should ideally be performed in a bloodless field. In addition to a thorough debridement of obviously necrotic muscle and contaminated tendon and bone, nonessential vessels are ligated. My colleagues and I prefer not to excise any skin at this stage even if obviously nonviable, because these contused skin flaps may be used as a donor site for skin graft. Although debridement of grossly contaminated tissue is obvious, several more accurate methods are available to determine tissue viability, including fluorescein labeling, cutaneous capillary circulation using laser Doppler flowmetry, and STSE.

Fluorescein is a phenolphthalein dye that, in the presence of an intact capillary circulation, fluoresces when exposed to ultraviolet light (15–17). Fluorescence is a type of luminescence in which light energy is absorbed without the dissipation of any energy. Ultraviolet light affects the fluorescein molecule by raising an electron to a higher energy level, releasing a photon as the electron returns to its prior energy level, resulting in a green fluorescence. The intensity of the fluorescence depends on the extracellular

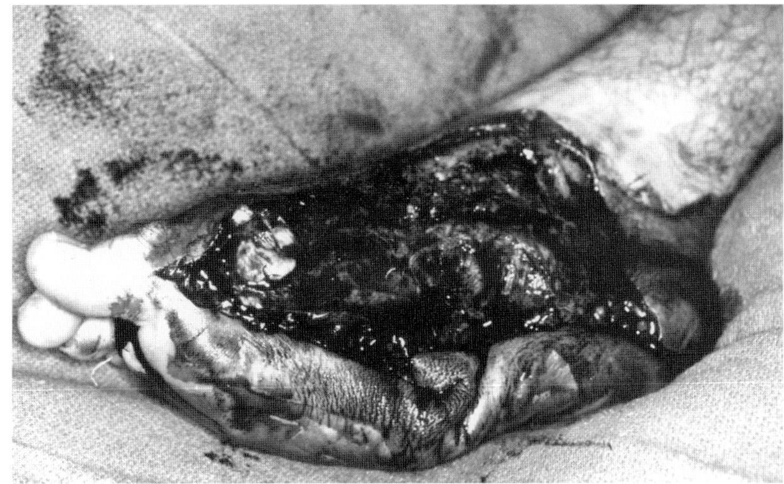

A

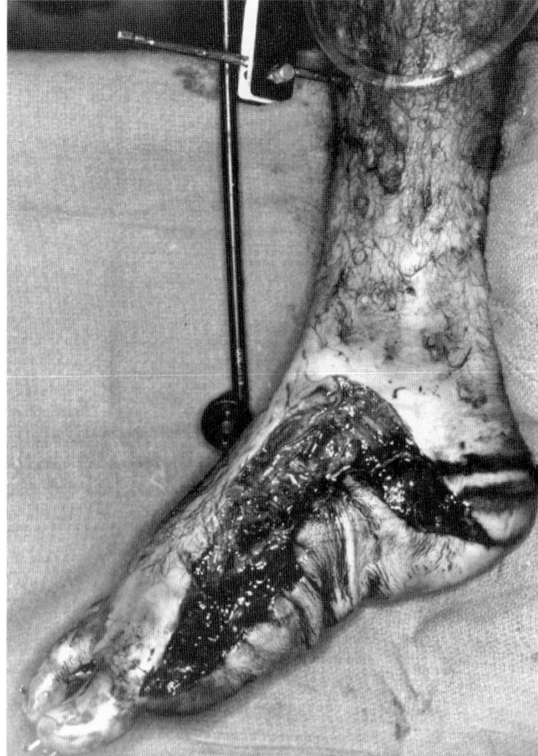

B

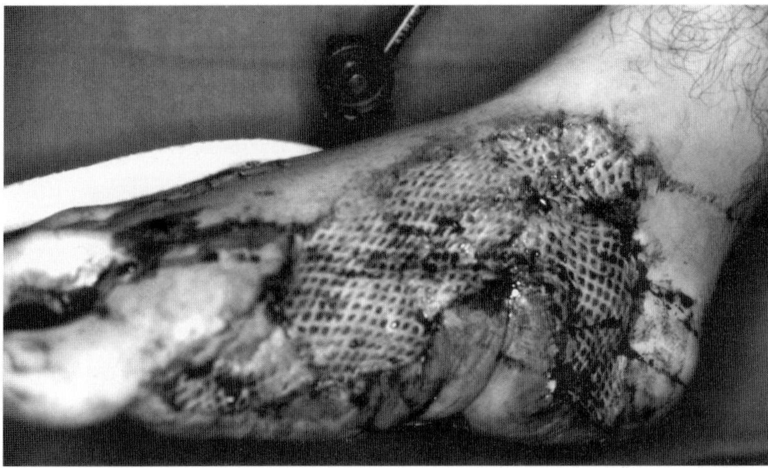

C

Figure 9. This foot was crushed in an industrial injury. **A:** Note the substantial soft tissue loss and plantar skin flap. After debridement and lavage, this injury was treated with immediate application of an external fixator and rotation of intrinsic muscle flaps. **B:** The skin was not reattached to its original location but was sutured without any tension to the muscle bed. **C:** A skin graft was immediately applied to obtain wound coverage but not closure.

concentration of fluorescein in the skin rather than on the absolute amount of blood flow or intravascular concentration. Fluorescein is quite nontoxic in the usual dose range of 10 to 15 mg per kilogram, and allergic reaction is rare. I would recommend giving 1 ml intravenously as a test dose and the balance over 5 minutes. Fluorescence is checked 15 minutes later when the peak extracellular concentration is reached. Fluorescein is rapidly excreted by the kidneys, and the intense yellow discoloration of the skin that occurs usually dissipates after 24 hours. I have frequently used fluorescein testing and have found it to be quite useful in delineating the extent of muscle and skin necrosis.

As an alternative to fluorescein, the technique of STSE is very useful in determining viability of tissue and the zone of injury; I now routinely use it to manage crush injuries of the foot associated with shearing and degloving of skin and subcutaneous tissue (18,19). This technique can delineate avascular tissue margins, predicting areas of deep tissue necrosis and providing graft material for early soft tissue coverage of open wounds (20–22).

STSE commences by suturing the avulsed or sheared flap of skin temporarily down to its original bed. A 0.010- to 0.015-in. thick split-thickness skin graft is then harvested from the potentially nonviable skin flap as well as the adjacent normal skin (Fig. 10). Because the extent of the skin viability is unclear, one can estimate the amount of skin graft that will be required and remove more potentially "normal" skin. The STSE technique also works with a closed crush injury with devitalized skin; the skin graft is

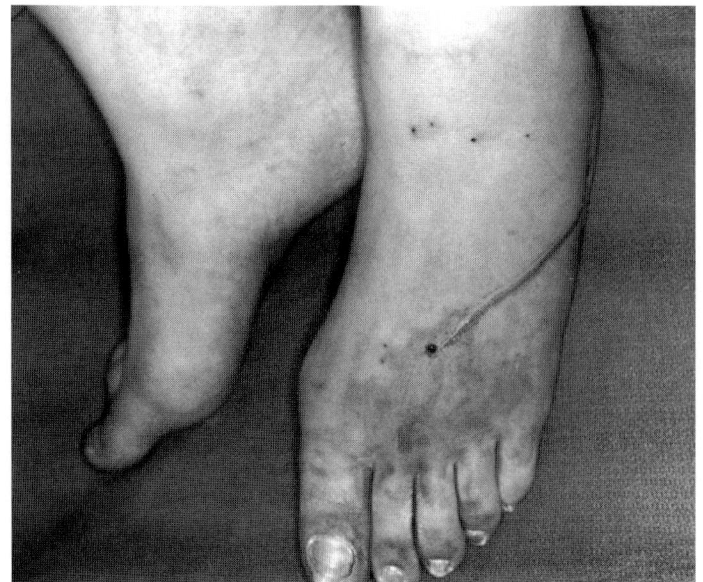
A

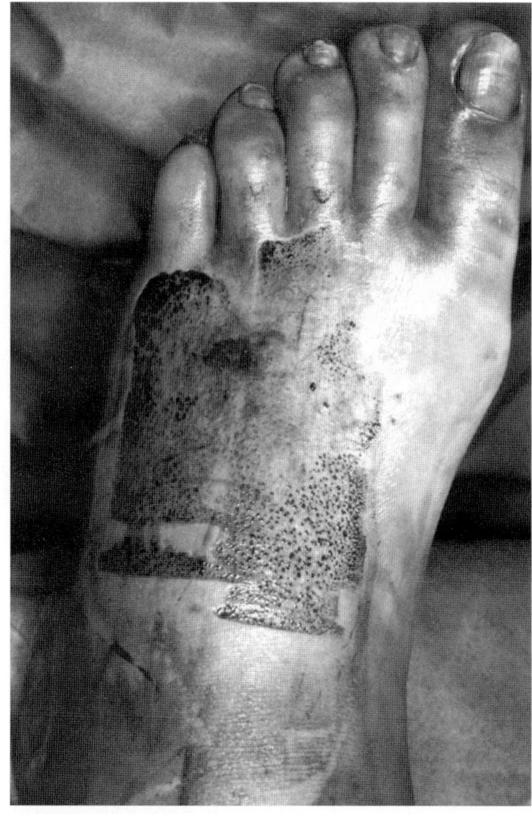
B

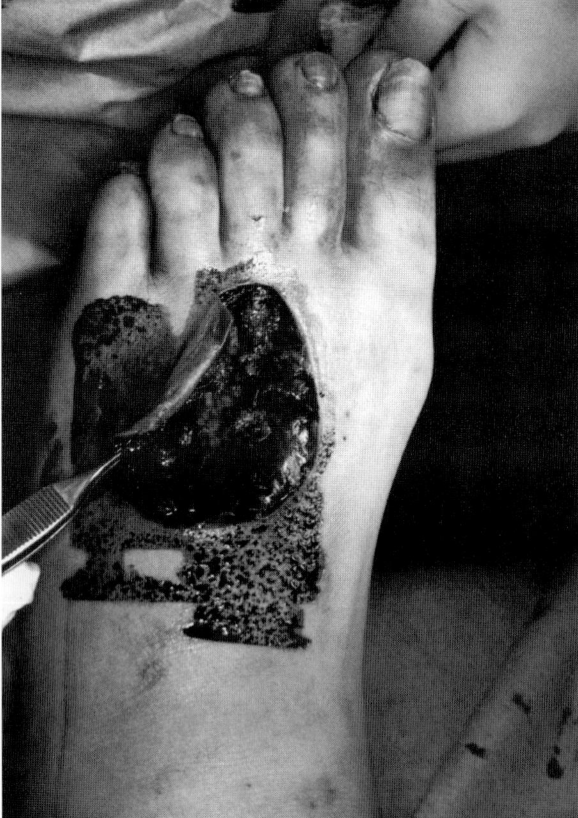
C

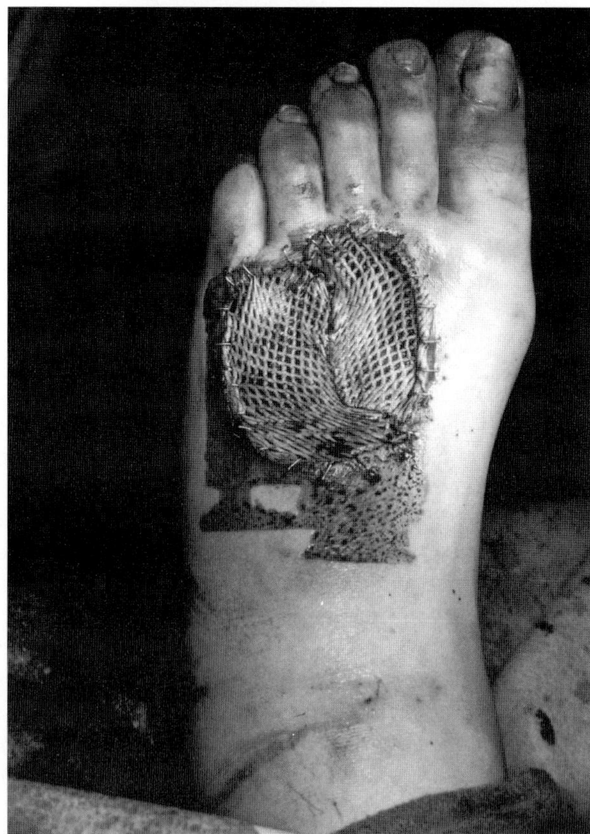
D

Figure 10. This crush injury demonstrates foot swelling and the extent of the zone of injury. **A:** Localized ecchymosis. To determine this zone of injury more accurately and obtain skin graft for immediate coverage, a split-thickness skin graft was harvested from the dorsal surface of the foot. **B:** Capillary bleeding indicates viability. **C:** The tissue in the center of the wound was removed as demarcated by the surrounding capillary bleeding. **D:** The skin graft harvested from the dorsum of the foot was applied immediately to cover the nonviable central area of full-thickness skin loss.

harvested similarly. Although the contour of the dorsal surface of the foot is irregular, the smaller electric dermatomes work well enough to harvest the graft. Because the nonviable areas do not bleed, dermal capillary bleeding is used as an indicator of skin viability. The nonviable skin flap, which is clearly demarcated by the zone of capillary bleeding, is then excised. The skin that was harvested across both the normal and nonviable skin may be used; it is meshed 1:1.5 and reapplied to the denuded area. This technique is ideally suited to definitive management immediately after injury, because cellular necrosis occurs after 24 to 48 hours, and the epidermal layers would probably no longer be suitable. Although the skin harvested from the nonviable portions of the flap would not be suitable under these circumstances, the STSE technique can nevertheless still be used to delineate the margin of viability.

Both split- and full-thickness grafts used during the initial surgical procedure have been shown to be superior to techniques in which salvage of the skin flap is attempted. Immediate reapplication of the flap and fixation with compression dressings usually fails, with necrosis of at least part of the flap likely. Delayed coverage of the wound is, of course, an alternative and may be achieved with grafting 7 to 10 days after injury. This procedure has the potential for secondary infection of the wound, compounded by the delayed treatment and prolonged hospitalization. Primary wound coverage currently appears to be the treatment of choice in shear avulsion trauma of the extremities. These crush injuries are typically associated with motor vehicle injuries in which the foot is run over at lower speeds, shearing the dorsal skin surface off its deeper fascial planes and bone (18). Large skin flaps are created, often with questionable viability. In these shear injuries, the STSE technique accurately determines the extent of viability of the flap and provides additional skin for immediate coverage. The technique may also be used in crush amputation injuries, in which the amputated part is temporarily reattached, the graft is harvested, and, after appropriate debridement and bone trimming, the graft is applied as a one-stage procedure. The common surgical goal in managing these complex crush injuries of the foot is to provide optimum skin coverage with minimum morbidity. Alternative methods for attaining these goals are clearly available, but they are associated with increasing complexity and morbidity. My colleagues and I have applied these techniques of STSE to harvesting the graft in both open and closed injuries, as well as those where the foot is clearly nonviable and is amputated.

The results of primary wound coverage depend on thorough debridement of the devascularized flap and wound bed, an observation in keeping with current philosophy that the fresh wound is a suitable site for donor tissue. The success of this procedure also depends on careful delineation of the viable and nonviable portions of the flap, particularly when dealing with crushing injuries of the foot involving shearing or avulsion of tissue. In these circumstances, the subcutaneous segmental vessels are disrupted, the dermal circulation is compromised, and accurate assessment of the flap becomes critical.

Techniques such as STSE and fluorescein testing that enhance identification of tissue viability and predict flap survival are integral to aggressive primary wound care. Other methods, such as visual inspection of the flap and clinical judgment, are satisfactory but clearly lack accuracy. I have found that fluorescein testing is a useful modality but that, on occasion, it has proved to be unreliable in predicting flap viability, perhaps as a result of altered perfusion of the dermal plexus in the flap due to arteriovenous shunting. The STSE technique cannot, however, be optimally utilized in all crushing injuries of the foot. In farm injuries or others in which substantial contamination is present, immediate coverage may be injudicious. There are other situations in which the bed is not suitable for application of a split-thickness graft of any nature, e.g., in which bare bone is exposed or the deeper tissues are nonviable. Such injuries may be better suited to application of a free flap.

CONTAMINATED WOUNDS AND SKELETAL STABILIZATION

Contaminated wounds should be treated with serial debridements and delayed closure. The decision to close the wound is based on its appearance, the mechanism of injury, the initial contamination, and the viability of adjacent tissues (Fig. 11). Over the past decade, my colleagues and I have attempted to close or cover wounds as early as possible, which has led to the development of aggressive protocols for wound management that include primary coverage and closure of wounds. There is, however, a marked difference between primary coverage with, for example, splitthickness skin graft, and primary wound closure. A skin graft is a biologic means of providing optimum coverage and decreasing colonization of the wound, edema, and pain. These grafts are all meshed to allow free drainage; an occlusive dressing should not be applied over a contaminated wound. This form of coverage is notably different from primary closure of a wound that may be contaminated. With aggressive wound debridement and irrigation, however, my colleagues and I have been able to close some wounds primarily that are potentially and highly contaminated, for example, those resulting from lawnmower accidents. However, because such injuries predominantly involve the hallux and toes, there are no large fascial and muscle defects, which may be the source of pathogens. If the plantar fascial spaces are involved and muscle is devitalized, then careful serial wound care is necessary.

Skeletal stabilization should be used for both wound management and fracture fixation. The role of skeletal stabilization in the management of the soft-tissue component of the injury is important. This concept is contrary to traditional experience because skeletal fixation is used routinely for fracture care. However, it is clear that some form of rigid fixation, whether internal or external, enhances wound management (9,23).

The fixation devices I use are simple and easy to construct; they utilize half-pins, not transfixation pins. A tibiometatarsal fixator is constructed with 5-mm pins for the tibia and 4-mm pins for the first and/or the fifth metatarsal; it is often necessary to place pins in both the first and fifth metatarsals to avoid the varus and supination deformity associated with pin insertion only into the tibia and first metatarsal (Fig. 12).

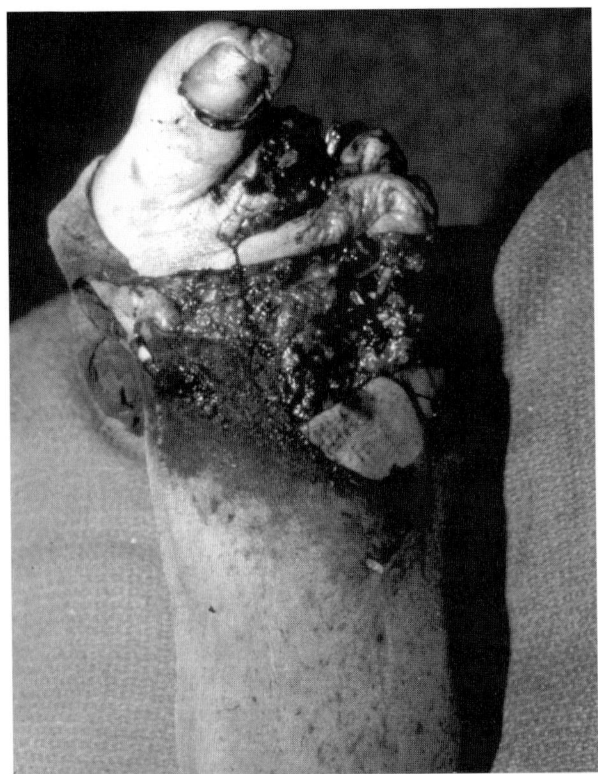

Figure 11. This mangling-type crush injury occurred in a 70-year-old woman in a farm injury. Although the first ray was viable and could be salvaged, it was felt that, due to her age and the extent of bone loss, a primary amputation would be preferable. This was performed with delayed primary closure due to the contamination of the injury.

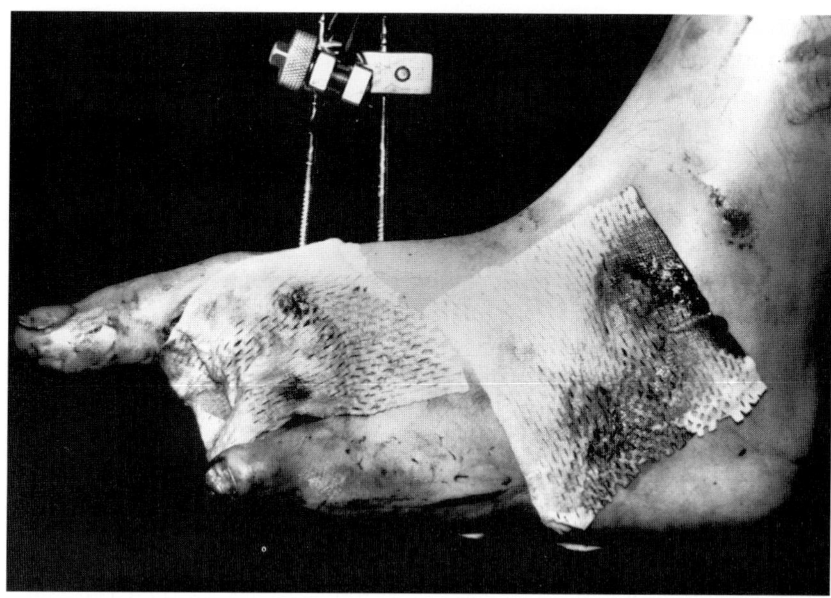

Figure 12. Temporary skeletal stabilization of severe crush injuries is important to allow access to the wound for dressing changes and support the soft tissues while healing; 4-mm half-pins are used in the first metatarsal, as demonstrated here.

Pin placement is occasionally determined by the type of wound and, in the case of a mangling injury, the presence or stability of the metatarsals. Although two pins in the fifth metatarsal are sufficient, if a more rigid frame is required, or for a longer period, lateral pins may be inserted into the fifth and fourth metatarsals. When inserting these pins, the coronal arc of the lateral metatarsals should be observed; otherwise, the pins will miss the fourth metatarsal. In this manner, the pins are inserted slightly toward the dorsal surface of the foot, instead of directly medially.

It is most important to maintain the flexibility of the toes while the foot is immobilized with an external fixator, even if it is applied only for a short time period. The intrinsic muscles of the foot atrophy rapidly and may result in fixed claw toe deformity, which is difficult to correct. Passive stretching exercises of the toes are therefore most important, and they should be done hourly by the patient and/or nursing staff, and at least daily under the supervision of a physical therapist. If the toes cannot be passively extended, or if a degloving of the extensor surface of the foot is present, including the extensor tendons, then some form of outrigger on the toes is necessary to prevent contracture. Rapid fixed flexion contracture of the metatarsophalangeal and interphalangeal joints occur if the extensor tendons are not functioning. An outrigger for the toes can be constructed with rubber bands attached either to a metal hook glued to the toenail or to straps around the distal toe.

RESULTS

In 1972, Omer and Pomerantz (24) reported that 50% of their patients who sustained crushing injuries of the foot required assisted ambulation or had residual pain. Despite improvements in the treatment of soft-tissue trauma (9) and increased attention to compartment syndromes of the foot, morbidity after these injuries remains high.

Over the past decade, my colleagues and I have managed crush injuries of the foot according to a standardized treatment protocol, with strict attention to skeletal stabilization and early soft tissue coverage (2). Despite what we considered optimal treatment, many patients had less than a satisfactory recovery.

The results of treatment for crush injuries of the foot are difficult to evaluate. The varying pathogenesis, mechanism, and severity of injury make comparison of one patient with another quite invalid. My colleagues and I have attempted to quantify our results of treatment, according to the type of injury, the presence of a compartment syndrome, the type of treatment initiated, delay between injury and treatment, work-related compensation, and ongoing litigation (2). By retrospective review, we evaluated 58 patients with crush injuries to the foot treated at our institution between 1986 and 1990 (2). All patients had received initial treatment according to a standardized protocol determined by the type and magnitude of the injury. Patients were examined at a mean interval of $3\frac{1}{2}$ years after injury, and the functional outcome was determined according to a foot trauma rating scale. Based on this scoring system, 46% of the patients had a good functional outcome, 29% had fair results, and 25% had poor results. There was a significant correlation between a good functional outcome and careful adherence to the treatment protocol; however, some patients fared poorly regardless of treatment. Poor results occurred if treatment was not immediately initiated or if soft tissue coverage was delayed, and particularly in those who experienced severe, mangling-type injuries that necessitated partial foot amputation. The patients who fared the worst were those who subsequently suffered from neuritis or reflex sympathetic dystrophy, or those involved in ongoing workers compensation and litigation (2).

The treatment protocol outlined here is based on the premise that aggressive fracture stabilization and early soft-tissue coverage can decrease the morbidity after crush injuries of the foot. It has been shown that early debridement and soft tissue coverage provide a lower infection rate and enhanced healing (13,14). The primary goal is therefore to stabilize the injury, so that early rehabilitation can commence. Soft tissue management begins with recognition of the zone of injury, which exists as an extended area of pathologic involvement surrounding the soft tissue and bone beyond the point of impact.

My colleagues and I have not identified a correlation between mechanism of injury and outcome. We found that the seemingly less severe compressive injuries carry their own inherent morbidity, because some of the worst results occurred in patients who sustained relatively trivial injuries. In these patients, the clinical findings at follow-up examination were unremarkable except for a constellation of neurologic findings, including dysesthesia and hyperesthesia, often beyond the point of impact. Neuroischemia may play a role in the development of chronic pain after crush injuries to the foot, either through direct trauma to the peripheral nerves or by intraneural or extraneural fibrosis after edema. A posttraumatic neuroma or resulting chronic neuritis may then serve as the trigger for reflex sympathetic dystrophy, because many of these patients sustained more minor compressive-type injuries. Regardless of the cause, the presence of ongoing pain limits the ability of the patient to pursue an active physical therapy program, resulting in further loss of motion and dysfunction.

In patients who are experiencing chronic pain, it is difficult to determine the origin of the pain, particularly if this has both a somatic and sympathetic origin. In these and in other patients with a suspected sympathetically mediated pain syndrome, a lumbar sympathetic block is a useful modality for both diagnostic and, in some instances, therapeutic purposes. The indication for this block is vague diffuse pain, particularly when associated with autonomic dysfunction. The diagnosis of reflex sympathetic dystrophy is confirmed if the pain is associated with positive scintigraphic findings on triple-phase bone scan (25) and is alleviated by this block; treatment is then accordingly initiated. The bone scan is more reliable in the adult.

My colleagues and I have found that the type of soft-tissue coverage used to treat crush injuries does not affect the outcome as much as the underlying condition that necessitated the coverage in the first place. Some mangling injuries necessitate partial foot amputations, and the results of treatment are determined by the magnitude of the deformity. The resulting disability may be a result of functional impairment more from partial foot amputation than from continued pain.

CONCLUSIONS

It is apparent that a variety of interrelated factors are probably responsible for the morbidity associated with crush injuries. For the severe shear, compressive, or mangling injuries, these factors are self-evident and include the loss of a viable soft tissue envelope associated with a difficult-to-stabilize fracture or dislocation. Less severe contusions to the foot, however, are also at risk secondary to nerve and other soft-tissue problems. When treatment does not follow this recommended protocol, poor results are more likely to occur; for example, delayed tissue coverage or incorrect assessment of the zone of injury can result in wound complications, dorsal scarring, and neuritis. Ongoing litigation or continuing workers compensation claims also seem to contribute to a higher number of poor results in this group of patients.

Despite a comprehensive treatment protocol, functional results in patients with crush injuries of the foot are not uniformly good. The prognoses after these injuries, particularly for compressive injuries, are unpredictable, and an injury classification scheme does not appear to be helpful in predicting outcome. These results may appear depressing and suggest that the ability to influence the course of these problems is beyond the clinician's control. However, institution of prompt, comprehensive care may limit the complications and sequelae of these injuries to an acceptable level, allowing clinicians at least to manage these patients more adroitly. Because these injuries are so diverse, it is not feasible to treat all of them routinely in a tertiary care center. It is important for the initial treating physician to recognize the problem and manage the injury according to the guidelines proposed here. Referral to a trauma specialist depends on good judgment as to the severity of the injury and the level of care available at the receiving facility.

REFERENCES

1. Myerson M. Crush injuries and compartment syndromes of the foot. *Int J Orthop Trauma* 1993;3:109–113.
2. Myerson MS, McGarvey WC, Henderson MR, Hakim J. Morbidity after crush injuries to the foot. *J Orthop Trauma* 1994;8:343–349.
3. Entin MA. Roller and wringer injuries. Clinical and experimental studies. *Plast Reconstr Surg* 1955;15:290–312.
4. Myerson MS. Management of compartment syndromes of the foot. *Clin Orthop* 1991;271:239–248.
5. Myerson MS, Ruland CM, Allon SM. Regional anesthesia for foot and ankle surgery. *Foot Ankle* 1992;13:282–288.
6. Myerson MS, Henderson MR. Clinical applications of a pneumatic intermittent impulse compression device after trauma and major surgery to the foot and ankle. *Foot Ankle* 1993;14:198–203.
7. Saxby T, Myerson M, Schon L. Compartment syndrome of the foot following calcaneus fracture. *Foot* 1992;2:157–161.
8. Myerson M, McGarvey WC. Crush injuries and compartment syndromes. In: Myerson M, ed. *Current therapy in foot and ankle surgery.* St. Louis: Mosby–Year Book, 1993:264–273.
9. Myerson MS. Soft-tissue trauma—acute and chronic management. In: Mann RA, Coughlin MJ, eds. *Surgery of the foot and ankle,* 6th ed. St. Louis: Mosby–Year Book, 1993:1367–1410.
10. Brown PW. The prevention of infection in open wounds. *Clin Orthop* 1973;96:42–50.
11. Levine NS, Lindberg RB, Mason AD Jr, Pruitt BA Jr. The quantitative swab culture and smear: a quick simple method for determining the number of viable aerobic bacteria on open wounds. *J Trauma* 1976;16:89–94.
12. Robson MC, Duke WF, Krizek TJ. Rapid bacterial screening in the treatment of civilian wounds. *J Surg Res* 1973;14:426–430.
13. Robson MC, Heggers JP. Bacterial quantification of open wounds. *Milit Med* 1969;134:19–24.
14. Godina M. Early microsurgical reconstruction of complex trauma of the extremities. *Plast Reconstr Surg* 1986;78:285–292.
15. McCraw JB, Dibbell DG. Experimental definition of independent myocutaneous vascular territories. *Plast Reconstr Surg* 1977;60:212–220.
16. McCraw JB, Dibbell DG, Carraway JH. Clinical definition of independent myocutaneous vascular territories. *Plast Reconstr Surg* 1977;60:341–352.
17. McCraw JB, Myers B, Shanklin KD. The value of fluorescein in predicting the viability of arterialized flaps. *Plast Reconstr Surg* 1977;60:710–719.
18. Myerson M. Split-thickness skin excision: its use for immediate wound care in crush injuries of the foot. *Foot Ankle* 1989;10:54–60.
19. Ziv I, Zeligowski A, Mosheiff R, Lowe J, Wexler MR, Segal D. Split-thickness skin excision in severe open fractures. *J Bone Joint Surg [Br]* 1988;70:23–26.
20. Papa J, Myerson MS. Soft tissue coverage in the management of foot and ankle trauma—Part I. *Contemp Orthop* 1991;22:509–520.
21. Papa J, Myerson MS. Soft tissue coverage in the management of foot and ankle trauma—Part II. *Contemp Orthop* 1991;22:657–665.
22. Papa JA, Myerson MS. Split-thickness skin excision for crush and degloving injuries of the foot. *Perspect Orthop Surg* 1991;2:77–85.
23. Myerson MS, Burgess AR. The initial evaluation and treatment of the acutely traumatized foot and ankle. In: Jahss MH, ed. *Disorders of the foot and ankle. Medical and surgical management,* 2nd ed. Philadelphia: WB Saunders, 1991;2209–2232.

24. Omer GE Jr, Pomerantz GM. Initial management of severe open injuries and traumatic amputations of the foot. *Arch Surg* 1972;105:696–698.
25. Holder LE, Cole LA, Myerson MS. Reflex sympathetic dystrophy in the foot: clinical and scintigraphic criteria. *Radiology* 1992;184:531–535.

EDITORIAL COMMENTS

Management Of Crush and Soft-Tissue Injuries of the Foot

Mark S. Myerson

Dr. Myerson has eloquently stressed the importance of addressing the soft tissue injury. Initial treatment of the soft tissue component can have significant impact on the results. The importance of the initial assessment and determination of the zone of injury and identification of devitalized tissue by fluorescein or STSE technique have been stressed. These are methods that will help us to determine devitalized tissue and be able to utilize it for biologic coverage. The earlier we obtain biologic coverage, not necessarily skin closure, the less fibrosis will occur around the zone of injury. It is important to note that skin grafting techniques can be applied to paratenon but not to bone and tendon. Poor results come from delay of soft tissue closure, inadequate debridement, and poor assessment of zone of injury. The use of elevation assisted by a pneumatic compression device on the plantar surface of the foot is a new and innovative approach to improvement of the soft tissue environment. We have found that the bladder pump used under foot splints is effective for almost all injuries to the foot and ankle and are tolerated well except for certain calcaneal injuries. The use of the foot pump in the face of elevated compartments is still in question and is being assessed.

The second feature of wound management is also fracture stabilization either by temporary external fixation methods or by initial reduction. Stabilization is felt to help in wound management. Proper skeletal management can certainly assist in wound care and possible flap management if needed. In the next chapter, proper applications of flap principles to soft tissue defects that remain uncovered are discussed.

In spite of aggressive fracture stabilization and proper treatment of soft tissue injuries, a large percentage of problems occur after soft tissue complications. The stiffness and injuries to the superficial nerves that result in these injuries cannot be overstressed. Compressive neuropathies and traumatic neuromas accompany severe injuries and will need to be addressed in the postoperative period.

If a sympathetic dystrophy syndrome should develop, early treatment is certainly necessary. Treatment should consist of a warm environment, elimination of nicotine and caffeine, a decrease in anxiety, peripheral nerve blocks, sympathetic blocks, judicious use of steroids, vasodilatators, peripheral nerve stimulation, graduated exercise program, elimination of the cause of pain, and knowledge that a premorbid personality profile often accompanies these situations. The early identification of these problems is the key to achieving an amelioration of the symptoms. In foot problems, particularly crush injuries, the treatment of focal nerve injury must be addressed.

Robert S. Adelaar, M.D.

Complex Foot and Ankle Trauma,
edited by Robert S. Adelaar,
Lippincott–Raven Publishers, Philadelphia © 1999.

16

Compartment Syndromes of the Foot

Mark S. Myerson

In the last decade, we have expanded our knowledge of compartment syndromes of the foot (1–4). Initial interest in this syndrome led to an identification of the anatomic compartments in the foot and an illustration of alternative approaches to fasciotomy in an experimental model (5). Since then, various reports have clarified the compartmental anatomy of the foot, described the clinical significance of these syndromes, and documented the potential for myoneural ischemia associated with calcaneus fractures. This chapter discusses the manifestations of acute and chronic compartment syndromes of the foot and highlights alternative treatments.

ACUTE COMPARTMENT SYNDROMES OF THE FOOT

Compartmental Anatomy

The foot has well-demarcated and anatomically identifiable compartments. For 60 years, it was thought that there were only four plantar compartments (medial, central, lateral, and interosseous) (6,7). These early findings were confirmed in a 1988 study that used methylene blue dye mixed with saline to identify four primary compartments of the foot; this study also presented the experimental basis for various fasciotomy incisions (5) (Fig. 1).

However, since then, research has identified numerous other compartments (8), although only five have major clinical importance: the medial, central, lateral, interosseous, and calcaneal compartments. The *medial* compartment, containing the abductor

M. S. Myerson: Department of Orthopaedic Surgery, The Union Memorial Hospital, Baltimore, Maryland 21218.

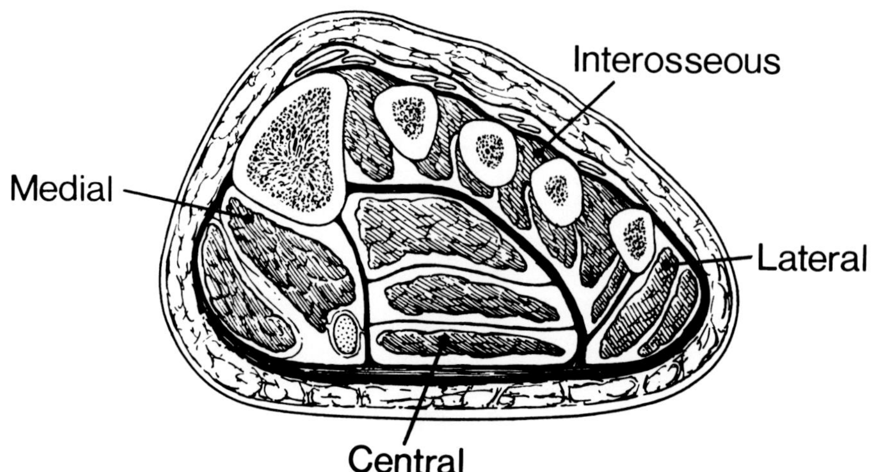

Figure 1. Coronal section through the base of the metatarsals demonstrates four of the compartments. Each interosseous muscle is anatomically a separate compartment; others, such as the adductor, are not demonstrated here. (From ref. 5, with permission.)

hallucis and flexor hallucis brevis muscles, is bounded medially and inferiorly by the extension of the plantar aponeurosis, laterally by an intermuscular septum, and dorsally by the first metatarsal (5). The *central* compartment contains (from plantar to dorsal) the flexor digitorum brevis, the lumbricales, the quadratus plantae, and the adductor hallucis muscles; its boundaries are the thick plantar aponeurosis inferiorly, the osseofascial tarsometatarsal structures dorsally, and the intermuscular septae medially and laterally. The *lateral* compartment contains the flexor, abductor, and opponens muscles of the fifth toe; its boundaries are the fifth metatarsal dorsally, the plantar aponeurosis inferiorly and laterally, and an intermuscular septum medially. The *interosseous* compartment contains the seven interossei and is bounded by the interosseous fascia and the metatarsal (5,9). In a recent injection study, nine plantar compartments were identified (8), including a deep central compartment that contains the quadratus plantae muscle and has particular relevance to calcaneus fractures (10). The *calcaneal* compartment contains the quadratus plantae muscle and the lateral plantar nerve; at times, the medial plantar nerve is also located more distally in this compartment (Fig. 2).

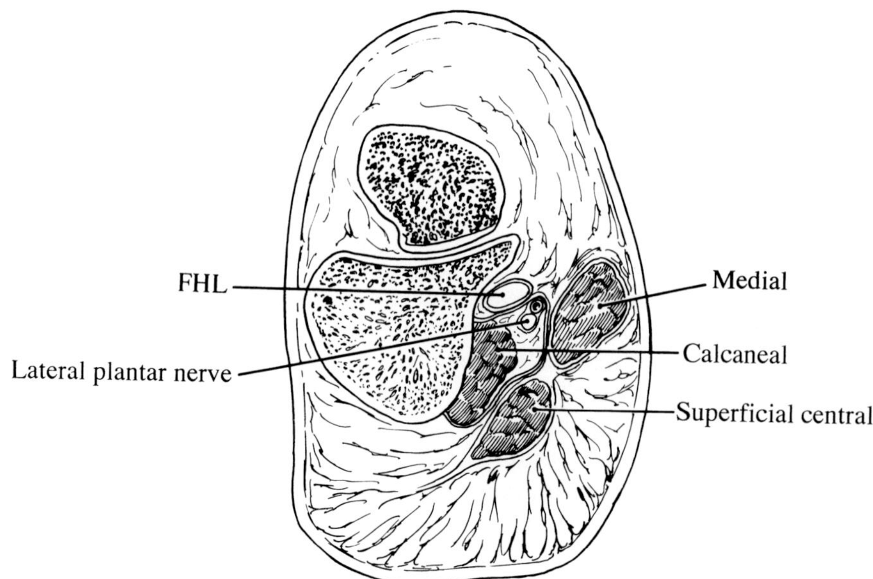

Figure 2. Coronal section through the hindfoot at the level of the calcaneus demonstrates the deep calcaneal compartment. The lateral plantar nerve courses through this compartment. FHL, flexor hallucis longus.

Under normal physiologic pressures, there is negligible communication or direct extension between the fascial spaces of the foot or with the leg. However, it has been shown experimentally that, under high pressures, dye can leak from one space into another (5); therefore, one might deduce that the normal minimal communication between compartments is increased at time of injury, whether from pressure or from disruption of fascial membranes. Nevertheless, this intercompartment communication does not preclude the development of a compartment syndrome.

Pathogenesis

When the foot is subjected to injury, its inelastic osseofascial structures confine bleeding and interstitial edema, causing compartment syndrome, i.e., elevation of the interstitial fluid pressure in local tissues and a decrease in the capillary perfusion to a point below that required to maintain tissue viability. Blood flow in the microcirculation stops when local tissue pressure equals the diastolic blood pressure; when pressures fall below diastolic levels, blood flow can no longer sustain local metabolic demands. Once established, the compartment syndrome complex will lead to vascular occlusion and myoneural ischemia, even in the presence of arterial flow and pulses. [Pulses in such injured areas are not generally palpable, predominantly because of soft tissue swelling, but they are always audible with Doppler ultrasound evaluation (4).] Clinicians have proposed many theories to account for the tissue injury to myoneural ischemia sequence of events, e.g., tissue hypertension and arteriovenous pressure gradients (11,12); however, all agree that if the elevated pressure is not dissipated by other means, the ischemic process will continue, resulting in irreparable damage, i.e., myoneural necrosis and fibrosis.

Clinical Presentation

The foot is in an extremely vulnerable location and is particularly prone to isolated injury. In my experience, most of the devastating foot injuries associated with compartment syndromes are caused by crushing forces, although the type of crushing force, and the population affected, may vary: my colleagues and I have identified compartment syndromes in children, who are obviously not "protected" from developing myoneural ischemia (Myerson, Herzenberg, and Sponsellor, unpublished data) and have managed some patients in whom a crush injury caused bursting of tissue on the plantar aspect of the foot, but did not preclude the development of a compartment syndrome.

Patients with crush injuries to the foot typically present with massive swelling and fractures and/or dislocations of the midfoot. Thus, the diagnosis is relatively obvious, but one should not be complacent with regard to the development of a compartment syndrome and the potential for myoneural ischemia. Although open foot fractures are usually less severe (grade I or II) than other open extremity fractures, it must be remembered that they are associated just as frequently with compartment syndrome complexes.

My colleagues and I have recently identified compartment syndromes associated with another type of foot injury that may involve less energy that the crush injuries described above: calcaneus fractures (1,13). Although some of these fractures and the resultant compartment syndromes occurred in falls from a great height, others were the result of falls from only a few feet. Calcaneal fractures are associated with profound pain and considerable swelling, far more so than with other devastating fractures of the foot and ankle. This is probably related to the large bleeding cancellous bone surfaces and the limited osseofascial compartments into which this hematoma may be dissipated; the amount of swelling may also depend on the duration from the time of injury and the intervening treatment before examination. The overall incidence of compartment syndromes associated with calcaneus fractures at this institution is approximately 10%.

Diagnosis

Although paresthesias and neurovascular deficits are helpful in forming a suspicion of compartment syndrome, these signs are not diagnostic and should not be used to determine either the presence of a compartment syndrome or the need for fasciotomy. The only reliable method of diagnosis is by clinical suspicion (based on the history of the injury and the findings of signs and symptoms compatible with myoneural ischemia) and measurement of raised intracompartmental pressures.

The earliest clinical finding of muscle and nerve ischemia is pain. Pain is present in all patients; however, pain secondary to compartment syndrome or ischemia is agonizing and out of proportion to the severity of the injury. I have examined patients who are writhing in pain and who could not get comfortable despite immobilization of the foot and adequate analgesia. The pain can be markedly exacerbated by gentle, passive dorsiflexion of the toes, which stretches the intrinsic muscles of the foot, the primary focus of myoneural ischemia.

Other findings, such as lack of sensation or absence of a dorsalis pedis or posterior tibial pulse, are not reliable diagnostic indicators. Sensation may be compromised by the swelling, and both pulses and normal capillary refill time may be present in a foot with compartmental ischemia.

Even when combined with a history of a crush injury associated with tense swelling and pain on passive dorsiflexion of the toes, the clinical findings and features may not be pathognomonic of a compartment syndrome of the foot (although, in fact, there may be little else clinically relevant). The only way in which compartment syndrome can be accurately diagnosed is by measurement of elevated compartment pressures. This is particularly important when the clinical findings are equivocal, but, even if the diagnosis is obvious, it is important to document the pressures. Raised pressures often precede the clinical findings of an incipient compartment syndrome, justifying liberal and routine use of pressure measuring devices.

We routinely measure the central compartment and, when clinically relevant, the calcaneal and other compartments potentially involved after injury. To measure the pressure in the central compartment, the surface landmark is the base of the first metatarsal; the needle is directed laterally immediately underneath the first metatarsal and through the abductor hallucis muscle (Fig. 3). (The medial compartment pressure can be measured as the needle advances through this muscle.) The needle is advanced 3.5 cm into soft tissue (not up against bone or tendon), the needle is cleared of soft tissue, and the reading is taken. The central compartment can also be monitored from

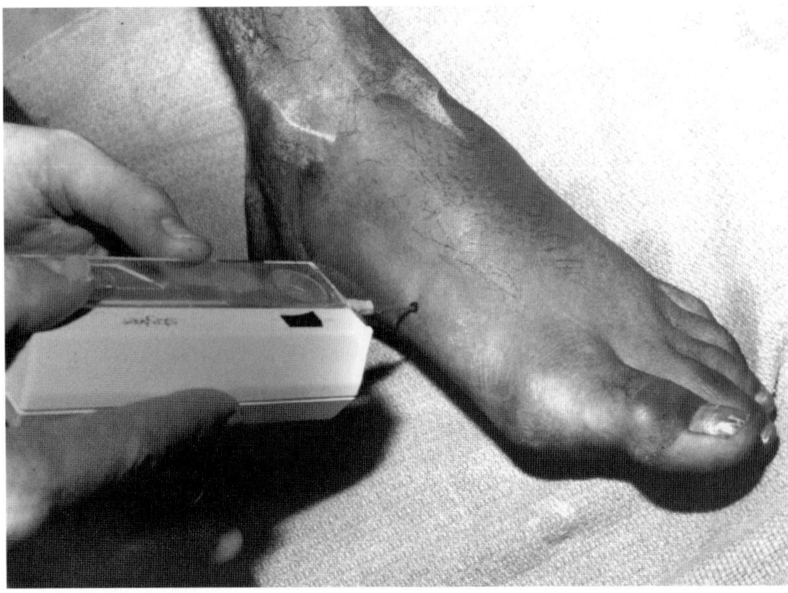

Figure 3. The pressure in the medial and deep central compartment is measured by inserting the needle through the abductor muscle immediately below the level of the first metatarsal.

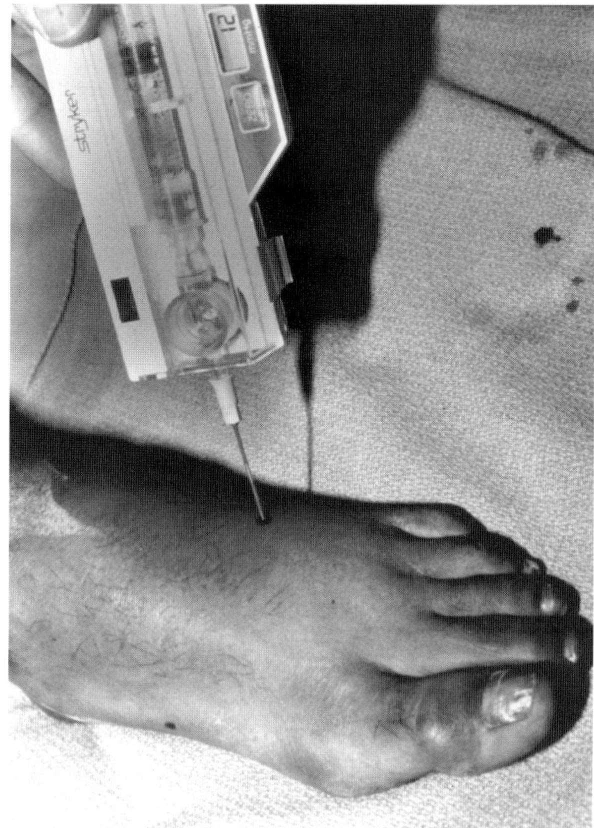

Figure 4. The pressure in the interosseous compartment is measured by inserting the needle in either the second or third web spaces and puncturing the extensor fascia.

a dorsal approach, measuring the interosseous compartment pressure when passing through it. The interosseous compartment pressure should be measured in more than one position by introducing the needle through the intermetatarsal space (Fig. 4). The second, third, and fourth web spaces are preferable, as these avoid inadvertent puncture of the dorsalis pedis or deep peroneal nerve. I do not routinely measure the lateral compartment pressure.

The calcaneal or quadratus compartment is measured by inserting the needle 5 cm distal and 2 cm inferior to the medial malleolus and advancing it through the abductor muscle, almost directly anterior and inferior to the calcaneus. Because swelling obscures the surface markings of the foot, the needle may be directed 3.5 cm directly inferior to the medial malleolus.

Treatment

General Principles

During the initial evaluation, all dressings should be removed. A circumferential cast should not be used if there is a potential for a compartment syndrome. The foot should be placed at heart level to ensure venous drainage without compromising local arteriolar pressures any further. Treatment should be based on a combination of clinical findings, pressure measurements, and time since injury.

Patients with a compartment syndrome begin to experience severe pain very soon after injury, presumably related to bleeding with the small muscle spaces, yet I have examined many patients who began to experience this unrelenting pain 12 or more hours after injury. Based on animal studies of muscle necrosis in experimentally induced compartment syndromes, fasciotomy should be performed within 8 hours after injury (14) and immediately once the diagnosis is made. However, because there is often a delay between the diagnosis of the compartment syndrome and the performance of a fasciotomy, I administer an ankle block, a safe way to keep the patient comfortable in the interim (15).

Management of the foot suspected of having a compartment syndrome depends on the level of increased compartment pressure. Although opinion varies about the absolute pressure above which fasciotomy should be performed, I recommend fasciotomy if the pressure is more than 40 mmHg, if the time since injury is less than 24 hr, as one is never quite certain when the pressure began to increase. If a patient is examined immediately after injury, and the pressures range between 30 and 40 mmHg, then fasciotomy may be performed, depending on the pattern of fracture or dislocation. For example, if a dislocation of the tarsometatarsal joint is present, and the pressure is 30 mmHg, fasciotomy is performed because its incision is used simultaneously to approach the dislocation; however, the foot not requiring surgical intervention is monitored closely but not treated with fasciotomy. If the pressures are within the 20- to 30-mmHg range, fasciotomy will not usually be required; I monitor the patient closely and apply an intermittent compression foot pump (AV Impulse, Kendall, Mansfield, MA) to decrease swelling and pressure. For patients in whom the diagnosis of a compartment syndrome is equivocal, particularly if the pressures are minimally elevated (less than 20 mmHg), I use the AV foot pump to reduce both the swelling and the compartment pressures (see Chapter 15 on crush injuries). These criteria may need to be adjusted depending on whether the patient is hypotensive or hypertensive.

To summarize the indications for fasciotomy: a foot with pressure more than 40 mmHg is treated with fasciotomy; one with pressures between 30 and 40 mmHg is closely monitored, unless open reduction of a fracture is required, in which case fasciotomy is performed; and a foot with pressure less than 30 mmHg is treated with a foot pump, with caution for those in the 20- to 30-mmHg range, in whom pressures may be increasing.

When is it too late to perform fasciotomy? Based on animal studies, fasciotomy should be performed no later than 24 hr after injury, before irreversible myoneural ischemia occurs. A dilemma occurs if a patient presents for evaluation 48 hr after injury, when a compartment syndrome has obviously occurred, and pressures are still markedly elevated. If these patients require operative treatment of the fracture, this is performed immediately, and the hematoma is decompressed when the incision is made. In these patients, however, one has to beware of the potential for increasing the risk of infection by converting a closed to an open injury. This is not a concern, for example, in midfoot injury, where adequate soft tissue is present and sufficient granulation tissue rapidly forms. With calcaneus fractures, however, the size of the incision and the lack of soft tissue coverage over the plate used for internal fixation make this form of treatment complicated.

Calcaneus Fractures

Reports of compartment syndromes associated with calcaneus fractures have appeared only recently, and controversy about the optimum treatment of this clinical problem still exists. Some clinicians maintain that the condition is not clinically significant, but my colleagues and I disagree, although I acknowledge that definitive management is as yet unclear: how can one accurately make this diagnosis and, once made, determine whether fasciotomy is necessary, whether immediate surgery will decompress the hematoma as well as the elevated compartment pressure, and how late after injury fasciotomy will treatment be clinically beneficial?

I have found that the deep, unrelenting pain in the foot dissipates immediately after fasciotomy, particularly in patients whose fasciotomies have been performed under local anesthesia. Although patients report discomfort from the fracture during the 24 hr after fasciotomy, the intensity of the pain is markedly improved. This pain relief, which is even more dramatic than that experienced after fasciotomy for crush injuries of the midfoot and forefoot, is probably related to relief of painful ischemia of the tibial nerve and its more major proximal branches, as well as relief of muscle ischemia.

Although in the past my colleagues and I have been quite aggressive about performing fasciotomy for elevated pressures associated with calcaneus fractures, this enthusiasm has been recently tempered by the remarkable success we have experienced in using the AV Impulse foot pump to decrease swelling. In treating patients who presented with massive swelling and findings suggestive of a compartment syndrome secondary to a fracture that occurred a week or more before evaluation, we measured the pressures and found them elevated; believing that fasciotomy would not be worthwhile after such a delay, we initiated the use of this foot pump to reduce the compartment pressures and noted that the swelling rapidly decreased as well. Since then, we have used the foot pump routinely to treat the swelling associated with calcaneus fractures and judiciously applied the principles of impulse technology to decrease elevated compartment pressures.

Fasciotomy Technique

The same principles that apply to fasciotomy elsewhere in the extremities apply to fasciotomy in the foot: no tourniquet is used, generous incisions are made, and subcutaneous fasciotomy is not advised. No debridement of muscle at the time of fasciotomy is performed because it is difficult to determine muscle contractility in the foot, and, once decompressed, the muscle may recover postoperatively. Skeletal stabilization, whether by external or internal fixation or a combination of the two, facilitates

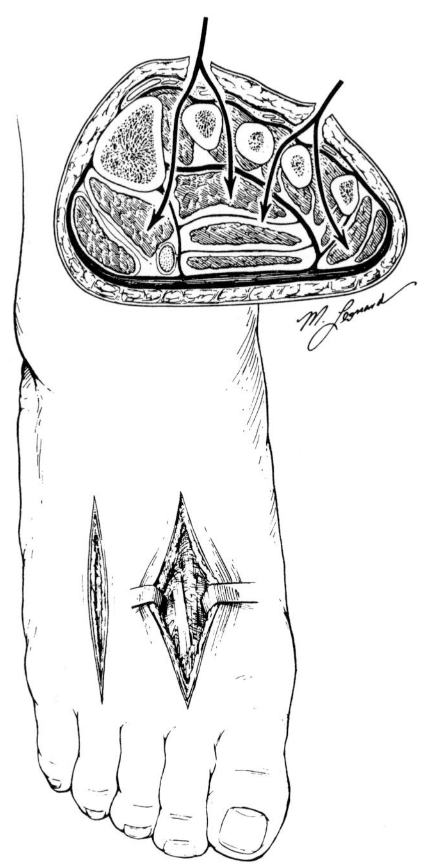

Figure 5. The approach to dorsal forefoot fasciotomy. Two incisions are made above the second and fourth metatarsals and deepened through the interosseous spaces into the deep central compartment. The *arrows* show the incision made and the direction of dissection. (From ref. 5, with permission.)

wound healing. Rigid skeletal stability enhances the environment for soft-tissue healing, decreases pain, and allows for more rapid mobilization of the extremity.

Several fasciotomy incisions may be used, including dorsal, medial, or a combination of the two. The decision to perform the fasciotomy dorsally or medially is based on the presence or absence of fractures amenable to open reduction and internal fixation. Many crushing injuries are associated with midfoot fractures and dislocations that are reduced with internal fixation after fasciotomy. Under these circumstances, the dorsal approach is used because it provides simultaneous access for fracture reduction and fixation. When a compartment syndrome is associated with a fracture pattern unsuitable for internal fixation, or when crushing occurs without fracture, then the medial incision is recommended. Regardless of the approach used, the pressures should again be measured after fasciotomy; if they are elevated, combined incisions should be used or the surgical decompression repeated.

For the dorsal approach for fasciotomy, two incisions are made, one over the second metatarsal and one over the fourth metatarsal (Fig. 5). These incisions should be placed slightly medial to the second metatarsal and lateral to the fourth metatarsal to ensure as wide a bridge of skin as possible. When the foot is swollen, the skin and subcutaneous tissues are also stretched and expanded; the skin bridge narrows considerably after fasciotomy when the skin resumes a more normal turgor. The skin incision is deepened to the bone, using a clamp to spread the tissue longitudinally. To avoid compromising the perfusion to dorsal skin, which is already tenuous, no subcutaneous dissection is performed (Figs. 6 and 7). When the bone is reached with the hemostat, further longitudinal dissection is performed in each interosseous space. From these dorsal incisions, reaching the medial and lateral compartments requires precise dissection and may not always be possible, despite the use of a curved clamp. I do not believe that complete release of these compartments is always necessary. Once the skin incision is made and the hematoma is decompressed, little needs to be done to decompress the

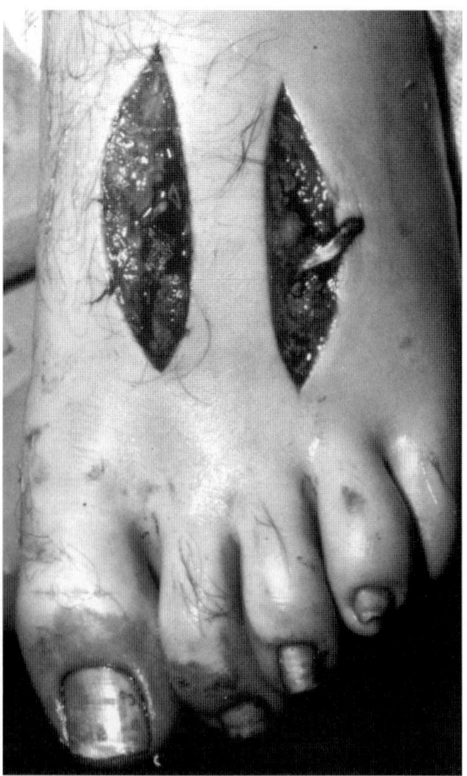

Figure 6. The dorsal skin bridge between the incisions may appear to be quite narrow after fasciotomy, but it will not become necrotic, provided subcutaneous dissection is not performed.

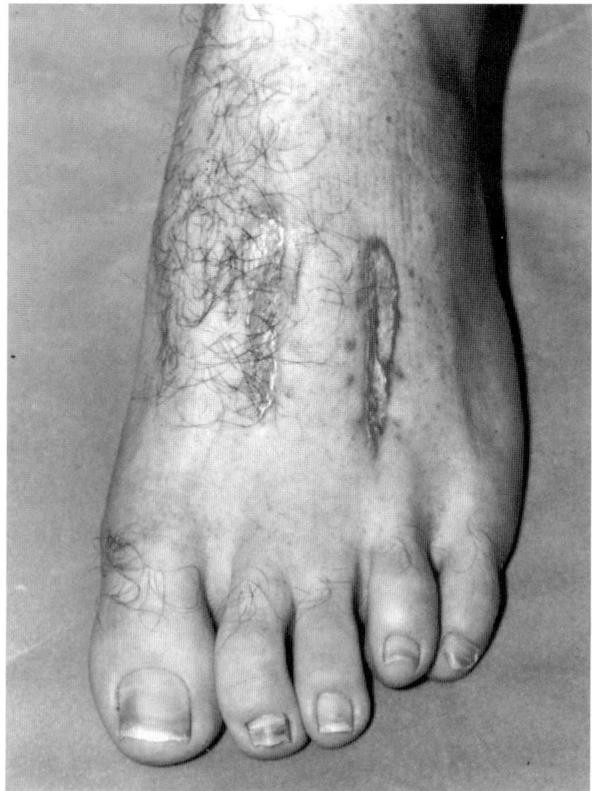

Figure 7. The fasciotomy incisions were covered with split-thickness skin grafts at 5 days and are demonstrated here at 4 months after injury. They contract after 2 to 3 months, at which time they may be excised and closed secondarily.

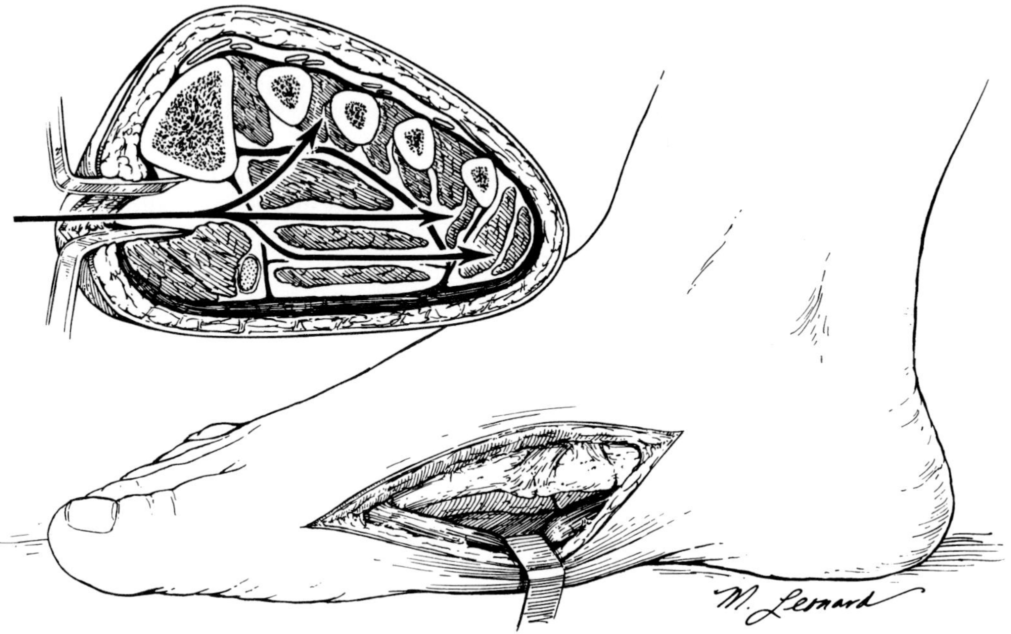

Figure 8. The medial fasciotomy incision is made immediately beneath the first metatarsal and releases the abductor compartment before entering the deep central compartment. The *arrows* show the incision made and the direction of the dissection. (From ref. 5, with permission.)

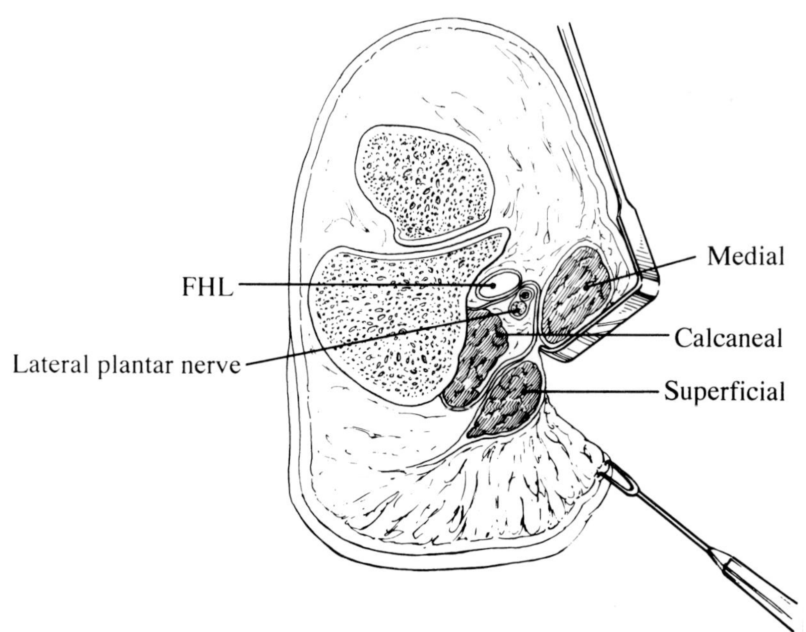

Figure 9. The fasciotomy for compartment release with calcaneus fracture is demonstrated. The abductor hallucis muscle is elevated dorsally, releasing its fascia, and the deep fascia overlying the quadratus muscle is opened, avoiding the lateral plantar nerve. FHL, flexor hallucis longus.

compartments further. Severe tearing of the limiting fascial planes between each anatomic compartment is usually present, and I have rarely needed to perform extensive dissection to complete the procedure.

The medial approach follows the length of the inferior surface of the first metatarsal, entering the medial compartment between the metatarsal and the abductor hallucis muscle and providing direct access into the other compartments (Fig. 8). Once the abductor hallucis muscle is retracted inferiorly, I prefer to gently spread the tissue longitudinally with a hemostat. The use of blunt finger dissection, rather than sharp instruments, will avoid injuring the neurovascular bundle when cutting across the central compartment. The skin incision can be extended more proximally to decompress the entire posterior tibial neurovascular bundle. This is occasionally required because patients may present with an acute tarsal tunnel syndrome. The presentation and pain is slightly different in these patients: they experience severe dysesthesias in the distribution of the medial and lateral plantar nerves.

The fasciotomy incision for treating a calcaneus fracture is made posteromedially, without performing a forefoot release, which is not necessary in cases of hindfoot injury (Fig. 9). The incision begins 4 cm from the back of the heel and 3 cm above the plantar surface. This incision extends distally, paralleling the sole of the foot for approximately 6 cm; if required, it may be extended proximally. Directly in line with the incision, the fascia overlying the abductor hallucis muscle is seen; this is opened, and the medial compartment is released. The abductor hallucis muscle is stripped from its overlying fascia and retracted superiorly. This reveals the dense white fascial layer of the medial intermuscular septum, which is opened longitudinally, and the calcaneal compartment is released. Care must be taken with this incision, as the lateral plantar nerve and vessels lie just below the septum. A more complete release for calcaneus fractures is rarely necessary, but if further dissection is felt to be warranted, then subcutaneous dissection is performed outside the previously opened medial compartment (1).

I do not recommend that the calcaneus fracture be fixed at the time of fasciotomy, because it is often difficult to close the skin at this stage, and the combined medial and lateral approaches to the foot may compromise the foot further. If the wounds are covered in 5 to 7 days, one can generally perform open reduction and internal fixation of the calcaneus at 10 to 14 days through a lateral incision. As stated above, my colleagues and I have begun to examine the effect of immediate open reduction through a lateral approach to treat a potential compartment syndrome simultaneously. This should be performed judiciously and planned according to the amount of swelling present and the time elapsed since injury.

Postoperative Care

Fasciotomy incisions are left open, and the wounds should not be closed before the fifth day. I frequently use porcine allograft to provide temporary coverage of the fasciotomy incisions, and these are changed at the bedside every 48 to 72 hours. The dorsal skin may still be tenuous; if so, the wounds are preferably closed with split-thickness skin grafts. These contract during healing, and the final cosmetic appearance of the foot is quite satisfactory. Closure of the dorsal incisions by suturing is possible, but should be performed judiciously because the skin edges may be tenuous and can necrose. The medial fasciotomy incisions approximate more easily with delayed primary closure than do the dorsal incisions, but split-thickness grafts can be used as well in this location.

CHRONIC COMPARTMENT SYNDROMES OF THE FOOT

Despite an increased awareness of the clinical spectrum of crushing injuries to the foot, the signs and symptoms of elevated compartment pressures within the foot are often overlooked (Fig. 10). The consequences of untreated compartment syndromes of the feet are serious, and these patients have substantial sensory and motor disturbances, e.g., chronic pain, stiffness, contracture, intrinsic atrophy, fixed

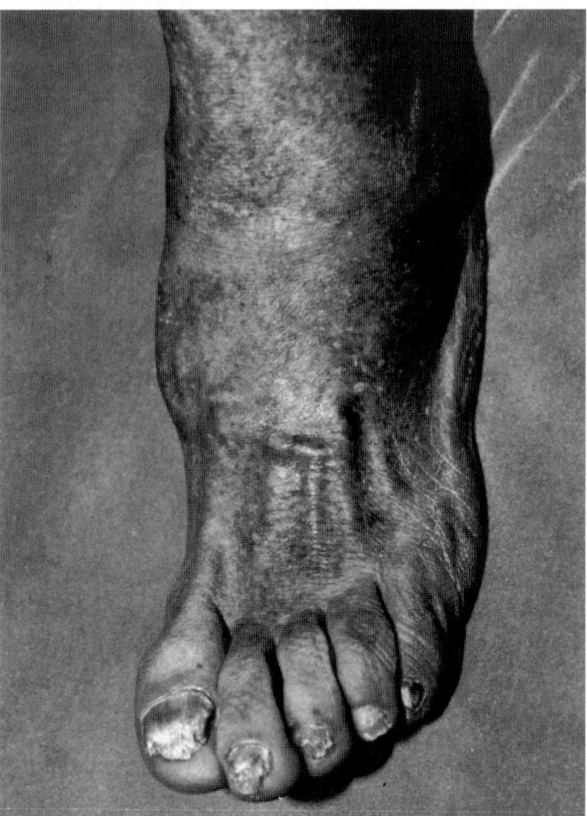

Figure 10. This patient sustained a dislocation of the transverse tarsal joint that was not initially diagnosed. Associated myoneural ischemia was present at the time of the injury, and the patient presented for late treatment of severe midfoot and forefoot stiffness, painful claw toes, and metatarsalgia.

clawing of the toes, soft-tissue dystrophy, and disuse atrophy with osteopenia. In many patients, these problems are compounded by chronic immobilization necessitated by the injury, further adding to the dystrophic changes in the juxtaarticular structures.

The end result of an untreated compartment syndrome is a foot that is dysfunctional and painful; it is certainly not a simple problem of claw toe deformities. If the intrinsic muscles of the foot atrophy, the balance between the intrinsic and extrinsic flexion of the toes is lost. The long extensor tendons then hyperextend the metatarsophalangeal joints, while the long flexor tendons flex both the proximal and distal interphalangeal joints. These deformities eventually become fixed, leading to further dysfunction. The remaining intrinsic muscles may also atrophy and, as the foot loses its contour and bulk, patients complain of discomfort from pressure around bony prominences. The foot is stiff, frequently from unresolved problems dating to the original injury. This ischemic process may also involve sensory deficits, a source of considerable additional debility.

There seem to be two types of toe deformity associated with chronic compartment syndromes: the toes can be clawed or stiff and hyperflexed. In some patients, diffuse claw toe deformities develop, with hyperextension of the metatarsophalangeal joints and flexion of the proximal and distal interphalangeal joints. Intrinsic atrophy is evidenced by wasting of the interossei, the abductor hallucis, and occasionally the extensor brevis muscles. This gives rise to a typical intrinsic minus deformity. The interosseous muscle, which attaches to the plantar base of the proximal phalanx, is the strongest flexor of the metatarsophalangeal joint, and when it undergoes atrophy the extensor digitorum longus tendon extends the metatarsophalangeal joint. The delicate balance between the intrinsic and extrinsic musculotendinous units at the metatarsophalangeal joint is lost, leading to further extension at the joint. The interosseous tendon subluxes dorsal to the axis of the metatarsal head, fixing the joint in extension and further perpetuating this imbalance. Alternatively, the toes are all acutely flexed at the metatarsophalangeal and interphalangeal joints. These joints are extremely stiff, and little active dorsiflexion of the digits is possible.

Both of these different forms of contracture of the digits occur as a result of acute myoneural ischemia. In the first group, the intrinsic minus deformity is due to atrophy of the involved muscles, probably as a result of neural ischemia. This is the same deformity identified in the upper extremity and hand, giving rise to an intrinsic minus deformity of the hand. The fixed flexion deformities in the second group are due to intrinsic muscle fibrosis, including the interossei, lumbricales, and flexor brevis. This sequence follows muscle edema, necrosis, and ultimate fibrosis after ischemia.

In some patients, a combination of unrecognized myoneural ischemia in both the foot and the deep posterior compartment of the leg occurs. In these patients, in addition to the forefoot deformities as described above, additional contracture occurs in the extrinsic flexors, including the posterior tibial, flexor hallucis, and flexor digitorum longus tendons. The entire foot is extremely stiff, the toes are immobile, and the foot exhibits equinovarus contracture. I have treated these deformities with excision of the involved musculotendinous units in the deep compartments. Although tendon lengthening may occasionally work, it is preferable to excise not only the tendon, but also the fibrotic muscle to prevent recurrence. The muscles no longer function, and full correction of the deformity is difficult to achieve without excision. Whether or not this should include the entire compartment or be limited to the contracted tendons in the foot and ankle is unclear. My colleagues and I have achieved satisfactory correction of the deformity by complete excision of the posterior tibial, flexor hallucis, flexor digitorum longus, and (occasionally) abductor hallucis muscles through a posteromedial incision that can be extended to include a lengthening of the Achilles tendon as needed. Although the incision is longer than that of a simple tenotomy, which may be performed percutaneously, excision is the mainstay of treatment.

Correction of toe deformities is difficult, and satisfactory function is never regained. Unfortunately, most of these feet are extremely stiff, and the goal in treating these patients is to maximize function and relieve pain. Arthrodesis of the proximal interphalangeal joints is the best form of treatment when combined with appropriate tendon lengthening or tenotomy. The soft-tissue releases will depend on which type of intrinsic deformity is present. For the fixed flexion contracture, both the short and long flexors are lengthened percutaneously by tenotomy through the proximal flexion crease. Passive dorsiflexion returns and, provided the extrinsic extensor tendons are still functioning, some active dorsiflexion is regained. In the presence of fixed hyperextension at the metatarsophalangeal joint, proximal interphalangeal arthrodesis is combined with soft-tissue releases at the metatarsophalangeal joint. If present, the long flexor tendons will function to flex the metatarsophalangeal joint.

REFERENCES

1. Myerson M, Manoli A. Compartment syndromes of the foot after calcaneal fractures. *Clin Orthop* 1993;290:142–150.
2. Myerson M, McGarvey WC. Crush injuries and compartment syndromes. In: Myerson M, ed. *Current therapy in foot and ankle surgery*. St. Louis: Mosby–Year Book, 1993:264–273.
3. Myerson MS. Diagnosis and treatment of compartment syndrome of the foot. *Orthopedics* 1990;13:711–717.
4. Myerson MS. Management of compartment syndromes of the foot. *Clin Orthop* 1991;271:239–248.
5. Myerson MS. Experimental decompression of the fascial compartments of the foot—the basis for fasciotomy in acute compartment syndromes. *Foot Ankle* 1988;8:308–314.
6. Grodinsky M. A study of the fascial spaces of the foot and their bearing on infections. *Surg Gynecol Obstet* 1929;49:739–751.
7. Loeffler RD Jr, Ballard A. Plantar fascial spaces of the foot and a proposed surgical approach. *Foot Ankle* 1980;1:11–14.
8. Manoli A, Weber TG. Fasciotomy of the foot: an anatomical study with special reference to release of the calcaneal compartment [see comments]. *Foot Ankle* 1990;10:267–275.
9. Sarrafian SK. *Anatomy of the foot and ankle. Descriptive, topographic, functional.* Philadelphia: JB Lippincott, 1983.
10. Manoli A II. Compartment syndromes of the foot: current concepts. *Foot Ankle* 1990;10:340–344.
11. Ashton H. The effect of increased tissue pressure on blood flow. *Clin Orthop* 1975;113:15–26.
12. Jennings AMC. Some observations of critical closing pressures in the peripheral circulation of anesthetized patients. *Br J Anaesth* 1964;36:683–692.
13. Saxby T, Myerson M, Schon L. Compartment syndrome of the foot following calcaneus fracture. *Foot* 1992;2:157–161.
14. Mubarak SJ, Hargens AR, Owen CA, Garetto LP, Akeson WH. The wick catheter technique for measurement of intramuscular pressure. A new research and clinical tool. *J Bone Joint Surg [Am]* 1976;58:1016–1020.
15. Myerson MS, Ruland CM, Allon SM. Regional anesthesia for foot and ankle surgery. *Foot Ankle* 1992;13:282–288.

EDITORIAL COMMENTS

Compartment Syndromes of the Foot

Mark S. Myerson

Dr. Myerson has given us a detailed account of the anatomy of the nine compartments of the foot and precise measurement techniques and criteria. A high index of suspicion must be used to diagnose compartment problems of the foot because these areas are not often the emphasis of primary investigation when the multitrauma patient arrives. With the advent of safety harnesses and air bags, there are more survivors of high-speed motor vehicle accidents, which unfortunately cause substantial trauma to both skeletal and soft tissue in the foot and ankle. Diagnosis of compartment syndrome requires clinical suspicion and the availability of simple accurate devices for measurement of compartment pressures. Histories of high-speed motor vehicle accidents or severe crush injuries should increase our suspicion without the presence of skeletal fractures. The measurement criterion of above 40 mmHg requires open decompression, 30 to 40 degrees of proper elevation, and pulsatile plantar pressure; for less than 20 mmHg, observation only is required. These criteria should serve as landmarks and not be rigid. One must also remember that the state of the patient, hypotensive or hypertensive, will affect these values and should be adjusted appropriately. When in doubt, we always favor a decompression of compartments because we believe that decompression can be performed by those schooled in proper anatomy without significant tissue destruction or significant morbidity with the wounds left open. In calcaneal fractures, there is usually a delay until the time of open reduction, and compartment problems should be treated immediately with the medial plantar incision because this will usually not interfere with the lateral extensile approach.

A missed compartment will usually result in contractures of the intrinsic and extrinsic musculature, leading to the fibrosis and foot deformities that will require further reconstruction. The goal is to prevent this from occurring and to treat the patient aggressively early. Judicious decompression of nerves is also indicated to prevent grade I and II compression-type injuries.

Robert S. Adelaar, M.D.

Complex Foot and Ankle Trauma,
edited by Robert S. Adelaar,
Lippincott–Raven Publishers, Philadelphia © 1999.

17

Treatment of Complex Forefoot Injuries

William M. Granberry and Michael J. Shereff

Forefoot injuries are relatively common and may lead to prolonged disability and residual dysfunction (1–3). These injuries are often overlooked, as in the case of the multiple-trauma patient (4). Alternatively, the severity of the soft tissue injuries is initially underestimated as in crush injuries of the forefoot (5). These injuries may result in malunion, nonunion, and joint stiffness; difficulties with ambulation can occur with abnormalities of lead distribution during the stance phase of gait. In spite of the potential disability and complexity of these fractures, very few reports describing evaluation and treatment are available in the literature (6). Anatomic reduction and adequate fixation combined with meticulous soft tissue management, however, can lead to optimum clinical results (7). This review emphasizes the application of fracture management principles to traumatic injuries of the forefoot.

FRACTURES OF THE METATARSALS

Functional Anatomy

Studies on the load-bearing characteristics of the forefoot during the stance phase of gait indicate that each of the lesser metatarsals supports an equal weight and that the

W. M. Granberry: Department of Orthopaedic Surgery, Baylor College of Medicine, Houston, Texas 77030; Section of Foot and Ankle Surgery, St. Luke's Episcopal Hospital, Houston, Texas 77030.

M. J. Shereff, Department of Orthopaedic Surgery, Medical University of South Carolina, Charleston, South Carolina 29425; Foot and Ankle Center, Orthopaedic Specialists of Charleston, Charleston, South Carolina 29414.

first metatarsal carries twice the weight of each of the lateral metatarsals. Displacement, especially in the coronal plane of the metatarsal fracture fragment, may lead to a non-anatomic metatarsal arch (4).

Lindholm (8) has emphasized that angulation of fractures through the metatarsal neck have a particular propensity to plantar displacement and subsequent increased loading (5,9), which may result in an intractable plantar keratosis at that site. Dorsal displacement of the distal fragment decreases the load applied to that metatarsal and may transfer greater pressure to the adjacent metatarsals (7). The coronal plane displacement becomes more apparent in the second and third metatarsals, as these have less motion of the tarsometatarsal joint and can accommodate less when malunion occurs.

Medial and lateral displacement of the fracture fragments toward an adjacent metatarsal may lead to mechanical impingement and interdigital neuromas. Medial displacement of the distal fragment of the first metatarsal fracture and lateral displacement of the distal fragment of a fifth metatarsal fracture may lead to prominent bony eminences that can rub against the toebox of the shoe (7). Deforming muscle forces result in typical fracture displacement. The strong flexor tendons and weaker intrinsic tendons will usually force the distal fragment of the metatarsal fracture in a proximal and plantar direction (5,7,8). Intraarticular fractures of the metatarsophalangeal or tarsometatarsal articulation may lead to decreased joint motion, early arthrosis, and gait abnormalities.

Incidence

Metatarsal fractures are relatively common injuries. A recent review stated that the metatarsal most commonly fractured in industrial injuries was the third (6). Fractures of the first and second metatarsals occurred with equal frequency, and the fourth metatarsal was the least commonly injured. It should be noted, however, that if one includes the common fracture of the base of the fifth metatarsal caused by inversion injuries to the foot, then the incidence of 23% makes the fifth the most commonly fractured metatarsal.

Mechanism of Injury

Fractures of the metatarsals may result from either direct or indirect forces (11). Direct injury, common in industrial accidents, often results from a heavy object falling on the dorsum of the forefoot. In addition, repetitive fatigue stresses to the forefoot can result in metatarsal stress fractures. Indirect injuries occur when the forefoot is held fixed and the leg or foot is twisted, a situation often seen in athletic injuries of the foot.

Clinical Manifestations

Patients describe pain on active motion of the foot as well as difficulty with ambulation. Physical examination reveals localized tenderness and swelling. Palpable motion may be present at the fracture site. Passive motion of the metatarsal distal to the fracture site may reproduce the patient's symptoms. This maneuver is particularly helpful for evaluation of stress fractures of the metatarsals. The neurovascular status should be evaluated because of the proximity of the arterial arch; the dorsalis pedis artery and the dorsal and plantar metatarsal arteries are particularly susceptible to injury associated with metatarsal fractures (12). In addition, in the case of crush injuries and multiple metatarsal fractures, the presence of a compartment syndrome should be determined.

Radiographic Evaluation

Radiographic evaluation of fractures of the metatarsals should include three standard views (7). The antero/posterior radiograph will reveal medial and lateral displacement of the fracture fragments. The lateral view allows evaluation of the dorsal and plantar displacement. Oblique views demonstrate the lateral metatarsals more clearly. Tomograms provide information regarding intraarticular extent and degree of fracture comminution in difficult situations. Each fracture should be assessed as to the location, extent of shortening, comminution, and rotation of the distal fracture fragments.

Treatment

Open Fractures

Treatment of open fractures of the forefoot should follow the same guidelines used for open injuries elsewhere in the musculoskeletal system (9,13). Appropriate initial irrigation and debridement should be performed as soon as possible. In addition, broad-spectrum antibiotics are instituted dependent on the wound type. Prophylaxis for tetanus is given. During debridement, all necrotic and devitalized tissue should be excised. Adequate fixation is essential to hasten bony union and allow adequate treatment of the soft tissue injuries. Fixation may be internal or external. Soft tissue debridements are performed every 24 to 48 hr as needed to ensure optimum wound management. Bone grafting may be required when there is extensive bone loss. All wounds are left open for delayed primary closure, skin grafting, or plastic reconstruction.

Closed Undisplaced Fractures

Numerous articles have described the various modalities of treatment for undisplaced metatarsal fractures (1,5,6,14,15). DeLee (1) described the use of adhesive strapping to the forefoot in combination with a wooden-soled shoe for a 3- to 5-week period. Morrissey (15) has recommended weight bearing as tolerated using a medial longitudinal arch support with elevation proximal to the metatarsal heads. The arch support and metatarsal pad are applied to the foot by means of adhesive strapping. Johnson (6) recommended initial treatment with a compressive dressing followed by return to weight-bearing status as tolerated in a stiff-soled work boot. He emphasized that immediate ambulation and weight bearing on the fractured foot are the keys to rapid return to work and minimal disability. Giannestras and Sammarco (5) describe the use of a short leg walking cast for 4 to 6 weeks. Garcia and Parks (14) describe the use of the short leg non-weight-bearing cast for 3 weeks followed by a walking cast for an additional 3 weeks. Non-weight-bearing treatment was emphasized, especially with fractures of the first or multiple metatarsals. There are many options. In general, adequate immobilization and avoidance of weight-bearing pressure to reduce the risk of displacement is best achieved by means of a non-weight-bearing short leg cast for 4 to 6 weeks. This is followed by removal of the cast and slow gradual return to weight bearing as tolerated (7).

Displaced Fractures

Displaced fractures often require reduction and immobilization. Dorsal or plantar displacement and/or of the fracture fragments is poorly tolerated. If left unreduced, these fractures may lead to a nonplantigrade foot and difficulties with ambulation. This is particularly true for younger, more active individuals. Although specific indications for open reduction of these fractures have not been described in the literature, it is recommended that an attempt should be made to improve alignment in any metatarsal fracture displaying displacement of greater than 3 to 4 mm or angulation of more than 10 degrees (7).

Consideration should be given to which and how many of the metatarsals are involved and the demands of the patient. Fractures of the first, second, and third metatarsals should be more aggressively treated; the more distal the fracture, the greater the likelihood for displacement (Fig. 1). The second and third metatarsals are the keystone, and displacement and angulation are not tolerated well.

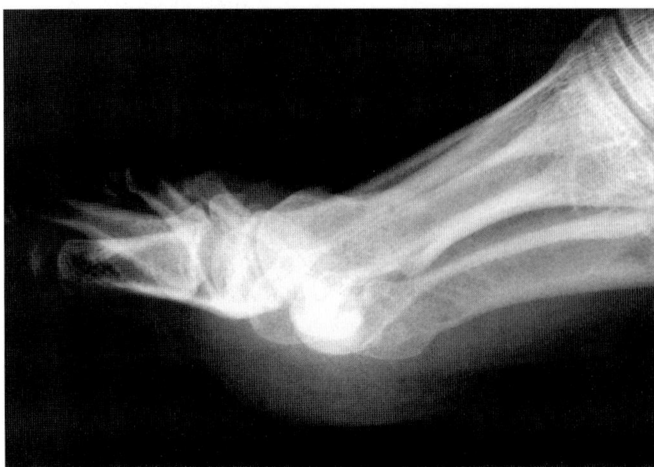
A

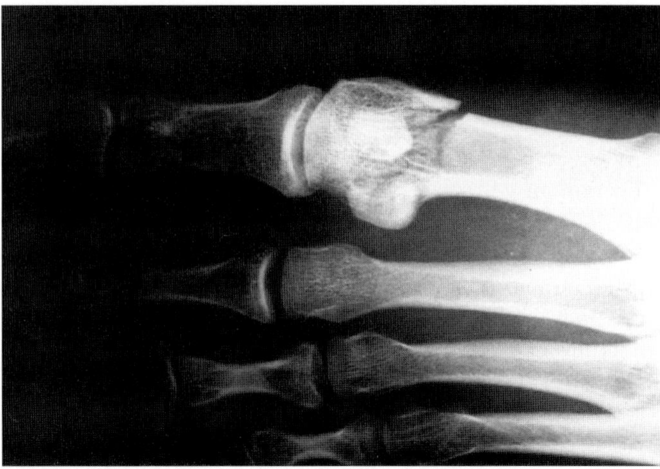
B

Figure 1. Anteroposterior (**A**) and lateral radiographs (**B**) showing dorsal displacement of first metatarsal. This minimally displaced fracture was treated with closed reduction and casting.

Reduction and immobilization can be achieved by various means. The use of Chinese finger traps applied to the toes with countertraction at the ankle has proved to be a most effective and safe method of reducing displaced metatarsal fractures (5,14). Anderson (4) reports that most displaced metatarsal fractures can be manipulated into satisfactory position under anesthesia and that position can be maintained with cast immobilization. A short leg cast from the tips of the toes to the tibial tubercle can be applied while the foot is still in the traction device. The patient is kept on crutches, non-weight-bearing for 6 weeks. After the cast is removed, the patient gradually returns to weight-bearing activity. If radiographs taken after the reduction show that the fracture is unstable, percutaneous pinning can provide excellent fixation of the fracture fragments. The 0.062 pins can be placed either transversely, transfixing the fractured metatarsal to an adjacent metatarsal, or, alternatively, cross pins can be placed within the fractured metatarsal across the fracture line itself (7,16). For pin fixation the second and third metatarsals should be utilized for stability. Johnson (6) has emphasized that if after closed reduction the fracture fragments are in any degree of apposition and are not displaced toward the sole, conservative treatment can be continued. Several authors (5,6,17) believe that displacement of the metatarsal shaft fracture with the exclusion of the first metatarsal is of no great clinical significance and does not require open reduction. Likewise, Johnson (6) suggests that shortening of single or multiple fractures of the middle three metatarsals is not significant. Dorsal or plantar angulation, however, cannot be accepted (Fig. 2). Rotation of the distal fragment is frequently not a consideration because of the strong distal ligamentous attachments between the metatarsal heads (2). Sisk (17) also emphasizes, however, that more distal fractures of the metatarsal are more likely to angulate and more often difficult to immobilize with external casting alone and that open reduction and internal fixation should be performed on these fractures (Fig. 3). For fractures not amenable to closed reduction, open reduction and internal fixation will provide optimum results. A dorsal longitudinal incision is centered over the involved bone. If multiple metatarsals are fractured, the incision should be placed in the interval between the metatarsals and two metatarsals can be exposed through the same incision. The fracture site is then exposed subperiostally. Special attention should be given to using atraumatic techniques in handling the soft tissues. After the fracture ends are cleaned with a curette, the bone is reduced and temporarily held in place with bone-holding forceps (18). The choice of fixation method depends on the fracture site and configuration. The type of fixation most commonly used is 0.45-mm smooth K-wire inserted in a crossed fashion (11). Alternatively, Johnson (6) has described a technique using intramedullary K-wire. Internal fixation with semitubular plate and bone screws along the medial or lateral aspect of the metatarsal

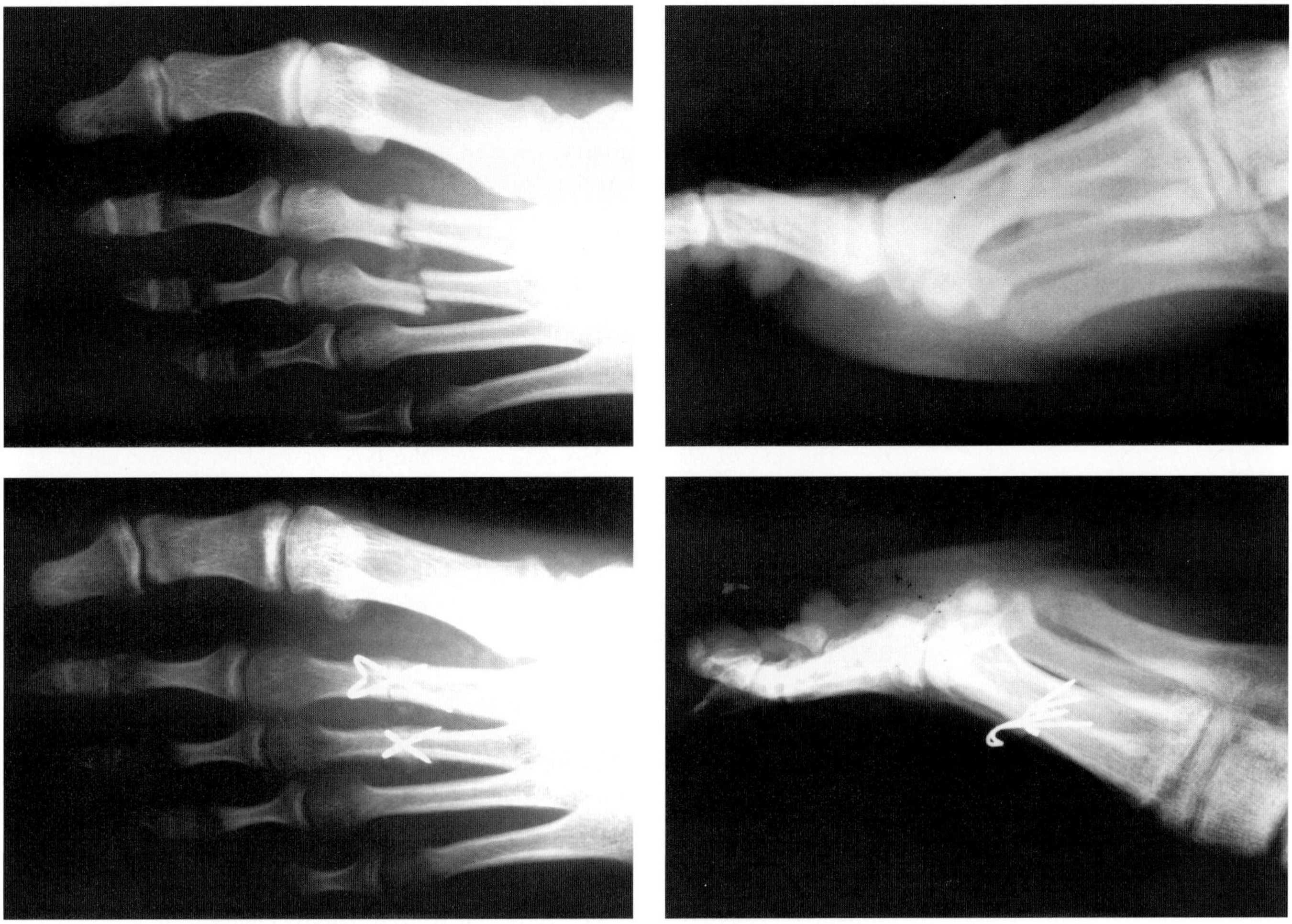

Figure 2. Dorsally angulated second and third metatarsal fractures (**A** and **B**), initially treated nonoperatively. Subsequent open reduction and pinning was required and produced an anatomic result (**C** and **D**).

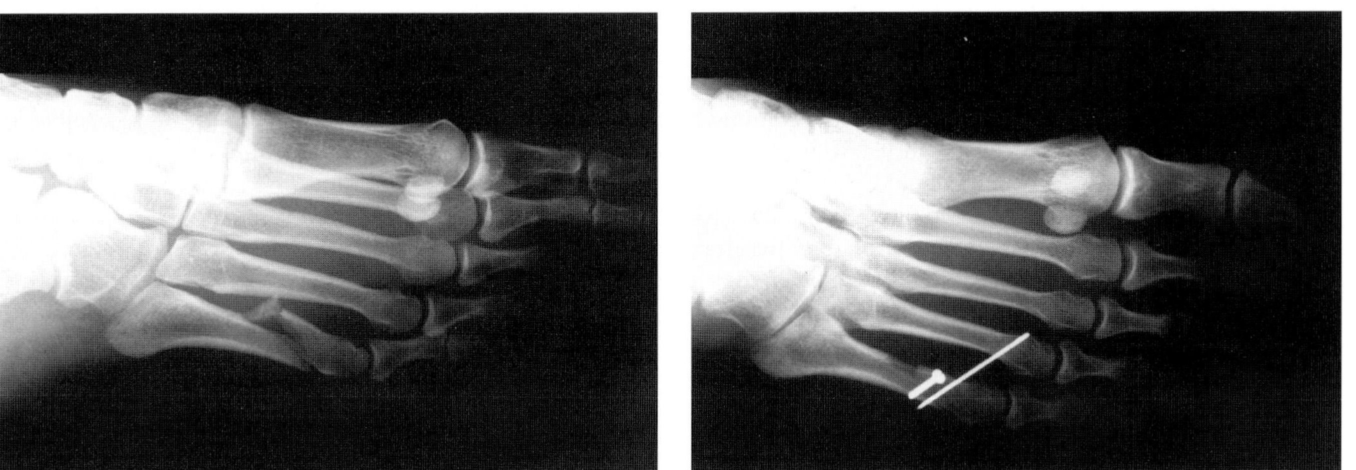

Figure 3. Displaced fifth metatarsal fracture (**A**) treated with open reduction and internal fixation (**B**).

has been advocated, as this method allows for early return to full weight bearing (1,19). If, however, K-wire fixation has been chosen, a short leg cast is applied, and the patient is placed on crutches and kept non-weight-bearing. After four to six weeks, radiographic evidence of union is present, the pins are removed, and a gradual return to weight bearing and ambulation is allowed. Patients with multiple displaced metatarsal fractures commonly require open reduction and internal fixation. Intraarticular fractures, especially those at the metatarsophalangeal articulation, require adequate reduction to restore articular congruity (1,6,7). This is most commonly performed using K-wire fixation but can be also performed using minifragment buttress plates and screws (19).

The configuration of internal fixation should be based on the configuration of the fracture (1,7,19). Transverse fractures are usually amenable to cross-pin fixation. Oblique and spiral fractures may be fixed with interfragmentary lag screws. Multiple K-wire fixation may be helpful in securing long spiral or comminuted metatarsal fractures. The site of fracture also determines the type of fixation device used. Small cancellous screws may be used in metaphyseal bone. Interfragmentary cortical lag screws are generally more effective in diaphyseal bone. When possible, one tries to avoid prolonged immobilization with percutaneous K-wire due to rehabilitation problems.

FRACTURES OF THE BASE OF THE FIFTH METATARSAL

Fractures of the base of the fifth metatarsal are the subject of much controversy. Numerous authors (1,20–23) have recommended a variety of treatments for this common metatarsal fracture, which have been classically termed the *Jones fracture* after Sir Robert Jones (24), who described the injury of his own foot in 1902. Jones described a transverse diaphyseal fracture of the fifth metatarsal that did not heal quickly. This fracture is less common than the avulsion-type fracture at the base of the fifth metatarsal or at the fifth metatarsal tuberosity caused by overpull of the peroneus brevis muscle.

In an effort to clarify fractures at the base of the fifth metatarsal, Stewart (22) introduced a classification of these fractures. Type I fractures are at the junction of the metatarsal shaft and base, subdivided into two groups, comminuted and noncomminuted. Type II fractures involve only the styloid process, also subdivided into two groups, those with and those without joint involvement.

DeLee (1) offers an updated classification scheme dividing the fractures at the base of the fifth metatarsal into three types. Type I includes nondisplaced acute fractures of the junction at the shaft of the base. Type I-B includes comminuted fractures at the junction of the metatarsal shaft and base. Type II fractures are at the junction of the metatarsal shaft and base with clinical and roentgenographic evidence of previous injury. Type III fractures are those involving the styloid process and are separated into two types, with and without joint involvement. This classification is important in that type II fractures often represent a more chronic situation and are more difficult to treat. Treatment recommendations are based on the location of fracture and whether the injury is acute or chronic. In general, undisplaced acute fractures at the base and shaft should initially be treated with non-weight-bearing short leg cast immobilization for 4 to 6 weeks or until union is present primarily. Consideration can be given to reduction and cross-pinning to stabilize the fracture and promote union, especially in active patients (25,26). In those fractures at the metaphyseal–diaphyseal junction with evidence of preexisting stress reaction of the bone, a more aggressive treatment plan should be undertaken. If nonoperative treatment is undertaken, the patient should be kept strictly in a non-weight-bearing short leg cast (8). If the patient continues to have pain or lack of union, evidenced by x-ray film, or if conservative treatment is not acceptable, internal fixation should be undertaken with either crossed K-wire pinning or intramedullary screw fixation (Fig. 4). Consideration should also be given to inlay bone graft or iliac crest cancellous bone graft during internal fixation (27). Due to the poor blood supply to this area of the fifth metacarpal, limited open or closed techniques are preferred.

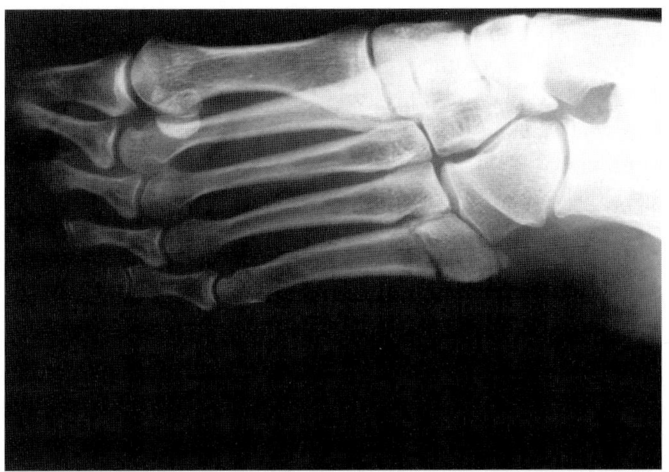
A

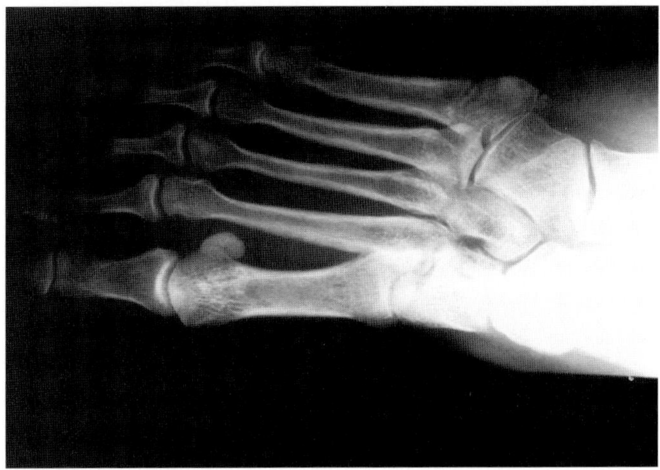
B

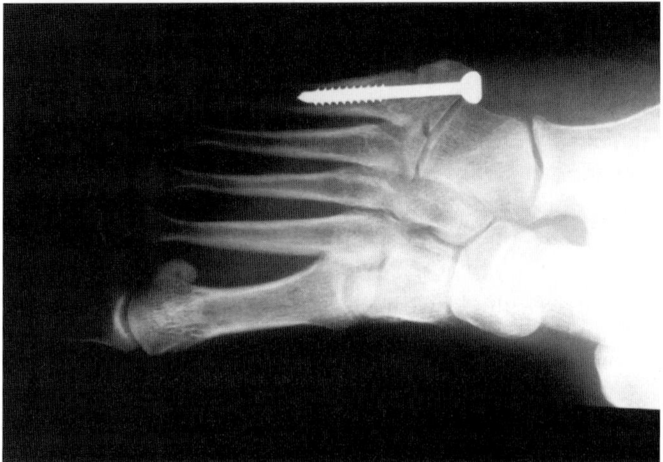
C

Figure 4. Proximal metaphyseal fifth metatarsal fracture. Failure to unite after 8 weeks of immobilization (**A** and **B**). Surgical treatment with internal fixation and bone grafting (**C**).

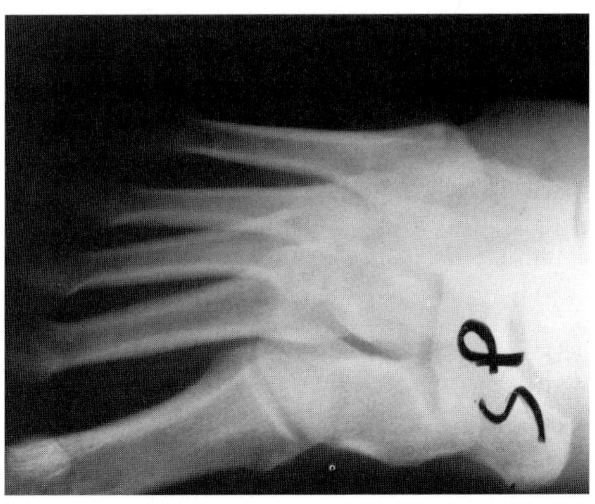
A

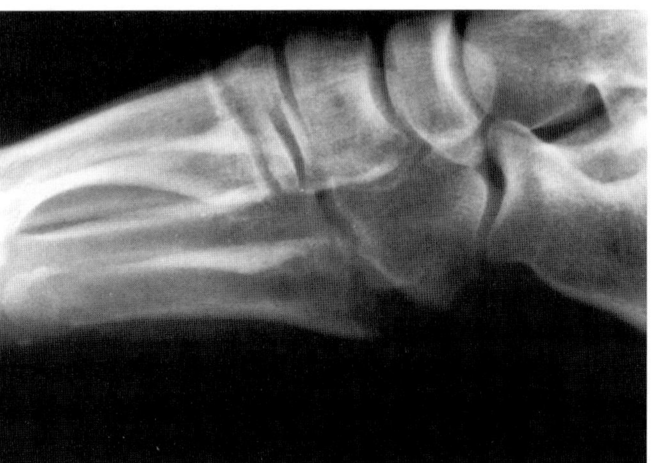
B

Figure 5. Symptomatic nonunion avulsion fracture of fifth metatarsal tuberosity (**A**). Surgical treatment with excision of fragment and advancement of peroneus brevis tendon (**B**).

Postoperatively, the patient is placed into a non-weight-bearing short leg cast for 3 to 6 weeks, and activity is increased as the fracture progresses toward union. Avulsion fractures at the base of the fifth metatarsal can be treatment symptomatically (6,7,22). Greatly displaced fractures with weakness or eversion can be treated with open reduction and internal fixation (28) or excision of the bony fragment and advancement of the peroneus brevis tendon into drill holes through the proximal aspect of the fifth metatarsal (7) (Fig. 5).

DISLOCATIONS OF THE METATARSOPHALANGEAL JOINTS

Traumatic dislocations of the metatarsophalangeal joints are relatively rare injuries because the joint is intrinsically stable and is strongly supported by extensive soft tissue attachments. Dislocations of these joints are usually caused by severe trauma and result from a combination of forces. The most common mechanism is hyperdorsiflexion of the toe. As the proximal phalanx is forcibly dorsiflexed, subluxation and finally dislocation occurs. Depending on the mechanism of injury, the sesamoids may remain attached to the proximal phalanx or fracture remaining under the metatarsal neck.

Jahss (29) has subdivided metatarsophalangeal dislocations into two basic types. In type I, the hallux dislocates dorsally with the sesamoids. There is no disruption of the sesamoid complex or intrasesamoid ligament. Diagnosis of type I dorsal dislocation can be made radiographically as the sesamoids appear unfractured and appear dorsal to the metatarsal shaft. In addition, they are not widely separated. These injuries are irreducible with attempted closed reduction as the plantar plate is interposed between the metatarsal head and the base of the proximal phalanx. Treatment of complex type I dislocations require open reduction, and the recommended approach is via a transverse plantar incision just over the prominent metatarsal head. After exposure of the metatarsal head with careful avoidance of the plantar nerves, a skin hook can be carefully placed over the metatarsal head dorsally to hook the plantar plate and deliver it distally and plantarly over the metatarsal head. Once the joint is reduced, it is stable and can be treated in a short leg cast or firm postoperative shoe with weight bearing as tolerated.

Type II dislocations of the metatarsophalangeal joint are different from type I in that there is damage to the intersesamoidal ligament with wide separation of the sesamoids. Type II injuries are further separated into type A and B. Type A injuries include a rupture of the intrasesamoid ligament. Type B injuries display a transverse fracture of one or both of the sesamoids. Distinct from the type I dislocations, type II dislocations can be reduced by closed means, which should be done as soon as possible. Once reduction is achieved, a careful check should be made for radiographic incongruity of the sesamoid or crepitus, with motion representing interarticular fragments. This type of dislocation is stable once reduced; however, it should be protected longer than the type I injury. If persistent instability is encountered, then percutaneous pinning can be performed.

Dislocation of the lesser metatarsophalangeal joints is an infrequent injury. This type of dislocation is distinct from the chronic dislocations at the lesser joints associated with claw or hammer toes. Attempted closed reduction should be performed as soon as possible. Irreducible dislocations have been reported. Once reduced, these joints are usually stable and can be treated with taping for comfort. Unstable joints can be pinned percutaneously to provide additional fixation.

FRACTURES OF THE PHALANGES

Fractures of the phalanges are the most common injury of the forefoot (1). The most common of these fractures is the so-called night-walker fracture involving the proximal phalanx of the fifth toe (5,6). Open fractures of the phalanges are not common but do occur in crushing-type injuries. Indirect mechanisms that apply forces to a fixed forefoot are less common. The phalanges of the hallux are larger and functionally more important than those of the lesser toes. In addition, injuries to the first digit are also frequent and more commonly lead to long-term disability. The proximal phalanx of the hallux is more commonly fractured (16). When the distal phalanx is fractured, it is most commonly from a crush injury and is often comminuted or dislocated (1). Fractures through the lesser toes most commonly occur at the proximal phalanx as it is the longest of the phalanges. Injuries to the lesser toes are often overlooked or dismissed as sprains (30).

Functional Anatomy

Fractures of the phalanges usually result in plantar angulation secondary to the combined effect of the extensor mechanism and intrinsic musculature. Functionally, the range of motion of the interphalangeal/metatarsophalangeal joints of the toes is not of great significance except when considering the hallux. Malunion of these fractures, however, can cause disability secondary to subsequent interdigital corns.

Clinical Diagnosis

Patients note swelling of the involved digit. Ecchymosis is quite common. Physical examination reveals localized tenderness and swelling in addition to pain and crepitus with attempted active motion of the toe. A subungual hematoma is associated with fracture of the distal phalanx. It should be noted that many of these injuries are secondary to direct trauma or crushing injury, and careful examination of the soft tissues and neurovascular status should be completed.

Anterior, posterior lateral, and oblique x-ray film are standard in the evaluation of phalangeal fractures. Coned-down views can also be informative.

Treatment

Open fractures of the phalanges receive the same treatment as has been described for the metatarsals. Treatment of closed fractures depends on which phalanx and which digit is involved. Because the hallux bears substantial force during the toe-off phase of gait, even undisplaced fractures of the proximal phalanx should be protected (7,30). Various means of immobilization have been described. ''Buddy taping'' of the hallux and second toe and protected weight bearing in a wooden-soled shoe have been recommended (16). Immobilization in a short leg walking cast may be appropriate for some patients (30). Displaced fractures of the proximal phalanx of the hallux may require closed reduction and immobilization in a non-weight-bearing short leg cast for 4 to 6 weeks. If reduction proves to be unstable, consideration should be given to percutaneous pinning. If the fracture is not amenable to closed reduction, or demonstrates significant interarticular stepoff, then open reduction and internal fixation may be appropriate, particularly in young and active individuals. Zrubecky (31) recommended open reduction and K-wire fixation for isolated medial or lateral condylar fractures or fracture dislocations, which are typically seen in stubbing injuries. Jahss (30) stresses that displaced fractures of the great toe phalanges, particularly those associated with dislocations of the adjacent joint, require anatomic reduction (Fig. 6). Undisplaced fractures of the distal phalanx of the hallux may be treated with buddy taping to the second toe and protected weight bearing in a wooden-soled shoe. Fractures of the distal phalanx of the hallux are rarely displaced due to strong periosteum and tendon insertions. Attempts at closed or open reduction with immobilization or fixation of these fractures has been described in the literature. Open reduction is appropriate for intraarticular fractures involving the interphalangeal joint (7).

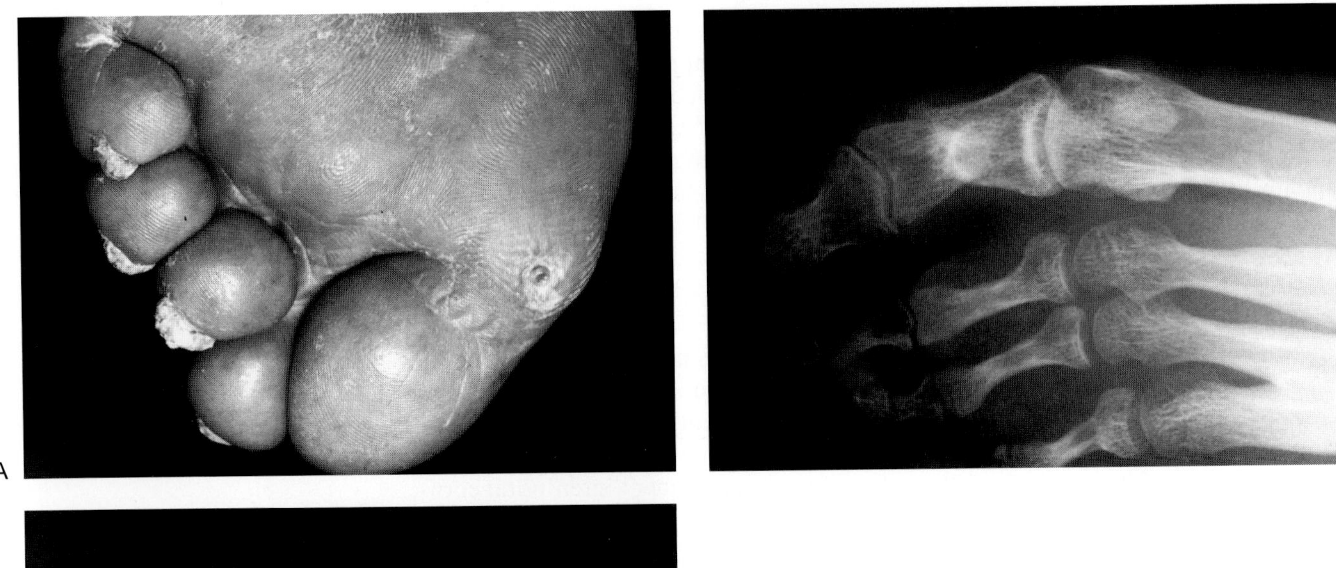

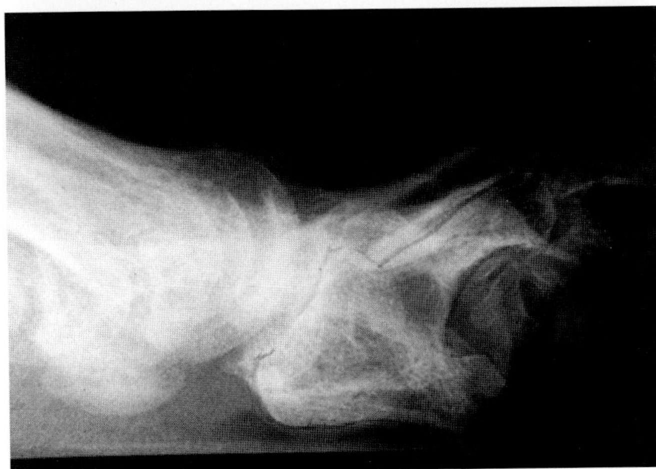

Figure 6. Clinical photograph (**A**) and radiographs (**B** and **C**) of symptomatic phalanx malunion.

Phalangeal Fractures of the Lesser Toes

Undisplaced fractures of the lesser toes may be treated with taping to the adjacent toe and protected mobilization in a wooden-soled shoe. In displaced fractures, closed reduction and buddy taping are often effective. K-wire fixation of the proximal phalangeal fractures may be appropriate in severe displacement or angulation not amenable to closed reduction and external fixation (5). In particular, one should attempt to reduce angulation or displacement leading to gross rotatory or angular deformities of the digits. Residual bony prominences may lead to interdigital soft corns. Mechanical impingement resulting from angulation against the adjacent toes may lead to hard corns in the areas of pressure from shoewear. Long-term sequelae from phalangeal fractures of the lesser toes are rarely reported (6).

REFERENCES

1. Delee JC. Fractures and dislocations of the foot. In: Mann RA, ed. *Surgery of the foot,* 6th ed. St. Louis: CV Mosby, 1993.
2. Lutter LD. Forefoot injuries. In: Kiene RH, Johnson KA, eds. *Symposium on the foot and ankle.* St. Louis, CV Mosby, 1983:81–88.
3. McKeever FM. Injuries of the forefoot. In: *American Academy of Orthopedic Surgeons Instructional course lectures,* vol 2. Ann Arbor, MI: JW Edwards, 1944:120–129.
4. Anderson LD. Injuries of the forefoot. *Clin Orthop* 1977;122:18–27.
5. Giannestras LJ, Sammarco GJ. Fractures and dislocations of the foot. In: Rockwood CA Jr, Green DP, eds. *Fractures,* vol 2. Philadelphia: JB Lippincott, 1975.
6. Johnson VS. Treatment of the forefoot in industry. In: Bateman JE, ed. *Foot science.* Philadelphia: WB Saunders, 1976.

7. Shereff MJ. Fractures of the forefoot. In: *American Academy of Orthopedic Surgeons instructional course lectures,* vol 29. St. Louis: CV Mosby, 1990:133–140.
8. Lindholm R. Operative treatment of dislocated simple fracture of the neck of the metatarsal bone. *Ann Chit Gynaecol Tenn* 1961;50:328–331.
9. Chapman MW. *Management of open fractures and complications: Part III, Role of bone stability in open fractures.* In: Frankel VH, ed. *American Academy of Orthopaedic Surgeons instructional course lectures,* vol XXI. St. Louis: CV Mosby, 1982.
10. Lehman RC, Torg JS, Parlor H. Fractures of the base of the fifth metatarsal distal to the tuberosity: a review. *Foot Ankle* 1987;7:245–252.
11. Blodgett WH. Injuries to the forefoot and toes. In: Jahss MH, eds. *Disorders of the foot,* vol 2. Philadelphia: WB Saunders; 1982.
12. Shereff MJ, Yang QM, Kummer FJ. Extraosseous and intraosseous arterial supply to the first metatarsal and metatarsophalangeal joint. *Foot Ankle* 1987;8:81–93.
13. Gustilo RB. Principles of management of open fractures. In: Gustilo RB, ed. *Management of open fractures and their complications.* Philadelphia: WB Saunders, 1982:15–54.
14. Garcia A, Parkes SC. Fractures of the foot. In: Giannestras NJ, ed. *Foot disorders: medical and surgical management,* 2nd ed. Philadelphia: Lea & Febiger; 1973:517–564.
15. Morrissey EJ. Metatarsal fractures. *J Bone Joint Surg* 1946;28:594–602.
16. Chapman MW. Fractures and fracture–dislocations of the ankle and foot. In: Mann RA, ed. *DuVries' surgery of the foot,* 4th ed. St. Louis: Mosby, 1978.
17. Sisk TD. Fractures. In: Edmonson AS, Crenshaw AH, eds. *Campbell's operative orthopedics,* 6th ed, vol 1. St. Louis: CV Mosby, 1980.
18. Sammarco GJ. Biomechanics of the foot. In: Frankel VH, Nordin M, eds. *Basic biomechanics of the skeletal system.* Philadelphia: Lea & Febiger, 1980:193–220.
19. Helm U, Pfeiffer KM. The foot. In: *Internal fixation of small fractures,* Berlin: Springer–Verlag, 1987:340–342.
20. Delee JC, Evans JP, Julian J. Stress fracture of the fifth metatarsal. *Am J Sports Med* 1983;11:349–353.
21. Kavanaugh JH, Brower TD, Mann RA. The Jones fracture revisited. *J Bone Joint Surg [Am]* 1978;60:776–782.
22. Stewart IM. Jones's fracture: fracture of the base of the fifth metatarsal. *Clin Orthop* 1960;16:190–198.
23. Torg JS, Balduini FC, Zelko RR, et al. Fractures of the base of the fifth metatarsal distal to the tuberosity: classification and guidelines for non-surgical and surgical management. *J Bone Joint Surg [Am]* 1984;66:209–214.
24. Jones R. Fractures of the base of the fifth metatarsal bone by indirect violence. *Ann Surg* 1902;35:697–700.
25. Arrangio GA. Proximal displaced fractures of the fifth metatarsal: two cases treated by cross pinning with review of 100 cases. *Foot Ankle* 1983;3:293–296.
26. Zelko RR, Torg JS, Rachun A. Proximal diaphyseal fractures of the fifth metatarsal—treatment of the fracture and their complications in athletes. *Am J Sports Med* 1979;7:95–101.
27. Dameron TB. Fractures and anatomical variations of the proximal portion of the fifth metatarsal. *J Bone Joint Surg [Am]* 1975;57:788–792.
28. Pritsch M, Heim M, Tauber H. An unusual fracture of the base of the fifth metatarsal bone. *J Trauma* 1980;20:530–531.
29. Jahss MH. Traumatic dislocations of the first metatarsophalangeal joint. *Foot Ankle* 1980;1:15–22.
30. Jahss MH. Stubbing injuries to the hallux. *Foot Ankle* 1981;1:327–332.
31. Zrubecky G. Bruche der Grosszehe, deren Behandlung und Behandlungsergebnisse. *Arch Orthop Unfallchir* 1955;47:591–611.

EDITORIAL COMMENTS

Treatment of Complex Forefoot Injuries

William M. Granberry and Michael J. Shereff

The goal with forefoot injuries is to maintain a foot whose plantar surface pressures with standing and walking will not result in forefoot disabilities. There should be no angulation or rotation that will be cosmetically unacceptable for shoe wear. When appropriate (with the exceptions of the Jones type II fracture and certain fractures of the proximal phalanx of the first toe that are intraarticular), closed treatments are usually most acceptable to preserve the precarious blood supply to the metatarsals and phalanges. When using closed methods one must be aware that the second and third metatarsal are the keystone, and they should receive privileged treatment: anatomic reduction with no malrotation. The first, fourth, and fifth metatarsals can accommodate more angulation, rotation, and displacement because of their hypermobility.

For the first metatarsal, an anatomic reduction in the sagittal plane should always be the goal, for continued even pressure over the sesamoid complex. If one is going to use open techniques then use minimal stripping and firm fixation. Screws and plates should be kept out of the weight-bearing surface area, and bone grafting should be considered when doing open reductions of metatarsals due to their precarious blood supply in the nonmetaphyseal area and the ease of harvesting bone graft from the medial malleolus and tibial tubercle. Like the hand fracture problems, cortical bone takes a longer time to heal than metaphyseal bone and usually requires 6 to 8 weeks of immobilization. Rehabilitation should often take preference over total bone healing. One should avoid utilizing external K-wires or external fixation methods if it will interfere with rehabilitation attempts. External fixators can be used for bone loss, particularly in the first metatarsal phalangeal joint, and should be considered for delayed reconstruction to preserve the hallux length. One should also be aware that severe crushing injuries of the forefoot accompanied by multiple fractures or no fractures may be prime candidates for causalgias and sympathetic dystrophies. Aggressive treatment and control of edema and pain control as well as awareness of this complication should accompany treatment. Injuries to the sesamoid ligament should be immobilized for lengthy periods, and orthotics should be utilized in addition to taping regimens to control the area until adequate ligamentous healing is possible.

Robert S. Adelaar, M.D.

Complex Foot and Ankle Trauma,
edited by Robert S. Adelaar,
Lippincott–Raven Publishers, Philadelphia © 1999.

18

Fractures of the Proximal Fifth Metatarsal

Alan S. Tuckman, Samuel S. Fleming, John G. Seiler, III, and Lamar L. Fleming

Although fractures of the proximal fifth metatarsal are common (1–3), few practitioners recognize the significant difference that variations in this fracture, occurring in such close proximity, have for treatment outcome. Unfortunately, these fractures are often grouped together when reporting study results, adding confusion to treatment recommendations. The differences between the various fractures of the proximal fifth metatarsal may appear subtle, but accurate assessment will guide treatment and optimize outcome.

HISTORICAL OVERVIEW

In 1902, Sir Robert Jones (4) reported on a series of six fractures of the proximal fifth metatarsal, including his own, sustained while waltzing. In this report, Jones provides a discussion of the anatomy and proposes a mechanism of injury. Although he offers no classification scheme or treatment recommendations, some fractures of the base of the fifth metatarsal have since become known as the *Jones fracture*.

A. S. Tuckman: Baltimore, Maryland 21208.
S. S. Fleming: Department of Orthopaedics, Emory University, Atlanta, Georgia 30322; Department of Orthopaedics, Kennestone Hospital, Marietta, Georgia 30060.
J. G. Seiler, III: Department of Orthopaedic Surgery, Emory University, Atlanta, Georgia 30309; and Department of Orthopaedic Surgery, Piedmont Hospital, Atlanta, Georgia 30309.
L. L. Fleming: Department of Orthopaedics, Emory University, Atlanta, Georgia 30322; Department of Orthopaedics, Emory University Hospital, Atlanta, Georgia 30322.

Jones' original article received relatively little attention, and 6 years later, Wharton (5) reported on three more proximal fifth metatarsal fractures that healed with plaster of Paris and strapping. That same year, Young (6) reported on a fracture that did not heal and was later treated with excision of the fragment.

In 1927, Carp (7), in an address to the Orthopaedic Section of the New York Academy of Medicine, was the first to focus attention on the frequency of nonunions in this region of the foot. He suggested that a poor blood supply in this area was responsible.

In 1960, Stewart (1) published a series of 51 fractures and clearly showed differences in the healing characteristics between fractures distal to the fourth–fifth metatarsal articulation and those of the tuberosity. In 1975, Dameron (8) reported on a series of 120 fractures of the proximal fifth metatarsal and, like Stewart, showed that a variety of clinical outcomes were predictable by the specific fracture pattern.

ANATOMY

Osteology

The fifth metatarsal is a small, tubular bone that has at its base a prominent tuberosity (or styloid process) that protrudes in a lateral and plantar direction. The base of the fifth metatarsal articulates with the lateral aspect of the base of the fourth metatarsal. Together they articulate with the cuboid to form the lateral portion of Lisfranc's joint (Fig. 1). Like the metacarpohamate joint of the hand, this cuboid–metatarsal articulation has significantly more mobility in a dorsal–plantar direction than in a medial–lateral direction (9).

A strong ligamentous complex secures the proximal fifth metatarsal. Plantar and dorsal intermetatarsal ligaments unite the base of the fifth metatarsal to the base of the fourth, and both are joined to the cuboid via plantar and dorsal tarsometatarsal ligaments. These ligamentous structures are reinforced by a stout slip of the plantar fascia, which arises from the calcaneus and inserts into the plantar aspect of the proximal fifth metatarsal (10) (Fig. 2).

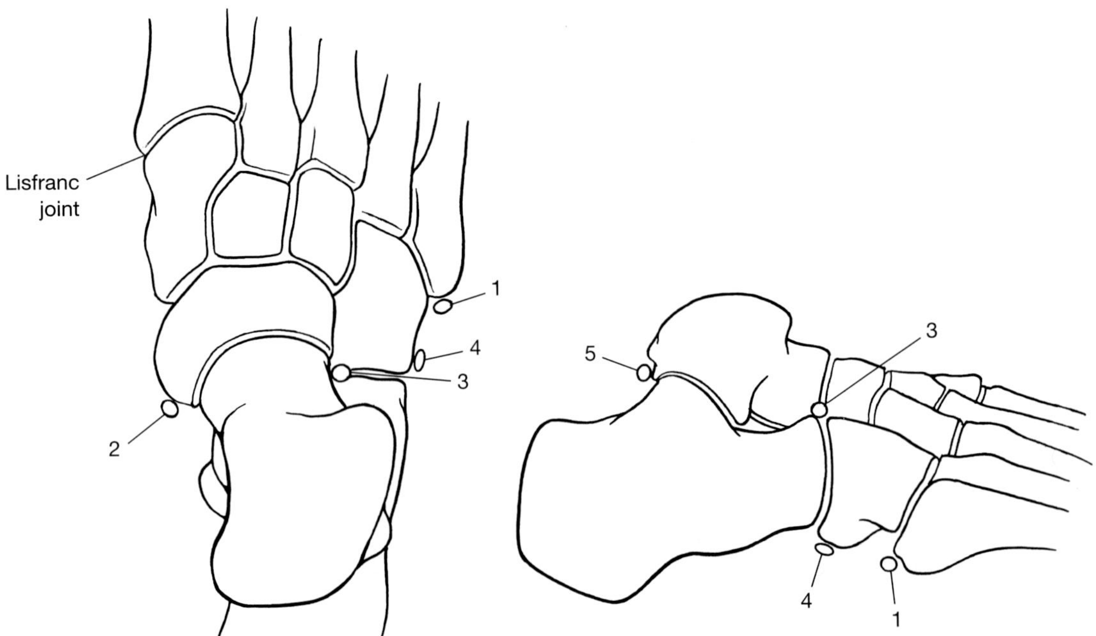

Figure 1. Accessory bones and LisFranc joint. *1,* os vesalianum; *2,* accessory navicular; *3,* os calcaneous secundaris; *4,* os peroneum; and *5,* trigonam.

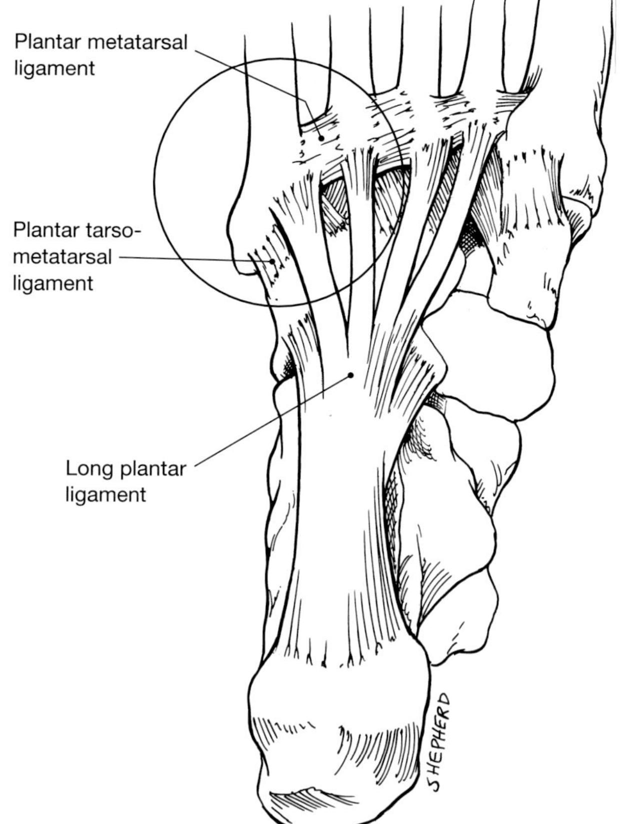

Figure 2. Plantar fascia connection to the fifth metatarsal.

The fifth metatarsal also serves as a point of insertion for several muscles (Fig. 3). The peroneus brevis inserts along the lateral aspect of the tuberosity, and the peroneus tertius attaches along the dorsal aspect of the base. The abductor digiti quinti originates from the lateral calcaneus and usually has a second attachment to the plantar aspect of the fifth metatarsal tuberosity before inserting on the proximal fifth phalanx. The peroneus longus will occasionally send a tendinous slip to attach to the base of the fifth metatarsal as it passes around the cuboid on its way to insert on the first metatarsal (11).

Growth and Development

Accurate radiologic assessment of the proximal fifth metatarsal is aided by an understanding of the normal ossification pattern. Like other tubular bones, the fifth metatarsal has a primary and a secondary center of ossification, separated by a physeal plate (Fig. 4). In addition, the fifth metatarsal may also have an apophyseal center of ossification. This appears as a flake-like calcification that is often confused for a fracture (Fig. 4). The incidence of this apophysis is controversial. Hoerr and colleagues (12) consider it a constant center of ossification, noting its appearance in 198 of 200 longitudinally studied children. Dameron (8) noted the apophysis in only 22% of 164 radiographs of children between the ages of 7 and 16 years old.

If present, the fifth metatarsal apophysis can usually be seen in girls 9 to 11 years of age and boys 11 to 14 years of age. Usually, this apophysis unites to the tuberosity within 2 years of its appearance (8). Rarely, the apophysis fails to unite and becomes a separate ossicle or accessory bone, termed the os vesalianum (13); it is seen in less than 1% of adults (8,13).

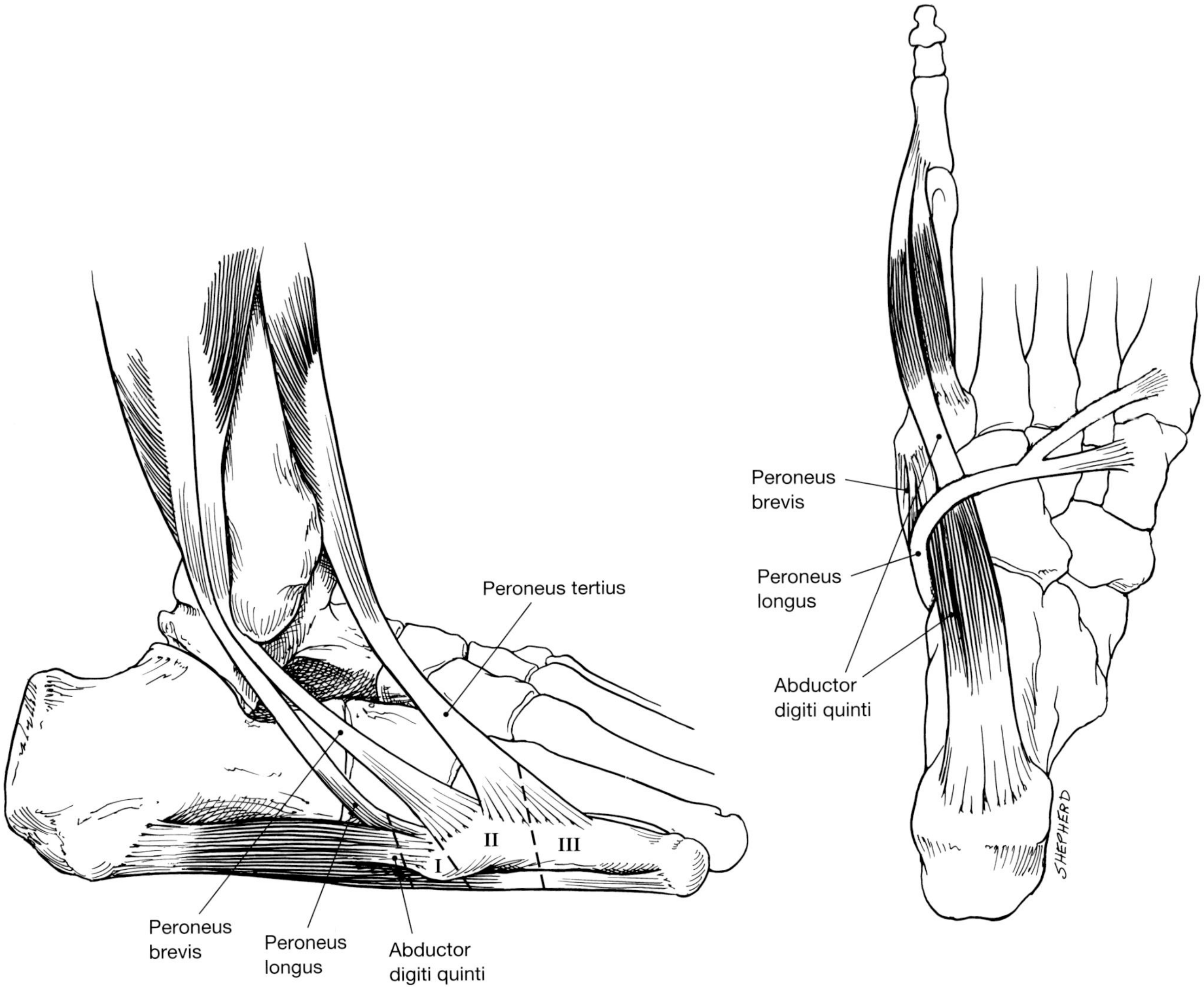

Figure 3. Tendon insertions on fifth metatarsal.

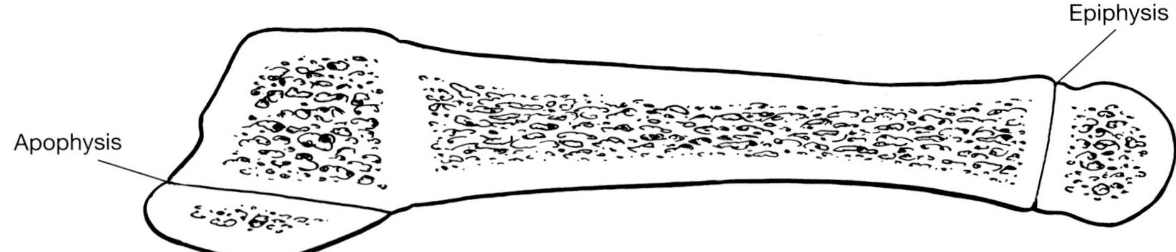

Figure 4. Apophyseal and epiphyseal centers of ossification on the fifth metatarsal.

As previously mentioned, the apophyseal ossification or the os vesalianum are often misinterpreted as an avulsion fracture. Several radiographic characteristics make differentiation easier. Both the apophysis and os vesalianum have smooth, well-corticated edges, whereas a fracture is characterized by irregular, ragged edges. The apophysis is located along the lateral plantar surface of the tuberosity and is oriented parallel to the long axis of the metatarsal. Oblique radiographs may highlight these features. The os vesalianum is located at the proximal tip of the fifth metatarsal (Fig. 1), the same location of an avulsion fracture. However, the fracture tends to involve either the metatarsal–cuboid or the fourth–fifth metatarsal articulation (8). The narrow age range of apophyseal appearance (ages 9 to 14 years) and the rarity of the os vesalianum should further aid in clinical assessment.

Vascular Anatomy

Two recent studies have evaluated the vascular anatomy of the proximal fifth metatarsal, increasing our understanding of the healing characteristics of this region. Shereff et al. (14) evaluated the extraosseous blood supply with an acrylic resin injection technique and the intraosseous blood supply using a modified Spalteholz technique. This study found that the extraosseous blood supply is provided by three main sources: the dorsal metatarsal artery, the plantar metatarsal arteries, and the fibular plantar marginal artery, an inconsistent branch of the lateral plantar artery (Fig. 5). These vessels supply variable numbers of branches that take part in the intraosseous blood supply (via the periosteal plexus). The medial aspect of the fifth metatarsal, just proximal to the fourth–fifth metatarsal articulation, was observed to have the highest concentration of these vessels (14).

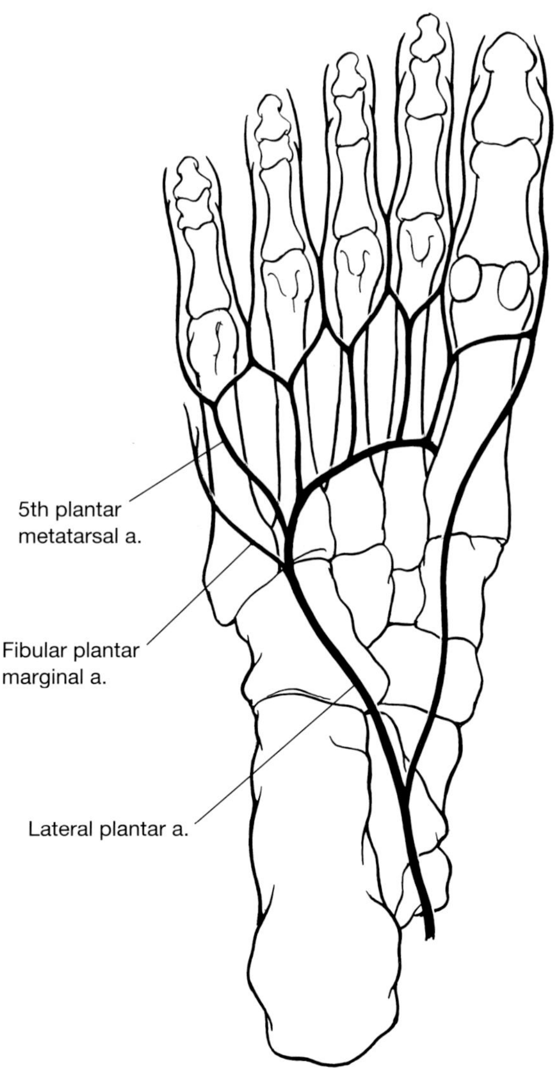

Figure 5. Extraosseous blood supply.

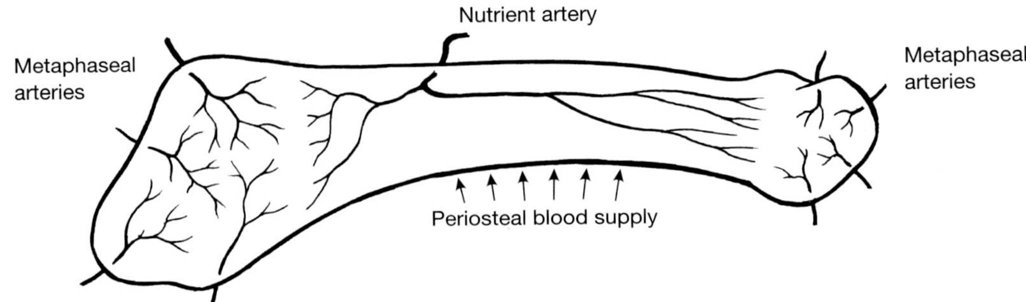

Figure 6. Intraosseous blood supply.

The intraosseous blood supply was found to consist also of three sources: a periosteal plexus, a nutrient artery, and metaphyseal vessels (Fig. 6). The periosteal plexus is supplied by the extraosseous vessels and is described above. A single nutrient vessel was found to enter the fifth metatarsal medially at the junction of the proximal and middle thirds. The metaphyseal blood supply is an extension of the extraosseous blood supply, which penetrates the bone via capsular vessels (14,15).

Smith et al. (15) also evaluated the intraosseous blood supply via a Spalteholz technique and found essentially the same three sources as described above. However, Smith et al. (15) were able to demonstrate a potential watershed region of bone, as first theorized by Carp (7) in 1927, between the abundant metaphyseal vessels and the nutrient artery. A fracture through the proximal diaphysis would disrupt the nutrient vessel or its proximal branch and create a ''zone of relative avascularity'' (15). This metaphyseal–diaphyseal fracture is notorious for slow healing, and often a nonunion results.

CLASSIFICATION

Although several authors have identified differences in clinical behavior of different types of proximal fifth metatarsal fractures (5–7), many physicians indiscriminately named all fractures of the proximal fifth metatarsal after Jones. In 1960, Stewart (1) proposed the first formal classification scheme intended to guide treatment and predict outcome. In this scheme, fractures were divided into two main categories: (a) fractures of the styloid, and (b) junctional fractures occurring at the junction of the shaft to the base. These were then further subdivided, depending on the amount of articular involvement and the amount of comminution. Recently, various authors have divided

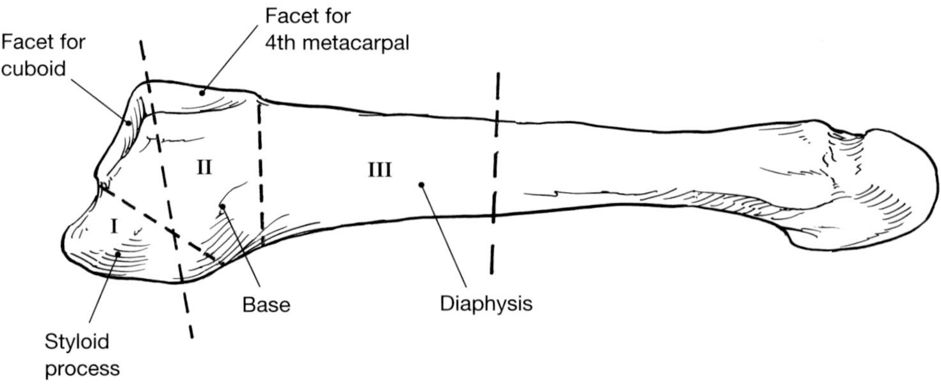

Figure 7. Bony anatomy of the fifth metatarsal.

these fractures into three subtypes based on anatomic zones (9,16). Zone I includes the cancellous tuberosity: fractures of this region usually involve the metatarsal–cuboid articulation. Zone II involves the distal aspect of the tuberosity, at the metaphyseal–diaphyseal junction. Fractures of this region involve the fourth–fifth metatarsal articulation. True Jones fractures are found in this region. Zone III fractures involve the diaphysis, beginning just distal to the intermetatarsal ligament complex and extending for approximately 1.5 cm (Fig. 7).

MECHANISM OF INJURY AND TREATMENT

Tuberosity Fractures

Several different mechanisms have been described for tuberosity fractures (also called avulsion fractures or zone I fractures). Until recently many authors concluded that tuberosity fractures were the result of an avulsion mechanism resulting from the pull of the peroneus brevis tendon on its insertion at the base of the fifth metatarsal during a sudden inversion of the hindfoot (Fig. 8) (2,8,13,17–19). This, however, was challenged by Richli and Rosenthal (20), who used selective sectioning techniques to show that with plantar flexion and an inversion stress, a fracture of the fifth metatarsal tuberosity could be produced only when the lateral band of the plantar aponeurosis was intact. This led to their conclusion that the avulsion is actually of the lateral band of the plantar aponeurosis (Fig. 2). This would also make anatomic sense, as the broad insertion of the peroneus brevis lies mostly distal to the region of zone I injuries (Fig. 3).

Due to the low morbidity of isolated fractures of the fifth metatarsal tuberosity, clinical series are infrequently reported. Pearson (19) reported on a series of 146 patients treated for styloid fractures with either a splint, an injection, or a bandage. Twenty-four of 26 patients who underwent injection with procaine were back to work within a week. Asymptomatic nonunions were seen in seven of the 53 patients (53%)

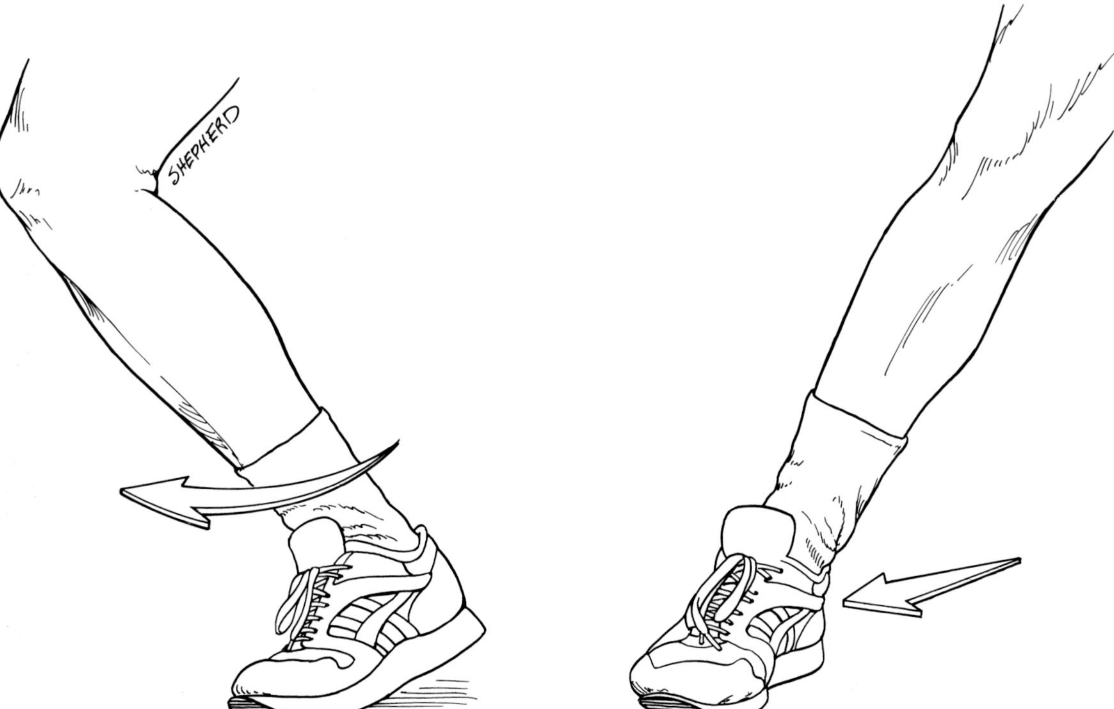

Figure 8. Mechanism of injury.

treated with injection and immediate weight bearing. Dameron's (8) series of 100 tuberosity fractures, treated with either elastic bandage or short leg walking cast, produced excellent results with either treatment. In this series there was a 99% union rate, with only one asymptomatic nonunion. A good long-term prognosis can be expected regardless of treatment method. The type of treatment is not felt to correlate with the length of time until the patient is pain free (21). Although the union rate for tuberosity fractures is high, asymptomatic nonunions require no further treatment.

Rettig et al. (22) reported on eight nonunions in young athletes. Five were treated with excision of the proximal fragment and three with screw fixation. All patients appeared to be improved postoperatively, but the authors have no preference between these treatments. Whether all the patients in the series of Rettig et al. (22) had acute fractures or nonunited apophysis was not clear, but this author has seen only two cases of a symptomatic nonunion in otherwise healthy middle-aged women. After approximately 8 months of conservative treatment, these patients complained of severely limiting lateral foot pain with ambulation, despite the use of prolonged casting. Radiographs demonstrated a nonunion of the tuberosity with sclerosis of the fracture edges. Because the proximal fragment included a large portion of the fifth metatarsal–cuboid articular surface (approximately 50% and 70%, respectively) open reduction, internal fixation with a 4.5-mm cannulated partially threaded cancellous screw, and local bone grafting were performed. Both patients were ambulating with discomfort 6 weeks postoperatively.

We prefer a hard-soled shoe and weight bearing as tolerated for initial treatment of fifth metatarsal tuberosity fractures.

Diaphyseal Fractures

Because most of the literature does not distinguish between zones II and III injuries, we will consider them together. The mechanism of injury for the diaphyseal fracture of the fifth metatarsal remains controversial and centers on whether these result from direct or indirect trauma. Although Carp's (7) observations of 21 fractures led him to the conclusion that six of 18 (33%) were the result of direct trauma, most of the literature supports an indirect mechanism. Jones' (4) original description proposed that a "cross-breaking stress directed anteriorly to the metatarsal base and caused by body pressure on an inverted foot while the heel is raised. . . ." was the responsible indirect force.

Stewart (1) made an important additional observation when he reported on two patients with bilateral fractures. These patients had symmetrical fracture patterns, suggesting the importance of local bone shape and strength in determining the effects of indirect trauma.

Kavanaugh et al. (23) evaluated 22 patients with a careful history of the initial incidence; none of his patients reported an inversion injury. Eleven of his patients recreated the position of their foot at the time of injury utilizing high-speed cinematology and force-platform analysis. These results show that forces are concentrated along the lateral column of the foot, in the region of the fifth metatarsal metaphysis, without an inversion injury.

The treatment of diaphyseal (zones II and III) fractures should be less cavalier than that of avulsion (zone I) fractures, as multiple studies have described a significant complication rate. In 1926, Carp (7) reported on one of the first large series of proximal diaphyseal fractures, including 13 fractures described to be at the base of the proximal phalanx. Four of these 13 fractures developed delayed unions, and Carp suggested that the limited blood supply was likely to be responsible.

Dameron (8) reported on the results of 20 fractures of the proximal metatarsal shaft, all initially treated nonoperatively. Fifteen fractures were "successfully" treated by nonoperative means, even though three fractures (20%) were still not radiographically healed at 1 year. Five patients (25%) eventually underwent a sliding bone grafting procedure for symptomatic nonunions; all healed by 10 weeks postoperatively.

Kavanaugh et al. (23) reported on a series of 23 proximal metaphyseal fractures. Eighteen patients were treated nonoperatively: 12 in short leg cases and six in soft compressive dressings. Twelve patients (67%) developed delayed unions, and nine eventually underwent intramedullary screw fixation at an average of 8 months after injury. Because of the prolonged healing time that characterizes these fractures, and the need for a timely return to activity, these authors recommended operative intervention for the athlete with a proximal fifth metatarsal fracture. Nonoperative treatment of a compressive dressing and weight bearing as tolerated was recommended for the nonathlete.

Torg and colleagues (24) reported on 46 fractures distal to the tuberosity of the fifth metatarsal. Clinical history and radiographic criteria were used to divide these fractures into three categories: 25 acute fractures, 12 delayed unions, and nine nonunions. Acute fractures were characterized by distinct radiographic fracture lines and absence of intramedullary sclerosis. Delayed unions showed a widened fracture line with intramedullary sclerosis. Nonunions were characterized by intramedullary sclerosis, which completely obliterated the medullary canal. Of the 15 acute fractures treated with a non-weight-bearing cast, 14 healed uneventfully at an average of 7 weeks. By contrast, of the ten acute fractures allowed to bear weight, only four went on to uncomplicated union. Six developed symptomatic nonunion, necessitating operative intervention with curettage and bone graft at an average of 11.5 months after the initial injury. Seven of ten delayed unions treated in a non-weight-bearing cast healed by 15.1 months. Three delayed unions required operative intervention to obtain bony union. The nine patients with nonunions were all treated with curettage and bone grafting. Eight of the nine (95%) healed at a mean of 12 weeks. One patient did not obtain radiographic union but was asymptomatic, and no further treatment was required. Torg et al. (24) concluded that an acute metatarsal diaphyseal fracture should be treated in a non-weight-bearing cast. Fractures with delayed union may eventually heal if treated conservatively, but active individuals and patients with nonunions should be treated by curettage and drilling of the medullary canal and bone grafting.

Josefsson and colleagues (25) reported on their treatment of 66 proximal diaphyseal fractures. Their series consisted of 27 acute fractures and 39 chronic fractures as determined by history and radiographic appearance. Forty-four patients were initially treated nonoperatively (35 bandaged and nine casted). Weight bearing was restricted in only six patients. With this treatment, only two of 17 (12%) of the acute fractures and eight of 27 (37%) of the chronic fractures eventually underwent operative fixation at an average of 7 months after their injury. All patients undergoing operative treatment eventually healed. Although medullary screw fixation had a 100% healing rate in this study, the authors felt that surgery was not necessary initially, because late surgical intervention still allowed complete functional recovery. Other series have had excellent results with nonoperative treatment. Zogby and Baker (26) had a 100% union in a series of ten diaphyseal fractures without any intramedullary sclerosis in non-weight-bearing short leg casts.

Clapper et al. (16) reported that of 25 diaphyeal fractures, seven eventually underwent operative treatment after failing treatment with a non-weight-bearing cast at an average of 25 weeks. These operative patients healed in half the time of nonoperative patients. These authors also believe that operative intervention is a ''low-risk'' procedure, with higher patient satisfaction than prolonged casting.

Mindrebo et al. (27) treated nine outpatients with acute proximal diaphyseal fractures with percutaneous intramedullary screw placement. They reported a 100% union rate, and patients were allowed to return to running at 5.5 weeks. There were no reported complications. Others have also reported similar rapid clinical healing with screw fixation (23).

Stress Fractures

The proximal portion of the fifth metatarsal is a region of high stress; this may lead to acute and chronic injuries. The chronic stress fracture is problematic (28) and is more likely to occur in the young, active individual. High-tensile stresses along the lateral border of the fifth metatarsal have been demonstrated by Roca et al. (29), using a photoelastic model. These stresses were accentuated by a 50-degree inclination of the position of the foot at toe-off. DeLee et al. (30) reported that 8 of 10 subjects in their series of stress fractures reported the pain was associated with pushoff.

Gross and Bunch (31) were able to measure stresses produced in the metatarsals of 21 runners. This analysis showed that the bending movements and shear stresses in the proximal fifth metatarsal were high, second only to those in the second metatarsal, another common location of stress fractures.

Although only one series in the literature looks specifically at patients with stress fractures (33), the reported delayed and nonunion rates are considered to be high (23,28). In the series of Kavanaugh et al. (23), nearly one-half of the patients reported prodromal symptoms suggestive of a stress injury. This series reported that 66.7% of the fractures treated nonoperatively (cast or elastic wrap) developed delayed union.

Similar to acute diaphyseal fractures, early operative intervention with screw fixation has led to rapid healing and fast return to activities. Delee et al. (30) reported on a series of ten athletes with stress fractures of the proximal fifth metatarsal. All ten patients described prodromal symptoms prior to the onset of acute pain and had radiographic evidence of a chronic injury (either medullary sclerosis or chronic periosteal reaction). Intermedullary screw fixation was utilized to achieve union by 4.5 weeks and return to competitive activities by 8.5 weeks. These results are similar to those of Kavanaugh et al. (23), in which the four patients treated with internal fixation returned to activities in 6 to 8 weeks, compared with 4 to 15 months in other patients in this series treated nonoperatively.

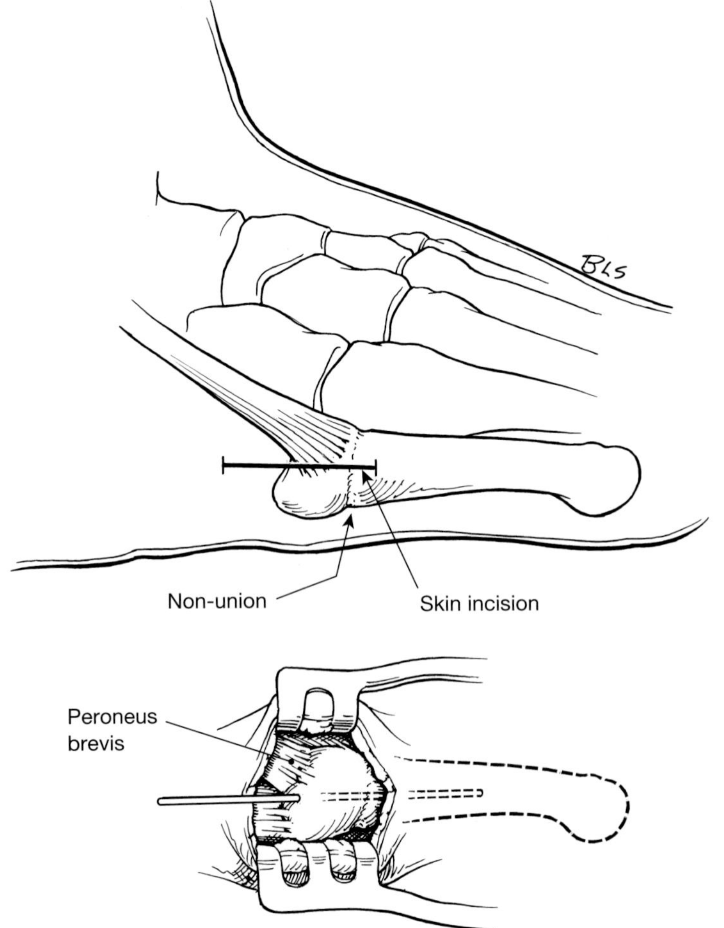

Figure 9. Basic operative technique.

SURGICAL TECHNIQUE

Although various techniques have been described for intramedullary screw fixation of fifth metatarsal fractures, we prefer a cannulated partially threaded cancellous 4.5-mm screw with fluoroscopic guidance.

Hardware selection is important, as smaller screws are subject to fatigue failure. If a partially threaded screw is not utilized, it is important to overdrill the proximal cortex. Screw head size is important, as the larger the head the more likely it is the screw will produce irritation with shoe wear, which may require removal at a later date.

The patient is placed in a supine position, with a bump under the ipsilateral hip to allow easy internal rotation of the leg. For nondisplaced fractures or stress fractures, a 2-cm incision is made dorsolaterally just proximal to the palpable fifth metatarsal tuberosity. The peroneus brevis tendon is located where it inserts into the fifth metatarsal. The tendon is either retracted superiorly, or divided in line with its fibers, to allow exposure of the proximal portion of the metatarsal. A guidewire is placed in the axilla where the tuberosity meets the metaphysis, similar to the starting point for a femoral rod in the piriformis fossa (Fig. 9). The guidewire is inserted down the medullary canal, checking the position with fluoroscopy using two views at 90 degrees to each other. The guidewire usually abuts the dorsomedial aspect of the distal metatarsal as it gently curves just proximal to the neck region. The guidewire is then measured and a 3.2-mm drill used for the entire length of the guidewire. The distal segment is tapped, the proximal segment is prepared with the countersink, and the appropriate screw is placed. Care is taken to ensure that all the screw threads have crossed the fracture site and that

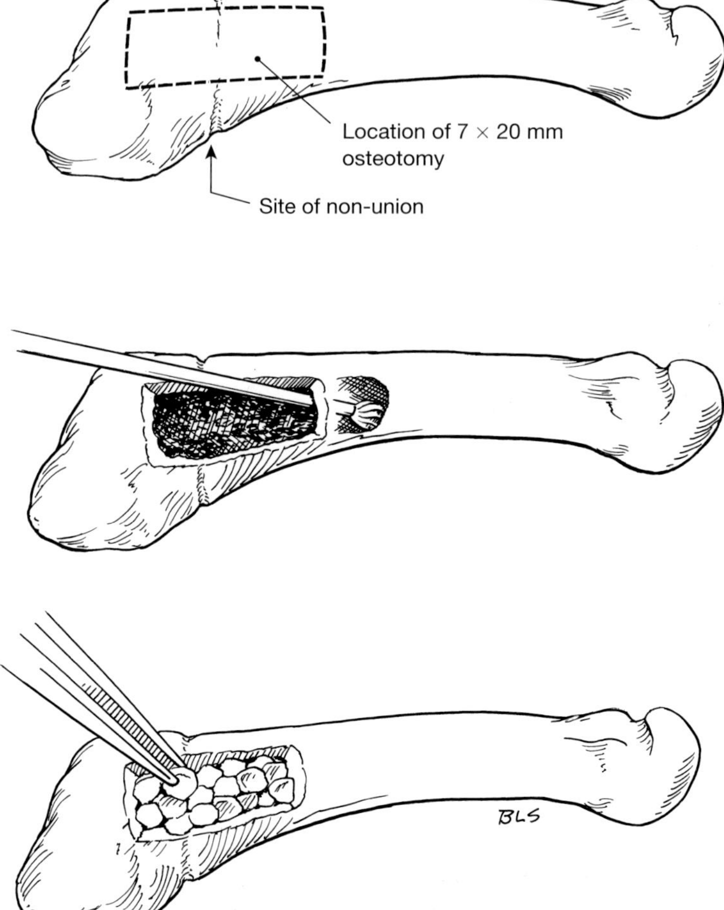

Figure 10. Bone graft technique.

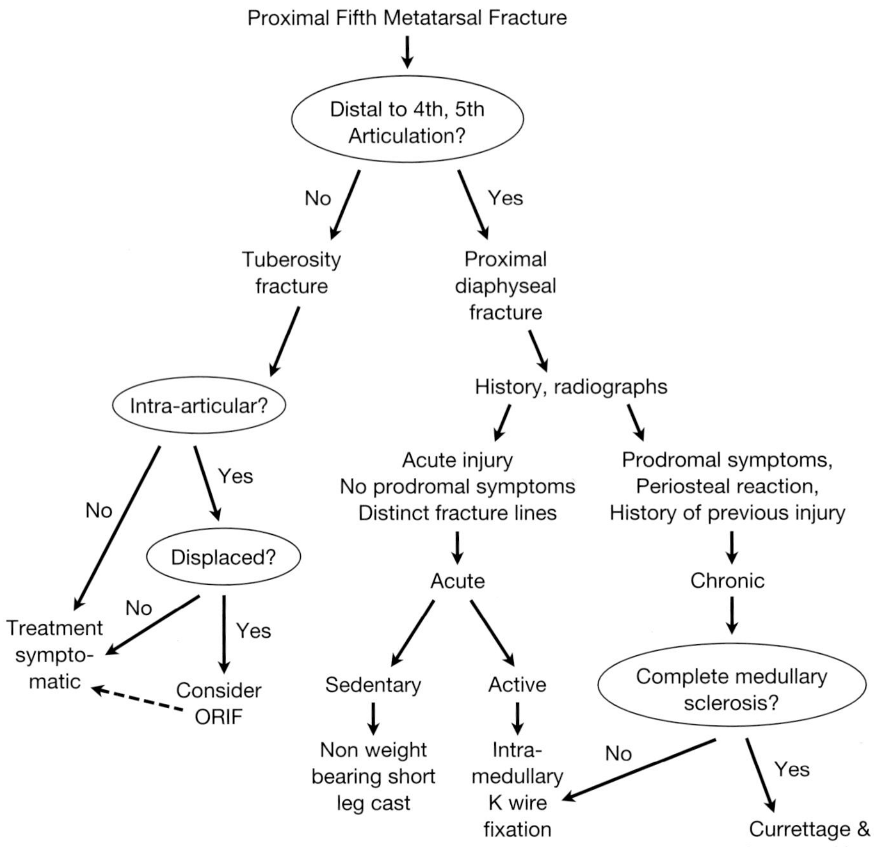

Figure 11. Algorithm.

overtightening of the screw does not result in stripping. In cases of nondisplaced or stress fractures, bone graft is supplied by the intramedullary canal reamings, and it is not necessary to open the fracture site (30). In cases of displaced fractures, the initial incision will often have to be extended more distally to allow exposure of the fracture site. In these cases, we prefer to make a longitudinal incision in the peroneus brevis tendon, which can be extended approximately 3 cm distally, in line with the tendon fibers, to allow exposure of the fracture. We debride the fibrous union, and sclerotic bone and recannulate the medullary canal with a drill or bur prior to screw insertion. A cancellous bone graft from either the medial malleolus or the cuboid is placed in and around the nonunion site prior to closure (Fig. 10). Dissection along the medial aspect of the metatarsal should be avoided so as not to disrupt the blood supply.

Postoperative care consists of non-weight-bearing treatment for 7 to 14 days until the wound heals. Weight bearing is then increased as tolerated in a hard-soled shoe, for a total of 6 weeks. Various weight-bearing schedules may be used, based on the patient's history, bone quality, and pain tolerance. Full return to activities is permitted with radiographic bony union.

CONCLUSIONS

We feel that most fractures of the proximal fifth metatarsal can be treated nonoperatively by limiting weight bearing in a wooden shoe for a period of approximately 1 month. A select group, classified as true acute Jones fractures or metaphyseal diaphyseal fractures, can be treated in non-weight-bearing casts for 6 weeks, and most will heal. In chronic cases or stress fractures, there is a higher incidence of nonunion, and these patients may be better treated with open reduction, bone grafting, and screw fixation (Fig. 11).

REFERENCES

1. Stewart IM. Jones's fracture: fracture of base of fifth metatarsal. *Clin Orthop* 1960;16:190–195.
2. Anderson LD. Injuries of the forefoot. *Clin Orthop* 1977;122:18–27.
3. Lichtblau S. Painful nonunion of a fracture of the fifth metatarsal. *Clin Orthop* 1968;59:171–175.
4. Jones R. Fractures of the base of the fifth metatarsal bone by indirect violence. *Ann Surg* 1902;35:697–700.
5. Wharton HR. Fracture of the proximal end of the fifth metatarsal bone. *Ann Surg* 1908;47:824–825.
6. Young JK. Discussion of Wharton H.R. Fracture of the proximal end of the fifth metatarsal bone. *Ann Surg* 1908;47:826.
7. Carp L. Fractures of the fifth metatarsal bone with special reference to delayed union. *Ann Surg* 1927;86:308–320.
8. Dameron TB Jr. Fractures and anatomical variations of the proximal portion of the fifth metatarsal. *J Bone Joint Surg [Am]* 1975;57A:788–792.
9. Lawrence SJ, Botte MJ. Jones' fractures and related fractures of the proximal fifth metatarsal. *Foot Ankle* 1993;14:358–365.
10. Hamilton WG. Surgical anatomy of the foot and ankle. CIBA Clin Symp 1985;37:1–32.
11. Clemente CD. *Anatomy, a regional atlas of the human body,* 2nd ed. Baltimore: Urban and Schwarzenberg, 1981:435–447.
12. Hoerr, Pyle, Francis. Regularly occurring and accessory bone growth center. In *Radiologic atlas of skeletal development of the foot and ankle.* Springfield, IL: Charles C. Thomas, 1962:41–42.
13. Coughlin MJ. Sesamoids and accessory bone of the foot. In: Mann RA and Coughlin MJ, eds. *Surgery of the foot and ankle.* St. Louis: Mosby, 1993:5, 530.
14. Shereff MJ, Yang QM, Kummer FJ, Frey CC, Greenidge N. Vascular anatomy of the fifth metatarsal. *Foot Ankle* 1991;11:350–353.
15. Smith JW, Arnoczky SP, Hersh A. The intraosseous blood supply of the fifth metatarsal: implications for proximal fracture healing. *Foot Ankle* 1992;13:143–152.
16. Clapper MF, O'Brien TJ, Lyons PM. Fractures of the fifth metatarsal: analysis of a fracture registry. *Clin Orthop* 1995;315:238–241.
17. Rockwood CA Jr, Green DP. *Fractures,* vol. 2. Philadelphia: JB Lippincott, 1975:1472.
18. Jahss MH. *Disorders of the foot,* vol 2. Philadelphia: WB Saunders, 1982:1456.
19. Pearson JB. Fractures of the base of the fifth metatarsal. *BMJ* 1962;1:1052–1054.
20. Richli WR, Rosenthal DI. Avulsion fracture of the fifth metatarsal: experimental study of pathomechanics. *AJR* 1984;143:889–891.
21. Dameron TB Jr. Fractures of the proximal fifth metatarsal: selecting the best treatment option. *J Am Acad Orthop Surg* 1995;3:110–114.
22. Rettig AC, Shelbourne KD, Wilckens J. The surgical treatment of symptomatic nonunions of the proximal (metaphyseal) fifth metatarsal in athletes. *Am J Sports Med* 1992;20:50–54.
23. Kavanaugh JH, Brower TD, Mann RV. The Jones fracture revisited. *J Bone Joint Surg [Am]* 1978;60:776–782.
24. Torg JS, Balduini FC, Zelko RR, Pavlov H, Peff TC, Das M. Fractures of the base of the fifth metatarsal distal to the tuberosity. *J Bone Joint Surg [Am]* 1984;66:209–214.
25. Josefsson PO, Karlsson M, Redlund-Johnell I, Wandeberg B. Jones fracture. Surgical versus nonsurgical treatment. *Clin Orthop* 1994;299:252–255.
26. Zogby RG, Baker BE. A review of non-operative treatment of Jones fracture. *Am J Sports Med* 1987;15:304–307.
27. Mindrebo N, Shelbourne KD, VanMeter CD, Rettig AC. Outpatient percutaneous screw fixation of the acute Jones fracture. *Am J Sports Med* 1993;21:720–723.
28. Monteleone GP Jr. Stress fractures in the athlete. *Orthop Clin North Am* 1995;26:423–432.
29. Roca J, Roure F, Fernandez-Fairen M, Yunta A. Stress fractures of the fifth metatarsal. *Acta Orthop Belg* 1980;46:630–636.
30. Delee JC, Evans JP, Julian J. Stress fracture of the fifth metatarsal. *Am J Sports Med* 1983;11:349–353.
31. Gross TS, Bunch RP. A mechanical model of metatarsal stress fracture during distance running. *Am J Sports Med* 1989;17:669–674.

EDITORIAL COMMENTS

Fractures of the Proximal Fifth Metatarsal

Alan S. Tuckman, Samuel S. Fleming, John G. Seiler, III, and Lamar L. Fleming

In proximal fifth metatarsal injuries, the particular vascular and ligamentous anatomy makes appropriate classification of injury imperative. One needs to determine whether there is articular involvement, avulsion of the peroneus brevis, or a metaphyseal diaphyseal fracture with its inherent prolonged healing and decreased blood supply. Malangulation is usually not a problem with these injuries. Therefore, the key is to recognize when total immobilization is needed versus screw fixation or no immobilization at all. A zone of avascularity occurs in the metaphyseal–diaphyseal junction because the nutrient artery inserts medial into the junction of the proximal and midportions of the metatarsal tarsal. Therefore, fractures identified in this area should be treated by more prolonged immobilization or, if the situation warrants it, by appropriate screw fixation. In our hands, screw fixation can be done very well using percutaneous methods, with only exposure of the tuberosity of the fifth metatarsal. We do not believe that bone grafting acute fractures is necessary, and stripping the periosteal or extraosseous blood supply would not be appropriate in this area of relative avascularity. One must be careful that the screw remains in the intermedullary canal and does not create a stress riser in other portions, particularly in the athletic population. Dr. Lamar Fleming and his coauthors have covered this topic in great depth and have given it the attention that I believe it deserves. I do not believe that every ''athlete'' deserves open reduction, but this procedure should be used in particular circumstances that justify the prolonged healing and disability. We have seen many patients sent back to athletic events too quickly who went on to experience refracture or delayed union, even in the face of appropriate fixation techniques.

Robert S. Adelaar, M.D.

Complex Foot and Ankle Trauma,
edited by Robert S. Adelaar,
Lippincott–Raven Publishers, Philadelphia © 1999.

19

Athletic Injuries of the Great Toe MTP Joint

Michael W. Bowman

The great toe is capable of many tasks. During the pushoff phase of normal gait and walking down steps, it must bear up to two times total body weight. The great toe is capable of great dexterity, as seen in the prehensile ability of a patient with congenital absence of the upper extremities. Athletics also requires strength from the hallux in activities such as jumping and spring board diving (up to seven times total body weight), as well as speed (sprinting) and control (ballet, Tae Kwon Do, power weight lifting).

ANATOMY AND BIOMECHANICS

Joint Anatomy

The metatarsophalangeal joint (MTPJ) is a condylar, cam-shaped, hinge-like joint, allowing dorsiflexion and plantarflexion (Fig. 1). The shape of the MTPJ varies widely when viewed from the anteroposterior (AP) direction (1) and may range from flat (a cylindrical joint) to rounded (a spherical joint) (Fig. 2). Hardy and Clapham (2), others (3), and personal experience have shown that the ''flattened'' MTPJ often allows less dorsiflexion and plantarflexion and has greater stability, which may predispose it to athletic injury. The flattened MTPJs often allow only a few degrees of abduction and adduction, whereas the spherical joints may allow up to 15 degrees of abduction and adduction.

M. W. Bowman: Department of Orthopaedic Surgery, University of Pittsburgh Medical Center, Pittsburgh, Pennsylvania 15206; Department of Orthopaedic Surgery, Allegheny University of Health Sciences, Pittsburgh, Pennsylvania 15212; and Consultant, Pittsburgh Steelers Professional Football Club, Pittsburgh, Pennsylvania.

Reprinted with permission from Bowman MW. Athletic injuries of the great toe metatarsal joint. In: Monograph: *Disorders of the great toe.* Rosemont, IL: AAOS, 1997:1–22.

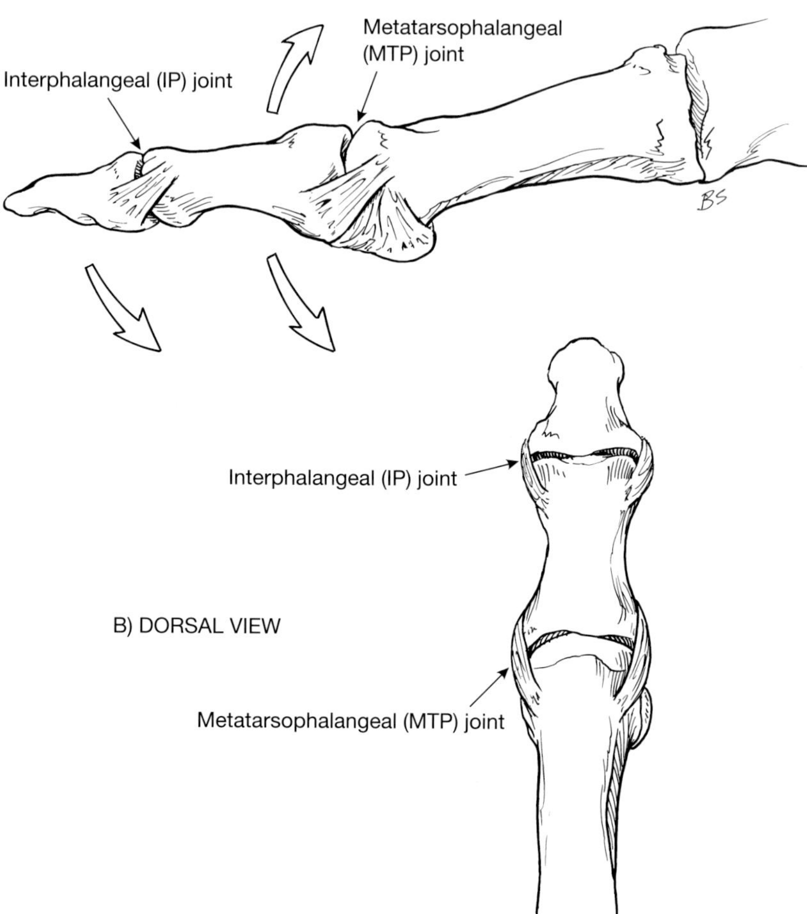

Figure 1. MTP joint and IP joint anatomy of the great toe. **A:** Dorsal view. **B:** Lateral view.

The absolute big toe MTPJ range of motion and distribution of that range of motion in an individual is highly variable. Joseph's (4) study in 1954 showed that the great toe MTPJ and interphalangeal joint (IPJ) were in mean resting positions of 16 and 12 degrees of dorsiflexion, respectively, during normal stance. The mean *active MTPJ dorsiflexion* was 51 degrees (10 to 80 degrees), and the mean *passive MTPJ dorsiflexion* was 84 degrees (40 to 100 degrees) during pushoff or a crouch-type position. The mean *MTPJ active plantar flexion* was 23 degrees (3 to 43 degrees). Note that passive dorsal flexibility of the first MTPJ in the standing weight-bearing position may be less than in the ''tip-toe'' or crouch position due to the windlass effect of the plantar fascia.

Thus, the mean total available MTPJ range of motion (active plus passive) during gait is 107 degrees (43 to 143 degrees). Approximately 60 degrees of MTP dorsiflexion is utilized during normal gait (5). Athletes, consciously or unconsciously, may accommodate up to 50% reduction in MTPJ motion due to hallux rigidus or stiff shoewear by various gait adjustments (foot/leg external rotation, shortened stride, increased ankle, knee, hip motion). As shown by Sammarco (6), the instant center of MTPJ motion is located within the metatarsal head (Fig. 3) near the isometric origin of the collateral ligament, changing slightly during dorsiflexion/plantarflexion due to the cam-like curvature of the metatarsal head. With increased flexion there is tightening of the collateral ligaments.

The IPJ of the great toe is a highly stable, condylar, hinge-like joint. Due to firm collateral ligaments and joint stability, only a few degrees of abduction/adduction are

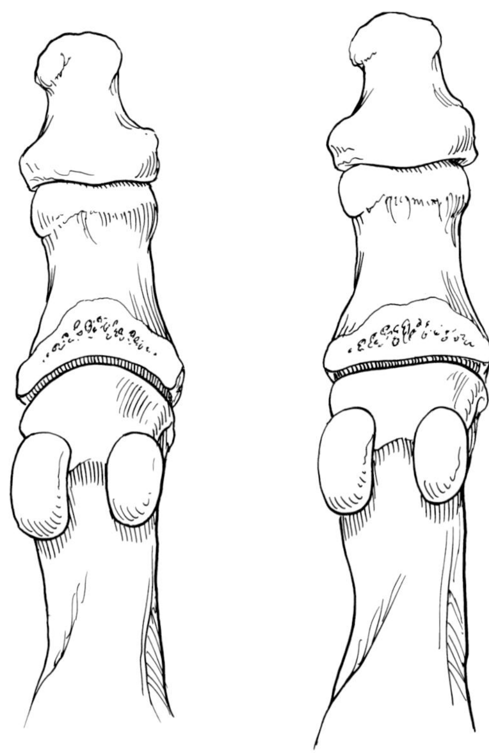

Figure 2. Variations in shape of the first metatarsal head. **A:** Spherical MTPJ. **B:** "Flattened" MTPJ. (From ref. 1, with permission.)

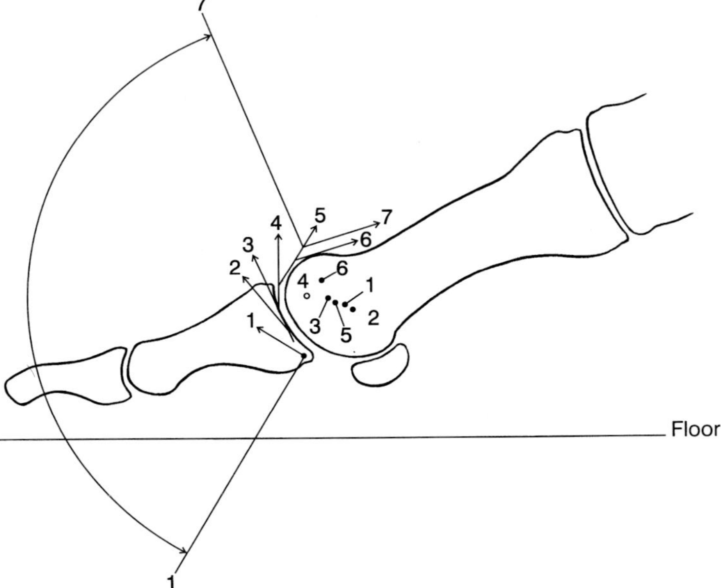

Figure 3. Biomechanics of the great toe MTPJ. Each *arrow* indicating direction from 1 to 7 (flexion to extension) corresponds to the instant center of motion in the first metatarsal head (*numbered dots*). MTPJ gliding takes place until MTPJ compression occurs near full MTPJ extension (6 and 7). (From ref. 6, with permission.)

permitted. As shown by Joseph (4), means of 12 degrees of *active dorsiflexion* and 40 degrees of *passive dorsiflexion* occur at the IPJ. A mean of 48 degrees (0 to 86 degrees) of *active plantar flexion* is possible at the IP joint. Some athletes with hallux limitus may have compensatory hypermobility of the IPJ.

Capsular–Ligamentous–Sesamoid Complex

The MTPJ has minimal stability provided by the normally spherical joint itself. Most MTPJ stability is provided by the ligaments and the capsular structure. The *medial capsular ligament* (MCL) and *lateral capsular ligament* (LCL) are fan-shaped structures originating from the dorsal aspect of the medial and lateral metatarsal heads, respectively (Fig. 1). The MCL and LCL insert into the medial and lateral base of the proximal phalanx, but also into the thick plantar MTPJ capsule or *plantar plate.* As is discussed later, the MCL and LCL are also attached to the abductor and adductor muscles, which aid in MTPJ stability. These medial and lateral capsular ligaments may be attenuated or injured by athletic injury, inflammatory arthritis, or repetitive stretching, resulting in hallux valgus or hallux varus deformity.

The dorsal capsule of the MTP joint is usually very thin and structurally weak. The plantar capsule, however, is a very thick and specialized structure with a firm attach-

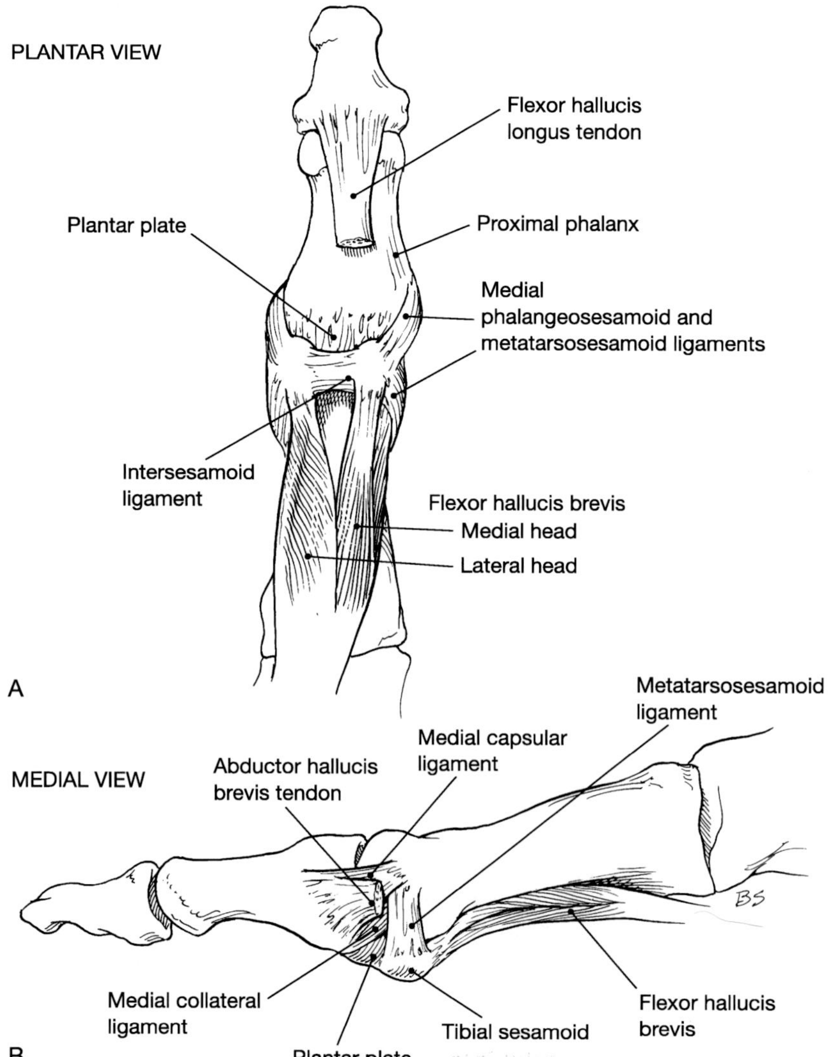

Figure 4. The capsulo–ligamentous–sesamoid complex of the hallux. **A:** Plantar view. **B:** Medial view.

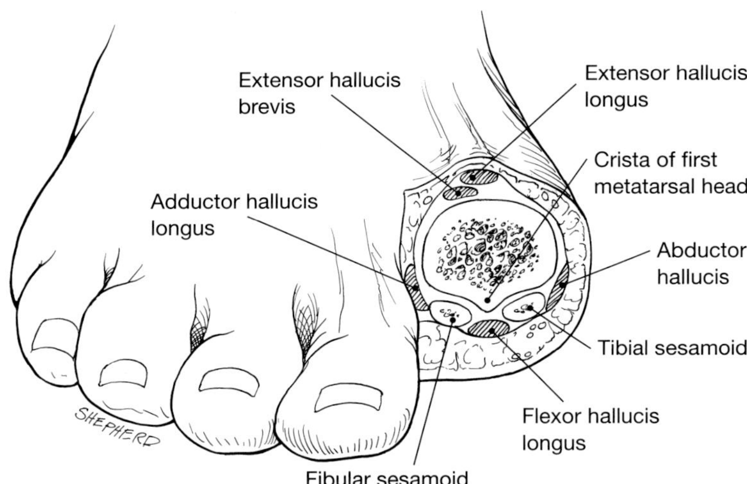

Figure 5. Cross section of the capsulo–ligamentous–sesamoid complex.

ment to the base of the proximal phalanx (plantar plate) and a thinner, more flexible attachment to the undersurface of the first metatarsal head (Fig. 4). Imbedded in this capsuloligamentous structure are the *medial and lateral sesamoids,* which are partially exposed, articulating with the undersurface of the metatarsal head. There are two shallow grooves in the plantar surface of the metatarsal head where the sesamoids glide, separated by a bony ridge or *crista* (Fig. 5). Several ligamentous thickenings of this capsular structure exist such as the *intersesamoidal ligament,* and the *metatarsosesamoid ligaments* (Fig. 4). The two heads of the *flexor hallucis brevis* muscle also insert into this capsuloligamentous complex, partially enveloping the sesamoids. The *flexor hallucis longus* runs in a tendon sheath between and slightly plantar to the sesamoids and medial and lateral heads of the flexor hallucis brevis.

It is this complex but sturdy musculocapsular ligamentous complex that provides the true stability to the MTPJ. As is discussed later, this complex also receives the brunt of athletic injuries to the great toe.

Muscular Attachments of the First MTP Joint

The *extensor hallucis longus* originates in the pretibial area and runs underneath the extensor retinaculum to lie dorsal to the MTPJ. Its insertion is the base of the distal phalanx. It primarily extends the IPJ and secondarily extends the MTPJ. This muscle usually extends fibers attaching to the extensor apparatus of the MTP joint (Fig. 6B), but variations exist in which a direct attachment of the extensor hallucis longus to the base of the proximal phalanx is seen (7).

The *extensor hallucis brevis* runs obliquely from the fascia covering the sinus tarsi to attach to the extensor apparatus on the dorsum of the MTP joint. Its primary function is extension of the MTP joint. Accessory extensor tendon slips are occasionally noted on the dorsum of the MTP joint.

The *flexor hallucis longus* (Fig. 6A) originates in the posterior medial calf, runs directly posterior to the ankle joint around the medial malleolus, crosses the flexor digitorum longus at the Master Knot of Henry, and then runs between the two heads of the flexor hallucis brevis, between the sesamoids to attach to the plantar surface of the distal phalanx. Its primary function is to flex the IPJ and secondarily flex the MTPJ. Interconnections can exist between the flexor hallucis longus and the flexor digitorum longus.

There are three intrinsic muscles of the great toe, the flexor hallucis brevis, the abductor hallucis and the adductor hallucis (Fig. 6A). The *flexor hallucis brevis* is divided into a medial and lateral head. The *lateral* portion originates from the plantar capsule of the calcaneocuboid joint and plantar surface of the lateral cuneiform and

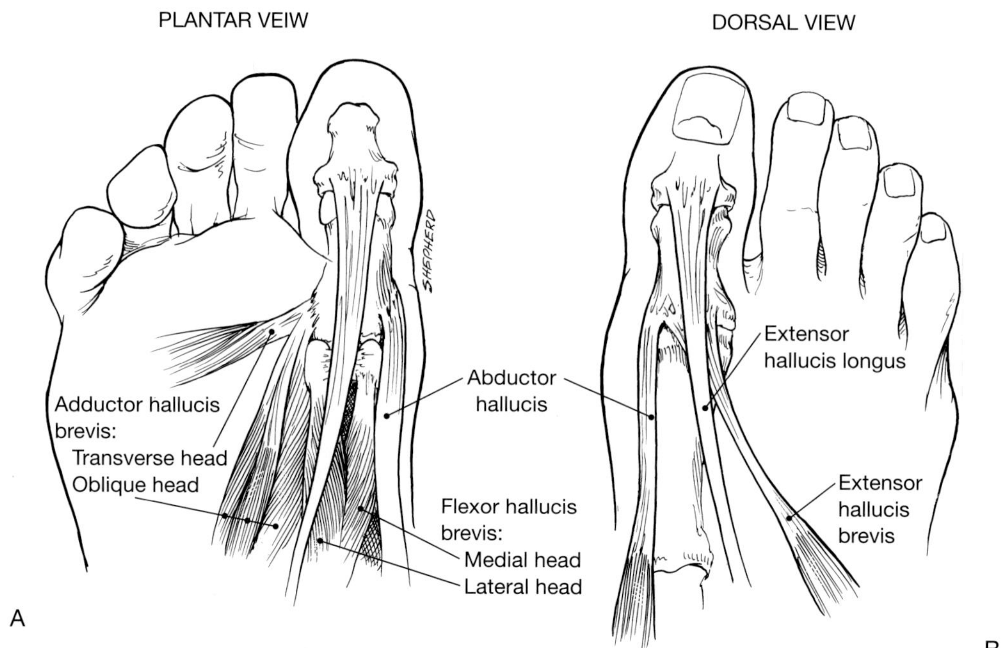

Figure 6. Musculotendinous attachments of the great toe. **A:** Plantar view. **B:** Dorsal view.

attaches distally to the lateral or fibula sesamoid complex, which, in turn, attaches to the base of the proximal phalanx. The *medial* half of the Y-shaped origin of the flexor hallucis brevis originates from the sheath of the posterior tibial tendon. The medial head of the flexor hallucis brevis attaches to the medial sesamoid and medial half of the plantar plate, along with fibers from the abductor hallucis. The flexor hallucis brevis provides important strong plantar flexion of the MTPJ, important for athletic activities such as jumping, spring board diving, sprinting, etc. It also provides critical stability to the MTP joint.

The *abductor hallucis* originates from the medial tuberosity of the os calcis, extending distally to cover the lower half of the tarsal tunnel and inserting into the MCL, the medial sesamoid complex, and the plantar plate. It provides abduction of the MTPJ and, more importantly, resistance to valgus stresses on the great toe.

The *adductor hallucis* is composed of an oblique head and transverse head. The *oblique head* originates broadly from the base of the second, third, and fourth metatarsals and corresponding tarsometatarsal plantar ligaments. It runs alongside the lateral head of the flexor hallucis brevis, dorsal to the deep intermetatarsal transverse ligament, and inserts into the lateral sesamoid, plantar plate, lateral base of the proximal phalanx, and LCL.

The *transverse head* of the adductor hallucis originates from the plantar plate of the third, fourth, and fifth MTPJs, corresponding deep transverse intermetatarsal ligaments, and part of the plantar aponeurosis to the third, fourth, and fifth toes. It runs dorsal to the deep transverse intermetatarsal ligament of the great toe and inserts into the lateral sesamoid, the extensor aponeurosis of the great toe MTPJ, and the fibrous sheath of the flexor hallucis longus and joins the fibers of the oblique head. Together, the two heads of the adductor hallucis provide for adduction of the great toe MTPJ and resist varus stress on it.

Neurovascular Supply to the Great Toe

Dorsally, arterial blood of the great toe is supplied by branches of the *first dorsal metatarsal artery* (Fig. 7) and perforating branches in the first web space. *Plantar medial* and *lateral hallucial arteries* (Fig. 8) exist in several variations, usually as

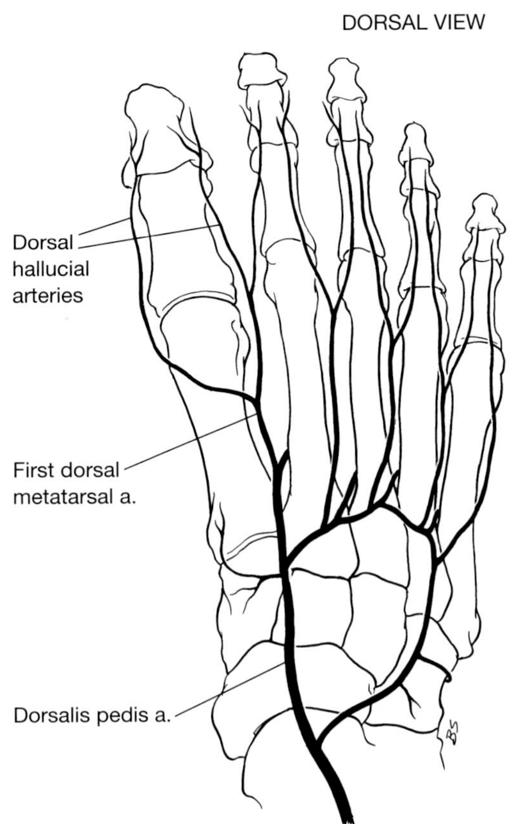

Figure 7. Dorsal arterial supply of the great toe.

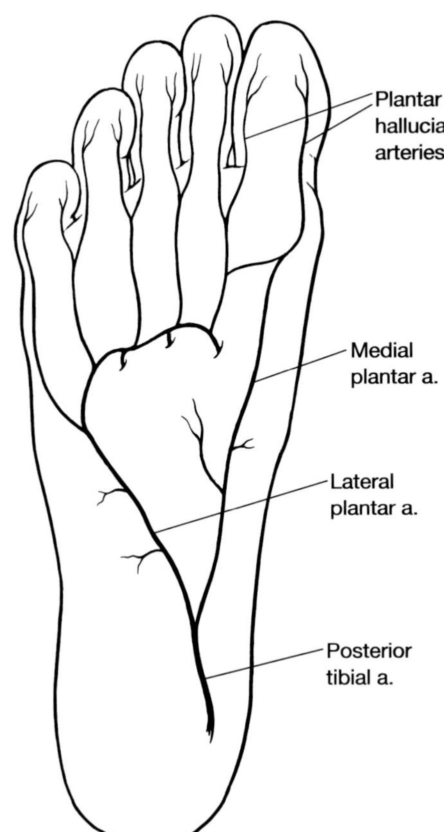

Figure 8. Plantar arterial supply of the great toe.

branches of the medial plantar artery. Various communications exist between the dorsal and plantar arterial supplies (7).

Sensation to the dorsum and dorsal medial aspect of the great toe (Fig. 9) is supplied by the *medial dorsal cutaneous branch* of the *superficial peroneal nerve.* Sensation to the first web space and dorsal lateral aspect of the great toe is usually supplied by the *deep peroneal nerve.* The *medial and lateral plantar hallucial nerves* (Fig. 10) run alongside the medial and lateral sesamoids, respectively, and supply sensation to the plantar aspect of the great toe. They may be stretched or compromised by injuries to the sesamoid–capsular complex and subsequent surgeries.

CLASSIFICATION AND MECHANISM OF INJURY

Most acute great toe athletic injuries occur during ''stop-and-go'' cutting, contact sports such as football, soccer, rugby, or basketball. However, athletic activities such as gymnastics, tennis, ballet, and basketball have also produced injuries of the great toe (8–13). Most reports of athletic great toe injuries concern National Football League (NFL) (14,15) and collegiate football players (3,5,16–19).

The incidence of athletic MTPJ injuries is significant, ranking third in games-missed injuries behind ankle and knee injuries at major universities (3,5,16–18). Coker et al. (3,18) noted six cases per year at the University of Arkansas. The ankle to toe injury ratio was 4:1, but both ankle and great toe injuries resulted in equal lost time, indicating that great toe injuries tend to be more disabling!

Athletic injuries of the great toe may be categorized as acute, subacute (acute injuries superimposed on chronic MTPJ pathology), and chronic (Table 1). The most common mechanisms of athletic MTPJ injury are hyperextension, hyperflexion, and valgus injury. A rare varus injury to the MTPJ has been noted (12). Preexisting conditions such

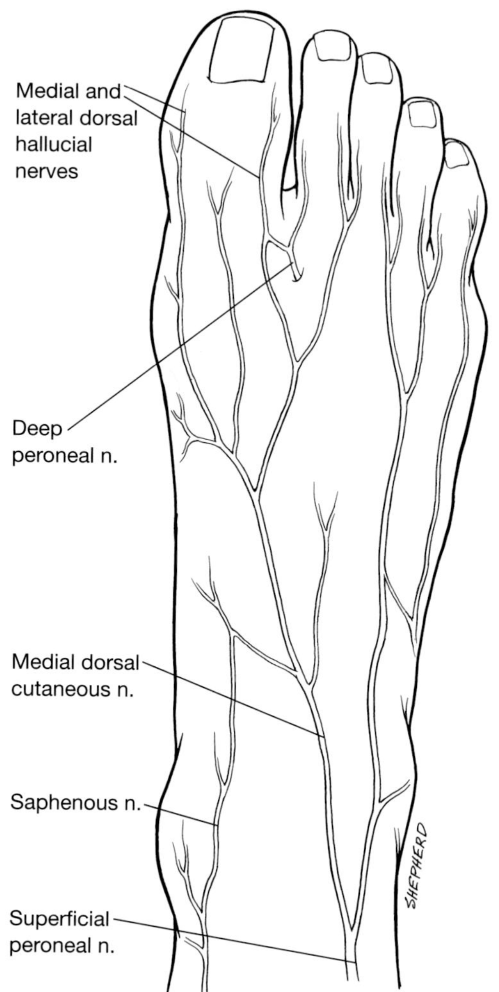

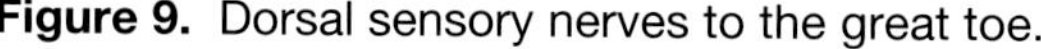

Figure 9. Dorsal sensory nerves to the great toe.

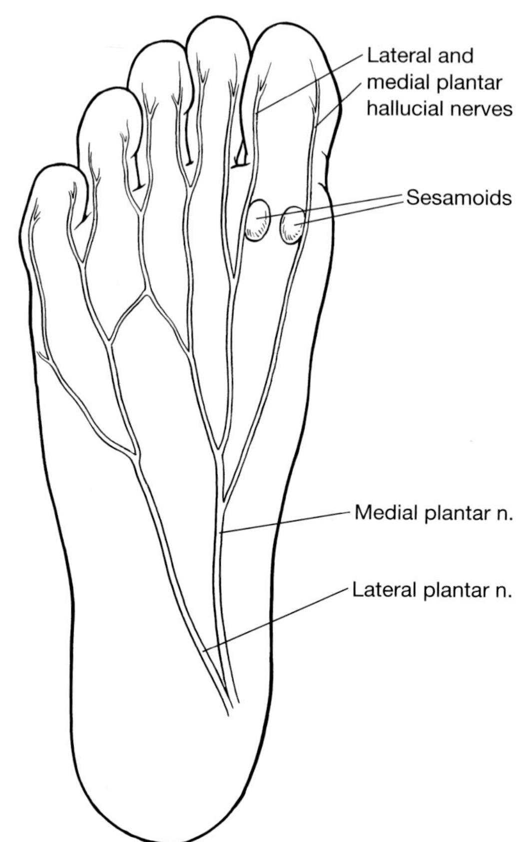

Figure 10. Plantar sensory nerves to the great toe.

Table 1. *Classification of athletic MTPJ injuries*

- I Acute MTPJ injuries
  - A. Soft tissue
    1. Capsuloligamentous tear
    2. Total MTPJ dislocation
    3. Cartilage "bruise"
    4. Cartilage avulsion/loose body
  - B. Soft tissue and bony injury
    1. Avulsion fracture
    2. Intraarticular fracture
    3. Sesamoid fracture
    4. Separation of bipartite sesamoid
    5. MTPJ fracture/dislocation
- II Subacute MTPJ injuries (acute on chronic injuries)/chronic MTPJ injuries
  - A. Hallux rigidus
    1. Cartilaginous
    2. Bony
  - B. Hallux valgus

as hallux rigidus or hallux valgus may render the great toe vulnerable to lesser or repetitive trauma.

The most commonly reported mechanism of injury to the great toe MTPJ is *hyperextension.* A very common scenario is a running athlete trapped under a ''pile-up'' with the MTPJ hyperextended, heel in the air, and another player or players falling on the outstretched leg, applying a severe dorsiflexion force (Fig. 11). Another scenario is a back-pedaling player, such as a lineman, forced backward onto a hyperextended MTP joint (Fig. 12). Runners may step into a pothole and suffer sudden hyperextension as well.

In these situations the normal gliding hinge-like motion of the MTPJ is stopped by the capsuloligamentous constraints discussed above. At this point, compression forces are applied to the dorsum of the base of the proximal phalanx and metatarsal head, resulting in either cartilage tears and bruising or an osteochondral defect. The plantar capsuloligamentous complex may be disrupted, the sesamoids may fracture, or bipartite sesamoids may be pulled apart with this injury (15,20,21) (Fig. 13). Instability may result, progressing in severe cases to frank dislocation. Bleeding, swelling, and a painful MTPJ results, limiting the ability to walk, run and push off. This soft tissue ''sprain'' of the MTPJ was termed *turf toe* by Bowers and Martin (16) and has come to represent all athletic capsuloligamentous injuries of the great toe.

Subacute or chronic cases of hyperextension injury to the great toe MTPJ may occur from repetitive hyperextension in sports such as running or tennis. Early hallux limitus with MTPJ tenderness, swelling, and stiffness may result. It is theorized that continuous MTPJ hyperextension exceeds the capacity of the normal gliding MTPJ motion and produces dorsal cartilage and bony compression. The dorsal base of the proximal phalanx is levered against the dorsal cartilage of the first metatarsal head. This probably produces the dorsal cartilaginous ''bump'' of the first metatarsal head seen in early or *cartilaginous hallux limitus* (Fig. 14), as well as cartilage erosion on both sides of the dorsal one-third of the metatarsal phalangeal joint (Fig. 15). Dorsal MTPJ synovitis is also noted on arthroscopy or arthrotomy.

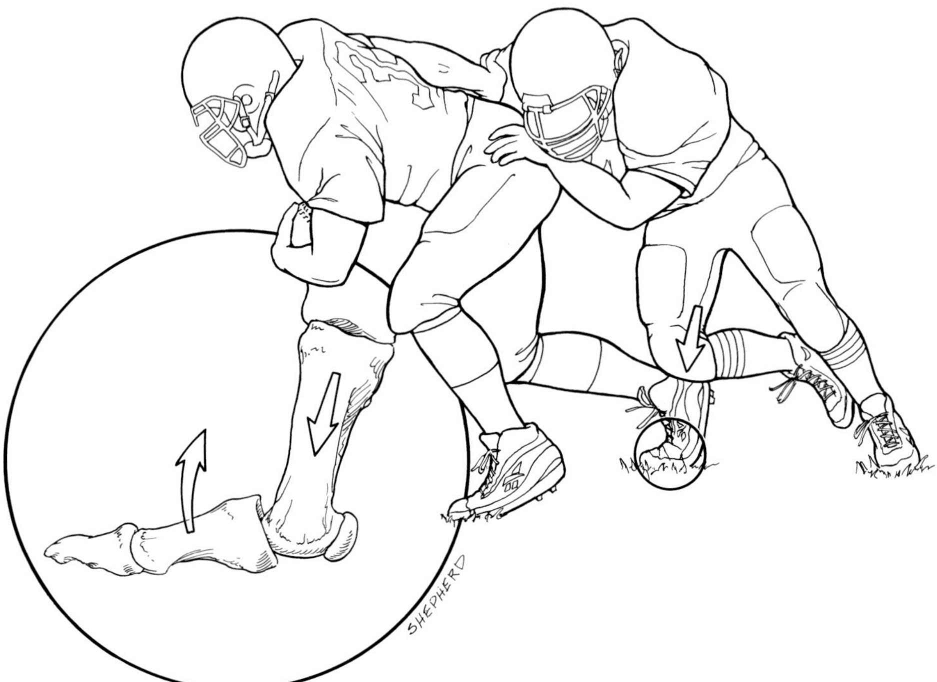

Figure 11. Hyperextension turf toe injury: a player at the bottom of a ''pile-up'' sustains an axial load to an already extended MTPJ.

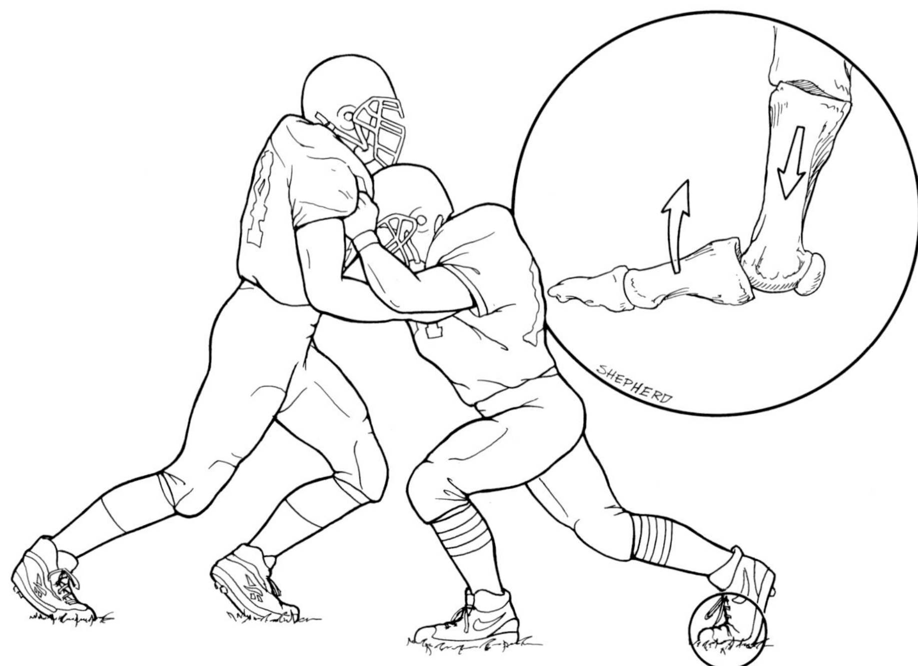

Figure 12. Hyperextension turf toe injury: forced back into a crouch position by an opposing lineman, the MTP joint becomes hyperextended.

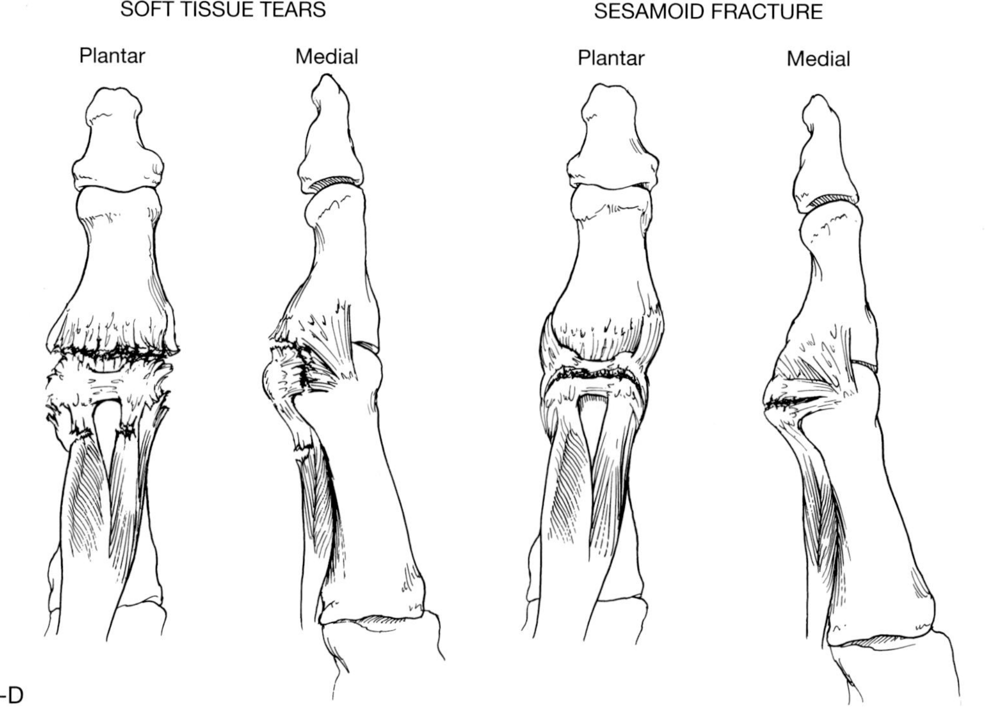

Figure 13. The pathology of turf toe injuries. **A,B:** Plantar and medial views of a soft tissue injury. **C,D:** Plantar and medial views of a sesamoid fracture.

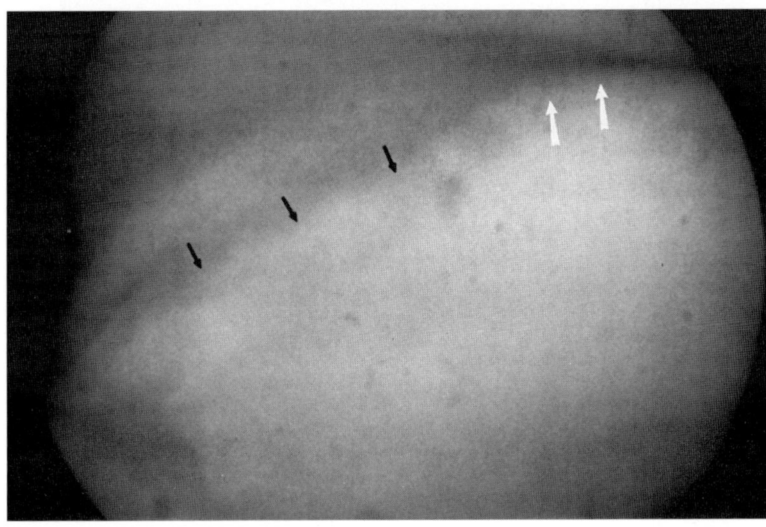

Figure 14. Arthroscopic view of cartilaginous hallux limitus. *Small black arrow,* cartilage depression in the first metatarsal head; *white arrows,* cartilaginous "bump."

Bony hallux limitus, an adult acquired condition, with bony spurs on the dorsum of the proximal phalanx and first metatarsal head, is probably a progression of the above problem (Fig. 16). Onset of symptoms is usually gradual but may be exacerbated by an acute upon a chronic injury.

The second most common mechanism of acute great toe MTPJ athletic injury is a *hyperflexion* injury. In this scenario, a player may be tackled from behind, pushing the player forward and producing flexion of the knee and plantarflexion of the foot (Fig. 17). In this particular case, the dorsal capsule may be torn and plantar cartilaginous compression injuries may result to the metatarsal head and proximal phalanx. Another possible scenario is a basketball, football, or rugby-type player landing on a plantar-flexed foot after a jump and either rolling over another player or being pushed forward on landing, resulting in hyperflexion of the MTPJ. Chronic or acute injuries of this sort may also be seen in young ballet dancers, who do not possess adequate strength and control while en pointe (9).

The third most common mechanism of acute MTPJ injury occurs when a *valgus force* is applied to the great toe MTPJ. Running backs, soccer players, basketball play-

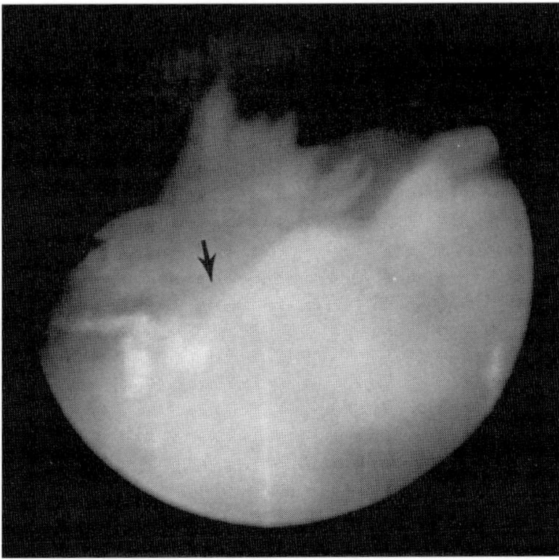

Figure 15. Arthroscopic view of osteochondral defect (*arrow*) and cartilage fibrillation on the dorsal surface of the first metatarsal head.

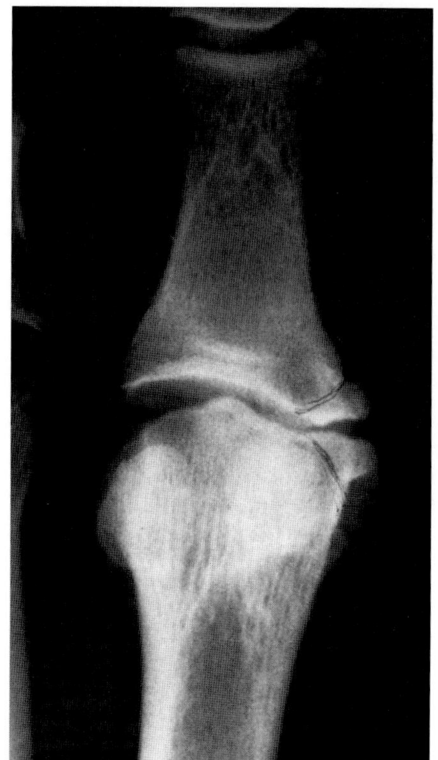

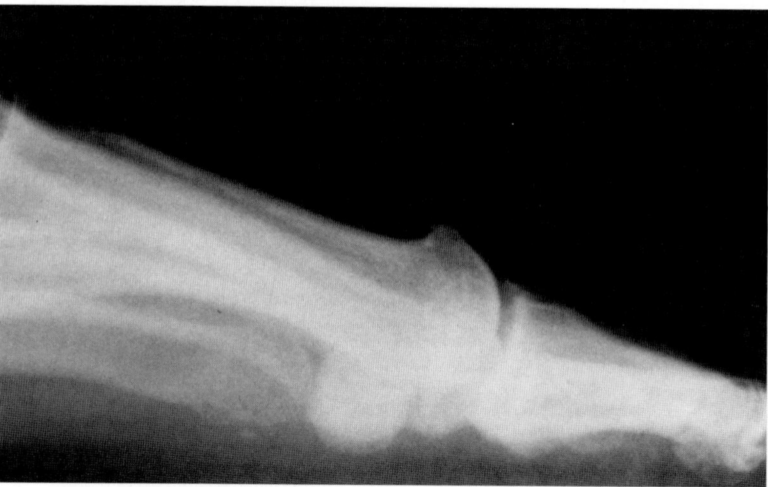

Figure 16. NFL Hall of Fame defensive linebacker with a history of "turf toe" injuries. AP and lateral radiograph showing MTPJ joint space narrowing and dorsal osteophytes.

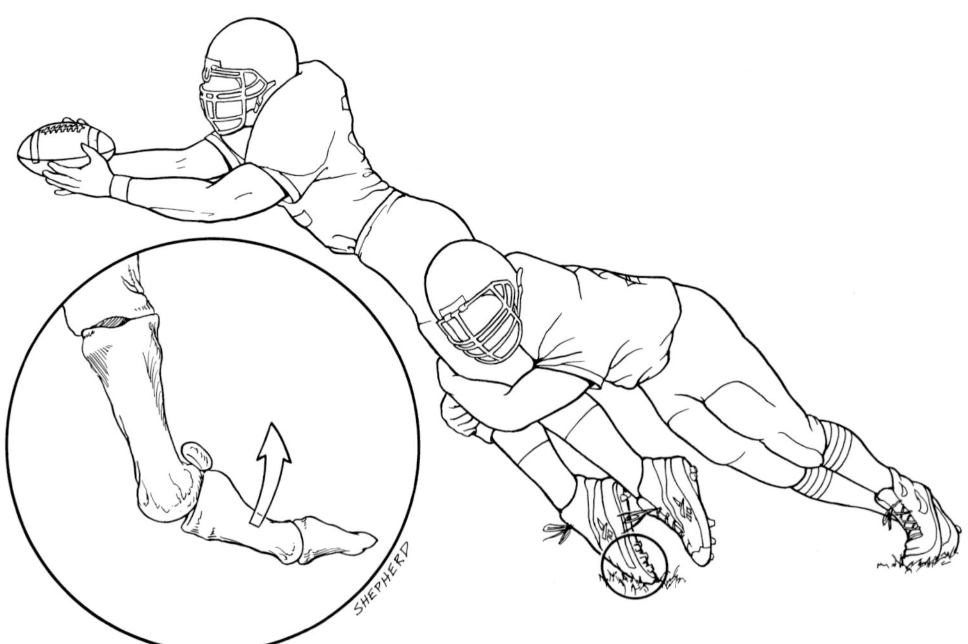

Figure 17. Hyperflexion turf toe injury: player is hit from behind, falling on flexed MTPJ.

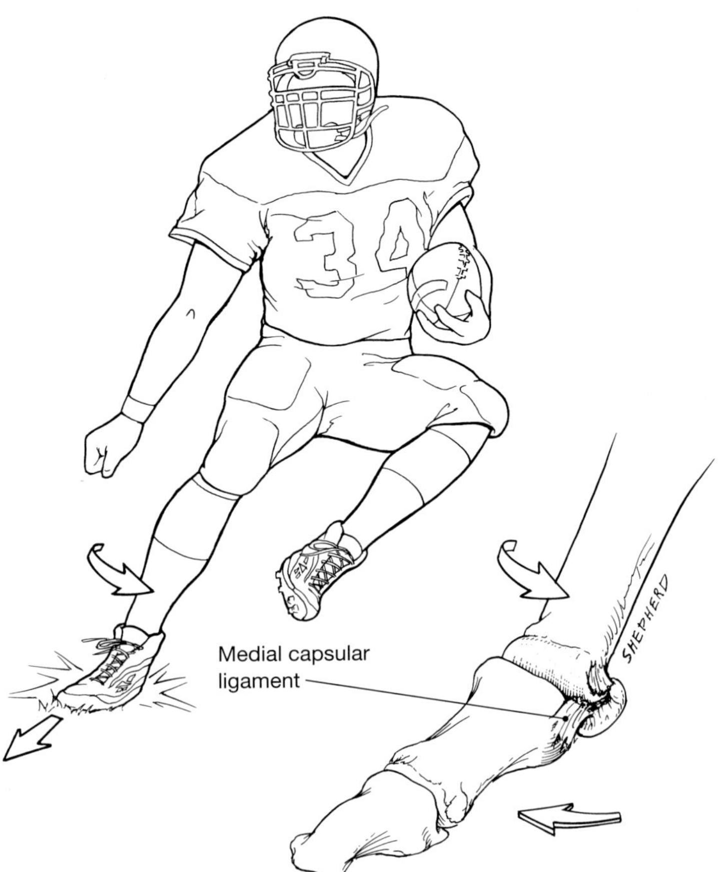

Figure 18. Valgus turf toe injury: player plants firmly on the foot and rotates internally to change direction, producing a valgus force on the hallux.

ers, and others who plant firmly on the forefoot and then internally rotate with pushoff to change directions acutely (Fig. 18), while running and deaccelerating at full speed, may produce a valgus twist type of injury to the great toe, tearing the MCL and medial metatarsosesamoid ligament. An avulsion fracture may occur off the base of the proximal phalanx, subluxation of the sesamoids may occur, or chronic hallux valgus may result. Jumping athletes, landing on another player's foot or on an uneven surface, may also fall to the side, producing this type of valgus strain.

This injury is also commonly seen in ballet dancers (9), occurring either acutely on landing or as a result of chronic attrition of the MCL. Athletes with preexisting hallux valgus or a planovalgus foot deformity with hyperpronation of the forefoot and great toe may complain of chronic MTPJ tenderness, pain, and swelling, especially in cutting and pivoting sports such as basketball or tennis.

Finally, a rare *varus stress* to the MTPJ has been reported by Mullis and Miller (12), who reported tear of the LCL and avulsion of the transverse and oblique head of the adductor hallucis. This occurred when a basketball player came down on his right foot and pivoted externally, rotating on a fixed forefoot. Swelling of the first–second web space occurred, followed by varus deformity of the first MTPJ.

ETIOLOGY

Many underlying causes have been felt to be responsible for the increase in MTPJ injuries seen in contact sports, especially football (5). Bowers and Martin (16) coined the term *turf toe* in 1976 to note that the advent of *artificial turf* in the late 1960s had led to an increase in MTPJ sprain type of injuries. In 1974 they noted that artificial turf ages poorly, becoming asphalt-like in hardness (22). Nigg and Segesser (13) and

Clanton et al. (5,17) felt that increased shoe–turf friction produced by artificial turf has resulted in increased MTPJ injuries. In the survey of trainers from 66 colleges and universities, by Coker et al. (3,18), 36% felt that turf was the primary factor in MTP joint injuries! Rodeo et al.'s (14) study of MTPJ injuries among two NFL teams found that 83% had the initial injury on artificial turf.

The increasingly *flexible forefoot of modern football shoes,* as players change from the seven-cleated shoe with a metal forefoot plate to the multicleated soccer-style shoes, has also been linked to increased MTPJ injuries. Bowers and Martin (16), Clanton et al. (5,17), Garrick (19), and Torg and Quendenfeld (23) have noticed increased frequency of MTPJ injuries with the newer style shoes. Coker et al. (18) reported that 24% of trainers felt that the shoe was responsible for MTPJ injury and 24% felt that both turf and shoewear were causative. Rodeo et al. (14) found no relationship in the NFL between shoes and MTPJ injury but noted that most players used the more flexible shoes, making comparison difficult. Scranton (personal communication) has also noted that the common practice of ''spatting'' or taping of football shoes decreases the friction on artificial surfaces. This may also have the effect of stiffening the midfoot and forefoot. Interestingly enough, lacrosse and soccer have not reported an increased MTPJ injury rate despite the same shoe–surface interface (5).

The relationship between *MTPJ range of motion* and acute turf toe injury has been carefully studied. Several authors, including Clanton and Ford (5) and Coker et al. (3) have suggested that previous MTPJ injury may predispose the MTPJ to repeat insult. Coker et al. (3,18) noted an increased incidence of ''flattened'' metatarsal heads among patients with MTPJ injury but could not ascribe cause and effect. Clanton and Ford (5) looked specifically at MTPJ range of motion prospectively and found *no relationship* between MTPJ range of motion and acute MTPJ injury. Coker et al. (3) and Rodeo et al. (14) also noted no relationship between range of motion in uninjured players and subsequent acute MTPJ injury. They did note decreased MTPJ range of motion *postinjury.* Our own anecdotal experience adds to the view that *previous MTPJ injury* is a predisposing factor to acute MTPJ injury.

There has been no study of the relationship between ''flat'' metatarsal heads or preexisting hallux limitus and chronic MTPJ injury. In my athletic foot and ankle practice, many athletes who present with chronic MTPJ swelling and pain have flat metatarsal heads and bony or cartilaginous hallux limitus. This group of patients represents the ''numerator'' without knowing the true ''denominator,'' or number of athletes with asymptomatic hallux limitus/''flattened'' metatarsal heads.

Various miscellaneous factors have been associated with increased incidence of turf toe-like injuries. Coker et al. (3,18) and Rodeo et al. (14) found *increased player weight* to be a significant factor in MTP joint injury, but Clanton et al. (5,17) did not. *Increased player age and length of NFL career* was found to be statistically significant by Rodeo et al. (14). Both Coker et al. (3,18) and Clanton and Ford (5) found *increased ankle dorsiflexion* to be a factor in increased MTPJ injury, suggesting that increased ankle range of motion may allow the toe to be placed in a more harmful position. Coker et al. (3,18) and Rodeo et al. (14) felt that running backs, wide receivers, and offensive linemen were at risk, whereas Clanton and Ford (5) felt that *offensive players* are most likely to end up at the ''bottom of the pile,'' increasing the chance of injury.

EVALUATION

Since athletic injuries of the great toe may vary greatly in severity, proper evaluation is essential to determine the degree of injury and therefore treatment and return to sports. The best time for evaluation of an athletic great toe injury (like many injuries) is immediately post injury, on the field or sideline. Swelling and discomfort may be at its minimum and may facilitate thorough evaluation. Prior to examination and removal of the shoe, it is important to obtain the history of athletic injury and mechanism, if possible. If the incident was not directly witnessed, often video tapes will later reveal the exact mechanism of injury.

Physical examination should note the amount of swelling and the ecchymosis present as well as the overall alignment of the toe. It is important to note whether the MTPJ is still located. Neurovascular status must be assessed, especially prior to any relocation efforts for a dislocated MTPJ. Points of tenderness are elicited, probing the plantar surface dorsally, especially around the sesamoids and the MCL and LCL. The presence of tenderness and its severity will often tell the examiner which structures have been injured.

Assessment of MTPJ stability is important in determining the type and speed of rehabilitation. Active range of motion by the patient prior to the onset of swelling is useful in assessing joint stability. Varus and valgus stress to the MTPJ is used to determine the status of the LCL and MCL, respectively. A dorsoplantar drawer test of the MTPJ is helpful in assessing the status of the dorsal capsule and plantar plate–sesamoid complex. Passive range of motion of the MTP joint is compared with the opposite uninjured side to find any limitations to motion caused by intraarticular fractures/loose bodies or whether hypermobility and joint subluxation exist due to a tear of the capsuloligamentous restraints. Another step in evaluation is to have the patient attempt MTPJ extension and flexion against resistance. This will demonstrate the presence of an intact extensor hallucis longus, brevis and flexor hallucis longus and brevis, as well as stability of the MTPJ under compression. Lastly, ability of the athlete to bear weight comfortably is an important consideration in determining the severity of the injury.

RADIOGRAPHIC EVALUATION

Regular radiographs should be taken on each patient to demonstrate reduction and congruency of the MTPJ, to rule out avulsion or intraarticular fractures, and to determine the presence of any preexisting intraarticular condition such as hallux rigidus. AP and lateral (weight-bearing, if possible), two obliques, and sesamoid views are obtained. There is some controversy on the utility of obtaining x-ray film of the contralateral and noninvolved side. Hallux valgus and hallux rigidus do not always exist to the same degree on each side. Bilaterality of bipartite sesamoids varies from 25% (15) to 85% (24).

Serial radiographs may be helpful to evaluate gradual proximal migration of sesamoids after a plantar plate tear, healing, or nonunion of sesamoid fractures, and separation of a bipartite sesamoid after injury to the synchondrosis (15). Progressive separation of the proximal and distal portion of a bipartite sesamoid (Fig. 19) may reveal inadequate healing of the surrounding tendon and capsule, requiring surgical intervention.

Rodeo et al. (15) have suggested a forced dorsiflexion lateral view, which may illustrate joint subluxation, sesamoid migration, or separation of an injured bipartite sesamoid. Varus and valgus stress AP views may demonstrate insufficiency of the LCL or MCL, respectively. AP and lateral tomograms are useful in evaluating intraarticular fractures, avulsion fractures, loose bodies, and healing of sesamoid fractures. A technetium bone scan is useful in evaluating a possible stress fracture of the sesamoids. Coker et al. (3,18) have reported use of an MTPJ arthrogram to help illustrate the presence of a capsuloligamentous tear and recently, magnetic resonance imaging (MRI) has been demonstrated to assess accurately the presence and severity of MTPJ capsuloligamentous injury (25).

In summary, as we would expect, the history and physical aided by regular x-rays are the most valuable tools in assessing MTPJ injury. Additional tests may be required when evaluating stress fractures and/or sesamoid injuries.

A 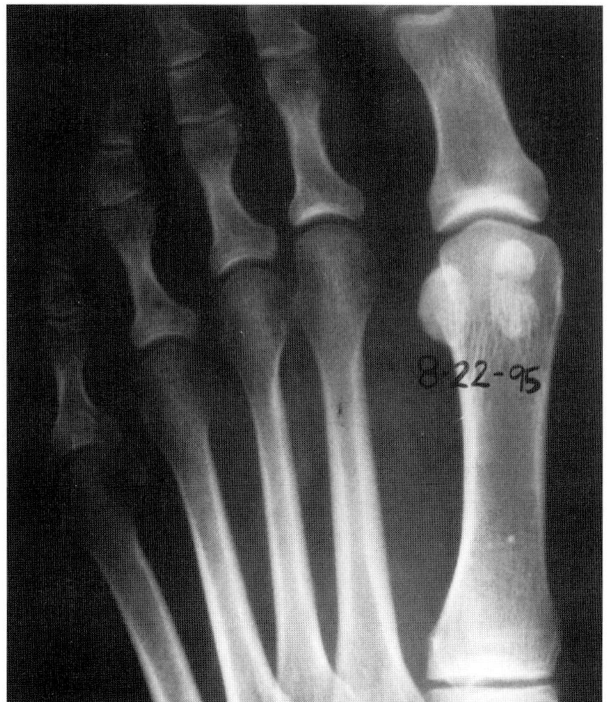

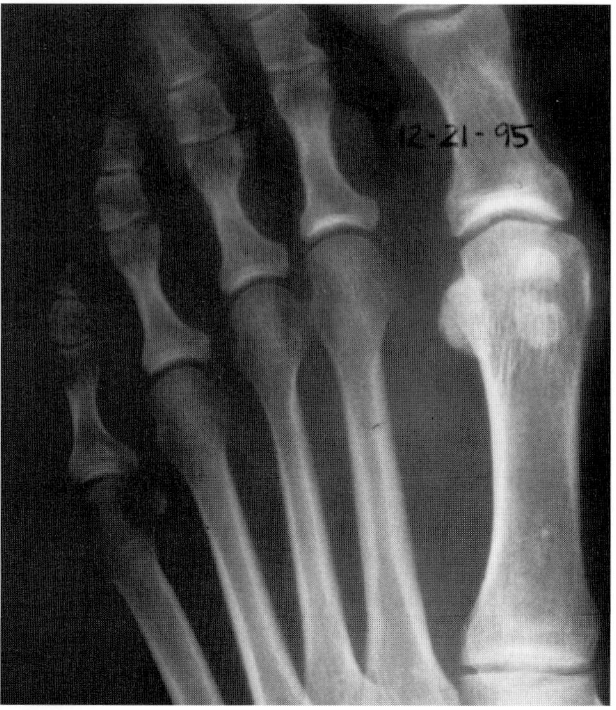 B

C 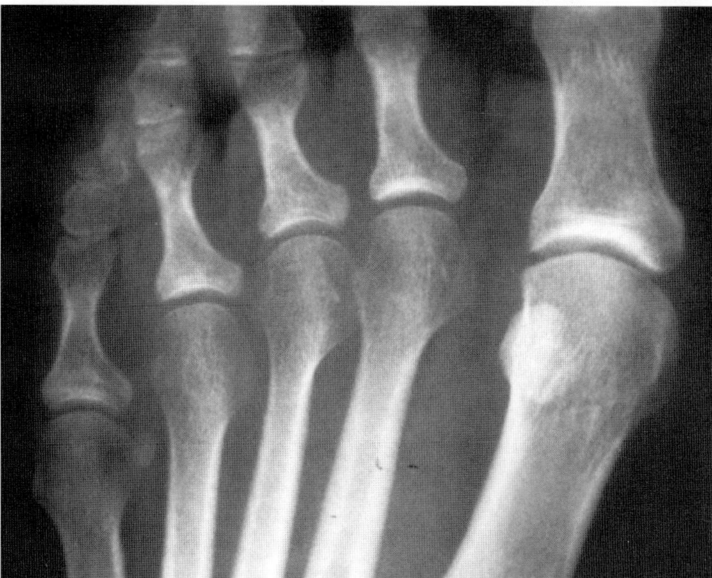

Figure 19. Injury to a bipartite tibial sesamoids in a 24-year-old professional skater. **A,B:** Progressive separation of the tibial sesamoid synchrondrosis despite conservative treatment (casting, shoe and skate modification). **C:** Tibial sesamoidectomy, which allowed the patient to return to skating.

TREATMENT

Treatment of athletic MTPJ injuries varies since the exact nature and severity of the injury may range from mild to severely disabling. However, as statistics in the reported studies above show, most MTPJ injuries involve soft tissue disruption and are best treated conservatively. Although specific elements may vary, most nonoperative treatment of MTPJ injuries, as outlined by Bowers and Martin (16), Coker et al. (3,18), Rodeo et al. (14,15), Clanton et al. (5,17), Sammarco (26,27), and our own experience, is similar.

After initial assessment is made and the appropriate studies performed, the exact nature of the injury and its severity are ascertained. The situations that require immediate surgical intervention are addressed later in this section. Most MTPJ injuries, however, may be treated as outlined in the algorithm of Fig. 20. First it must be estab-

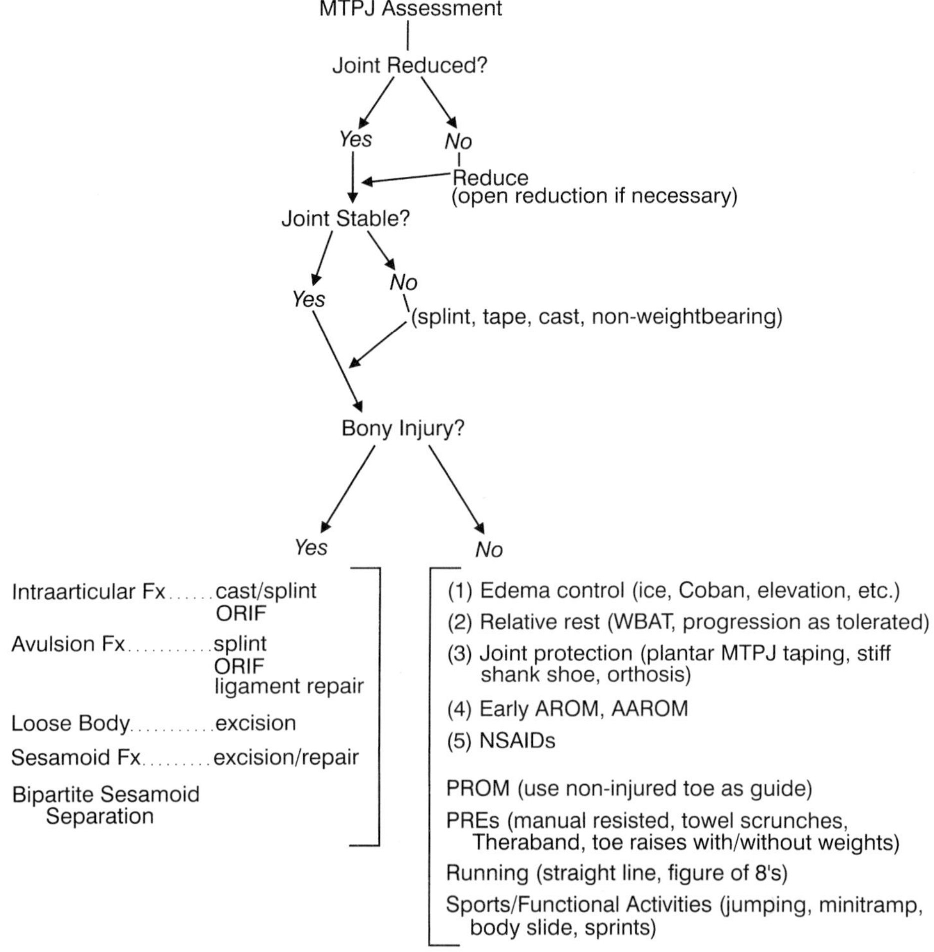

Figure 20. Algorithm for the treatment of athletic MTPJ injuries of the great toe.

Table 2. *Clanton "turf toe" grading system*

Grade I
Pathology
Stretching of capsuloligamentous structures
Signs and symptoms
Localized tenderness—plantar, medial
Minimal swelling
No ecchymosis
Treatment
May play with protection, conservative treatment
Grade II
Pathology
Tear of capsuloligamentous structures
Signs and symptoms
Diffuse tenderness
Mild to moderate swelling, ecchymosis, decreased range of motion
Treatment
Conservative treatment, may lose 1 day to 2 weeks of playing time
Grade III
Pathology
Capsuloligamentous tear plus articular compression injury
Signs and symptoms
Severe diffuse tenderness, maximal dorsally
Marked swelling, ecchymosis, and marked decreased range of motion
Treatment
Conservative treatment, may lose 3 to 6 weeks of playing time

Data from ref. 5.

lished that the joint is reduced. If not, reduction should be performed, either by closed means or operatively. Once joint reduction is established or produced, stability is assessed. Stable joints may be started on immediate rehabilitation. Joints that are unstable may need initial protection with either a splint, cast, or plantar taping. Stability is reassessed in 3 to 5 days, and rehabilitation is started once the joint is stable.

The initial rehabilitation varies in intensity depending on the severity of injury. Clanton and Ford's (5) grading classification, as noted in Table 2, is an excellent guide to initial therapy. However, my approach has been to individualize each injury. Relative rest, edema control, joint protection, range-of-motion exercises, progressive weight bearing as tolerated, and nonsteroidal antiinflammatory medication are the hallmarks of initial conservative treatment.

Weight bearing may be permitted as tolerated, ranging from non-weight-bearing crutch status to straight-ahead running as tolerated. Relative rest implies avoidance of aggravating activity to the MTPJ. In mild MTPJ injuries, this may mean avoidance of certain aggravating activities in practice. Absolute joint rest and non-weight-bearing treatment may be needed in severe cases. Edema control is aggressively pursued immediately. Ice slush baths and cryotherapy are used in the initial 48 h, followed by contrast baths and Coban or Ace bandage wrapping to reduce and control swelling.

Joint protection depends on the exact nature of the injury. For hyperextension injuries, which are most common, plantar taping is utilized. The athletic shoe may be stiffened with either a spring steel or carbon fiber plate, as shown in Fig. 21, or

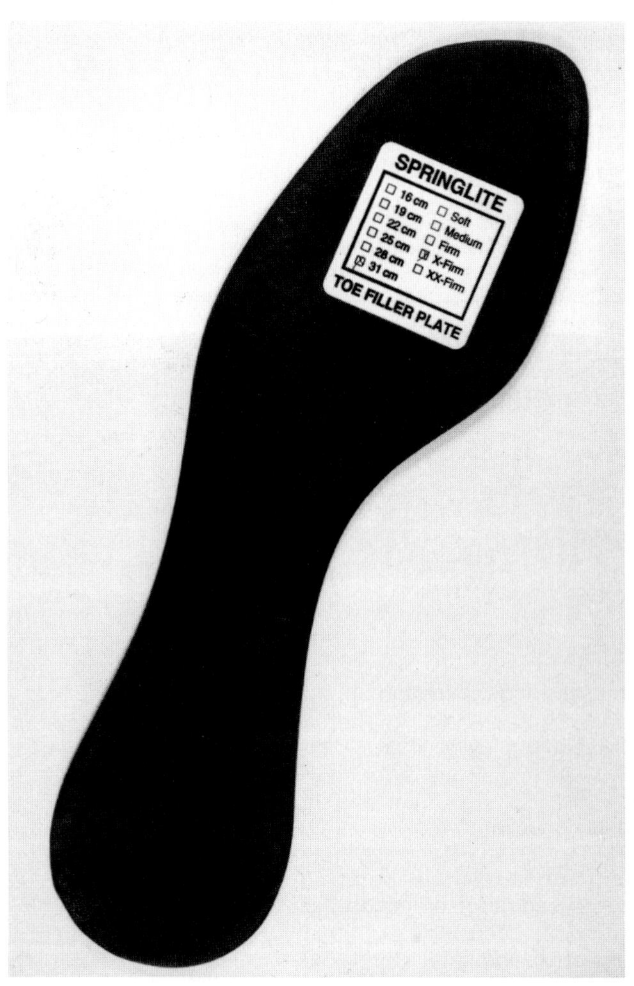

Figure 21. Lightweight carbon fiber plate for stiffening of the athletic shoe. (Courtesy of Bob Dougher, C.O., St. Francis Hospital, Pittsburgh, PA.)

by use of a custom molded orthoplast splint, initially suggested by Garrick (19) (Fig. 22). Valgus-type injuries may also be aided by figure-of-eight taping to prevent valgus MTPJ stress, as well as a molded toe spacer between the first and second toes to prevent valgus deviation. Simple buddy-taping of the first to second toe, separated by a small gauze or foam pad, will protect the MTPJ in cases of the rare varus MTP joint injury.

Oral nonsteroidal antiinflammatory medication is started early to control swelling and inflammation of the MTPJ. Joint mobilization is begun once the joint is determined to be stable and pursued aggressively as swelling and pain permit. Active range of motion is initiated, together with active assisted range of motion. Passive range of motion is instituted when tolerated, using motion of the opposite normal MTPJ as a guide to avoid hyperextension or hyperflexion.

When the swelling is controlled and range of motion has improved, progressive resisted exercises for the toe extensors and flexors are initiated. These exercises range from towel scrunches to manual resisted exercises to Theraband extension and toe flexion exercises. Functional exercises such as toe raises, stair dips and raises, and finally sport-specific activities such as sprinter/lineman type crouch, running, minitramp, jumping, side-to-side activities (body slide, baseline tennis drills, and figure-of-eight cutting type drills) may be used to guide return to sports.

Since MTPJ injuries may produce chronic symptoms, a maintenance program of ice/edema control, MTPJ taping or splinting, and shoewear modifications may be needed. We have found that increasing shoe size by one width or one length is very often helpful in avoiding pain since many players have become accustomed to wearing shoes that are actually undersized by traditional fitting techniques. MTPJ motion exercises are continued to avoid soft tissue hallux limitus due to scar formation from healing of the capsuloligamentous complex.

A 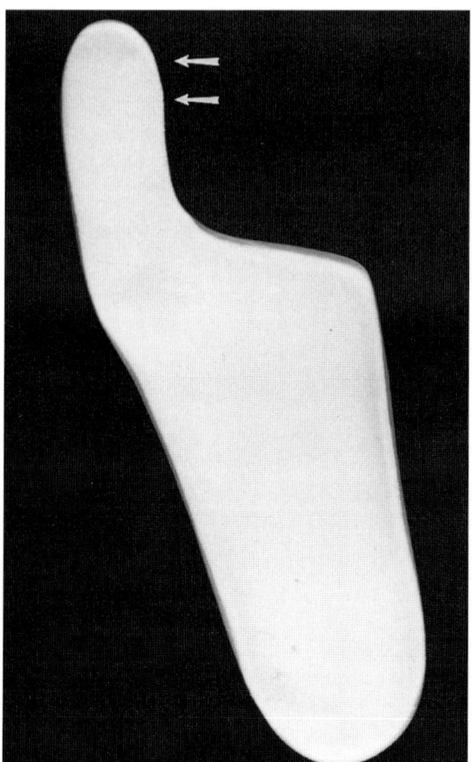

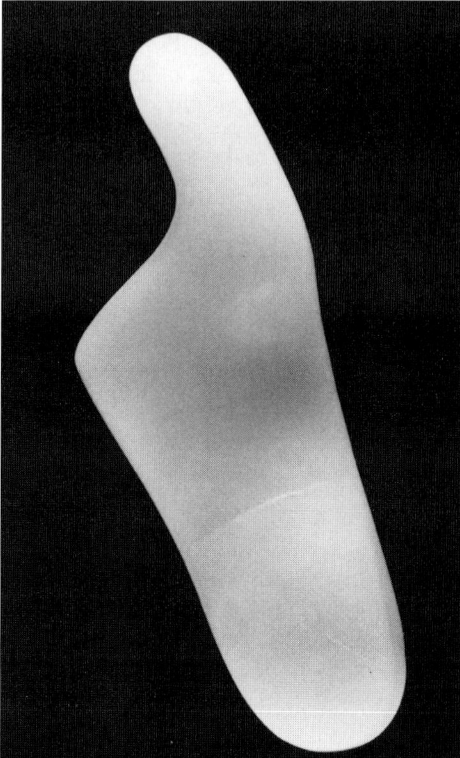 B

Figure 22. Custom-molded orthoplast or polyethylene shoe inlay with a Morton's extension (*arrows*) to limit great toe hyperextension. **A:** Top view. **B:** Bottom view. (Courtesy of Bob Dougher, C.O., St. Francis Hospital, Pittsburgh, PA.)

Some controversy exists concerning the use of cortisone MTPJ injections (28). Coker et al. (3,18) used corticosteroid injection in 24% of their turf toe cases, whereas Clanton and Ford (5) felt that cortisone injection was rarely indicated in the management of turf toe injuries. We feel that cortisone injections should probably be reserved for recalcitrant and chronic cases of MTPJ synovitis following initial conservative care. Repeated corticosteroid injections are also to be avoided.

SURGICAL TREATMENT

Occasionally acute surgical intervention is required for MTPJ injuries. Displaced intraarticular fractures may require internal fixation prior to rehabilitation. Avulsion fractures, if displaced, indicating instability, may require open reduction and internal fixation or excision of the bony fragment and ligament repair if the piece is small. Loose bodies (Fig. 23) require arthroscopic removal or arthrotomy and removal. Irreducible dislocations of the MTPJ are usually due to interposition of the plantar plate or ligament complex in the MTPJ and may require open reduction (11,29,30). Nonunion of fractures may require bone grafting and internal fixation. Displaced sesamoid fractures, sesamoid fracture nonunion or disruption, and diastasis of bipartite sesamoids, as described by Rodeo et al. (15), may require flexor hallucis brevis repair and excision of the distal sesamoid fragment.

Most situations requiring surgery are acute cases of MTPJ injury that failed to resolve with conservative treatment, producing chronic MTPJ pain. Cartilaginous or bony hallux rigidus that is preexisting may be aggravated by acute MTPJ injuries and may require either open or arthroscopic cheilectomy.

Osteochondritis dissecans or fracture nonunion of the sesamoids may require sesamoidectomy if not relieved by conservative measures such as shoe modifications and orthotic padding (20,21,31). Hallux valgus that is either aggravated or caused by acute MTPJ injury may require reconstruction of the MCL by isometric repair using suture anchors such as the ROC (Innovasive Devices, Marlborough, MA) anchor (Fig. 24). Postoperatively in each case, once stability is restored and with adequate soft tissue healing after the procedure, the above-mentioned rehabilitation program is begun.

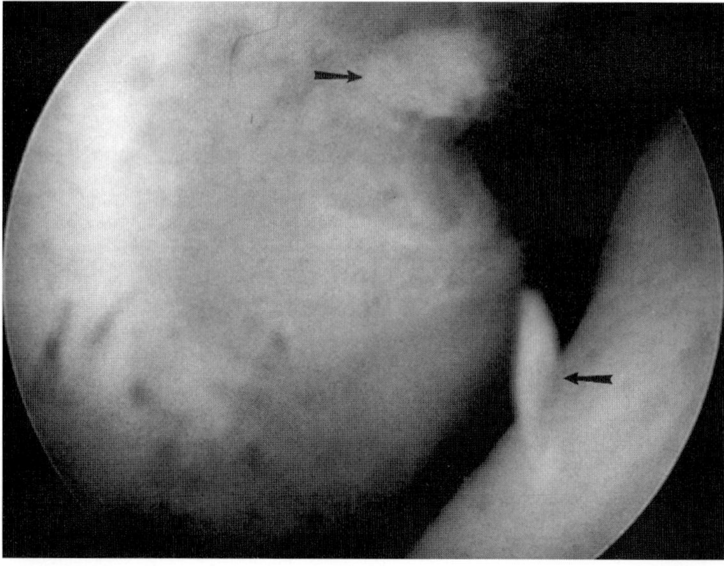

Figure 23. Arthroscopic view of loose osteochondral fragments (*arrows*) from the first metatarsal head after an MTPJ hyperextension injury.

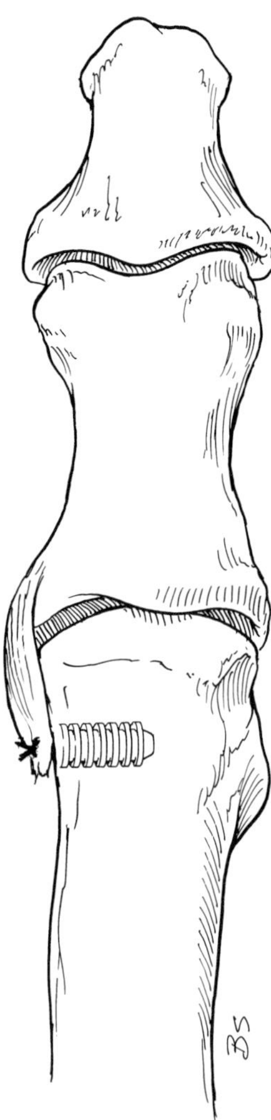

Figure 24. Isometric repair of the medial capsular ligament using a ROC anchor.

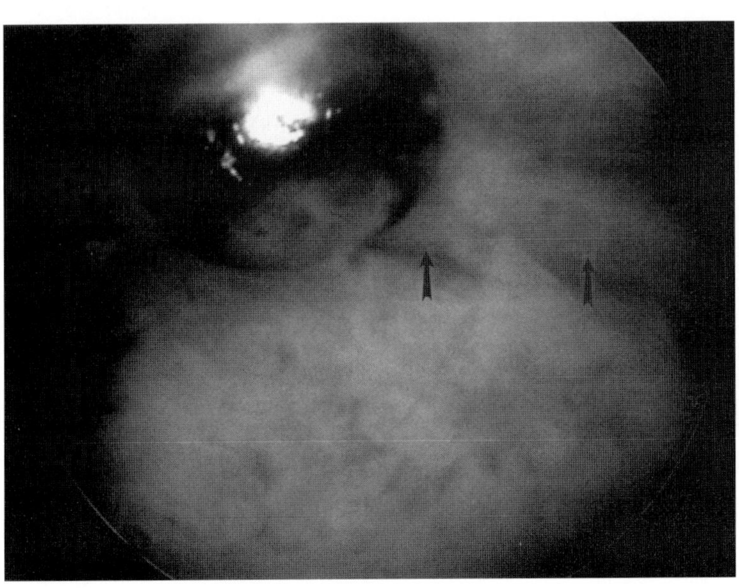

Figure 25. Adhesive capsulitis of the great toe MTPJ. Arthroscopic view showing intense dorsal capsular adhesions (*arrow*) being trimmed with a shaver.

CHRONIC MTPJ INJURY SEQUELAE

In our practice, I have noted that chronic cases of hallux limitus following acute MTPJ injury fall into two broad categories:

1. *Adhesive capsulitis:* the disrupted capsuloligamentous complex heals by intense scar formation, thereby limiting motion. Secondary wear of the articular cartilage may also be seen.
2. *Bony hallux limitus:* may have preceded the acute MTPJ injury. Often there are dorsal osteophytes on the metatarsal head and base of the proximal phalanx, as well

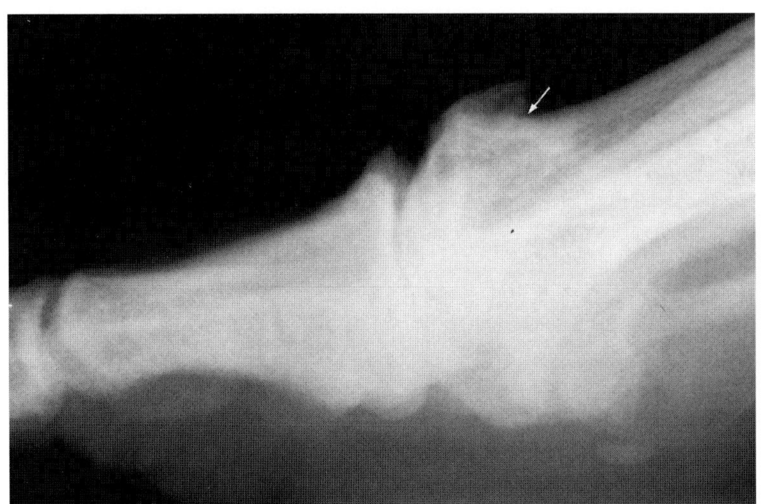

A

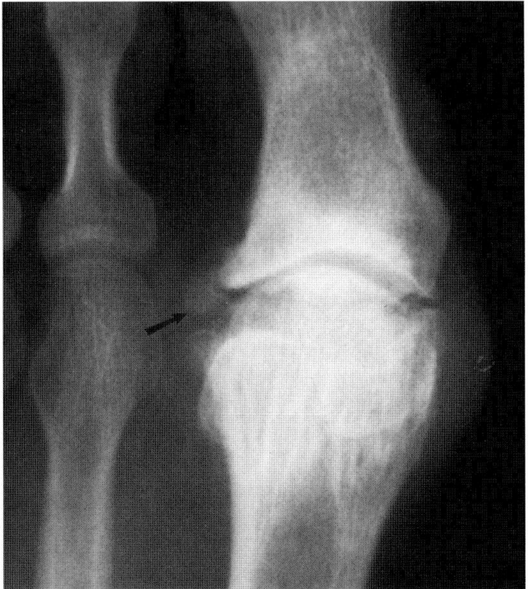

B

C

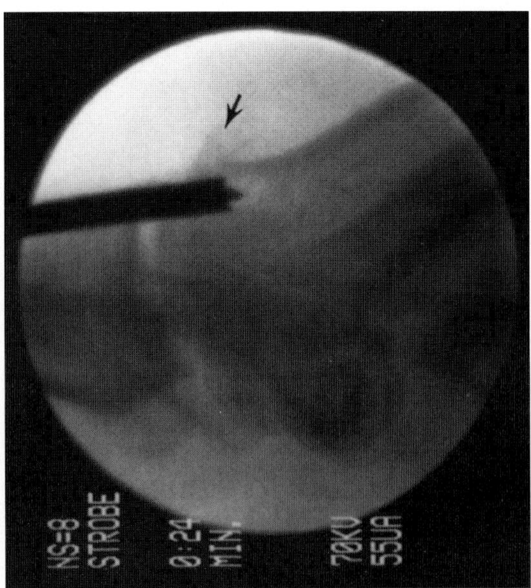

D

Figure 26. Arthroscopic cheilectomy. **A:** Preoperative lateral radiograph of bony hallux limitus showing dorsal osteophytes (*arrow*). **B:** Preoperative AP radiograph of bony hallux limitus showing lateral osteophytes (*arrow*). **C:** Arthroscopic view of a bur removing a dorsal osteophyte (*arrows*) partially obscured by the dorsal capsule. **D:** Fluoroscopic view of an arthroscopic bur removing the dorsal osteophyte (*arrow*).

as lateral metatarsal head spurs. Thinning of the dorsal articular cartilage of the metatarsal head, as described by Mann and Coughlin (32), may be present.

In both cases, arthroscopic evaluation and debridement has proved to be helpful in collegiate and professional athletes in our practice. Patients with adhesive capsulitis can be evaluated arthroscopically; if the articular surface remains in good condition, they can undergo synovectomy and lysis of the adhesions using the small arthroscopic shaver (Fig. 25) and a Freer elevator introduced through the dorsal portal to free up the capsular adhesions. This is followed by immediate aggressive range of motion and has produced good results in our practice.

Cases of bony hallux rigidus have benefited from arthroscopic synovectomy and debridement of the dorsal osteophytes, along with arthroscopic burring of the dorsal one-third metatarsal head (arthroscopic cheilectomy) (Fig. 26). This procedure, once again, is followed by edema control and immediate range of motion. In both cases, the patient will begin immediate active and active assisted range of motion with weight bearing on the heel for 2 weeks, followed by passive range-of-motion and progressive

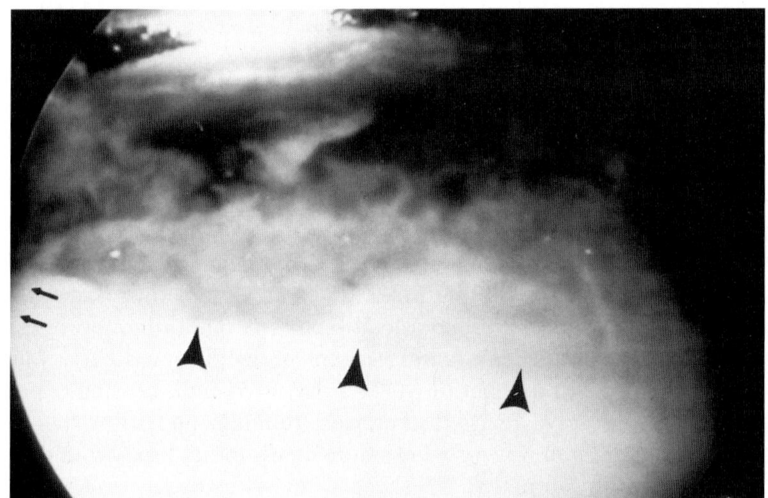

E

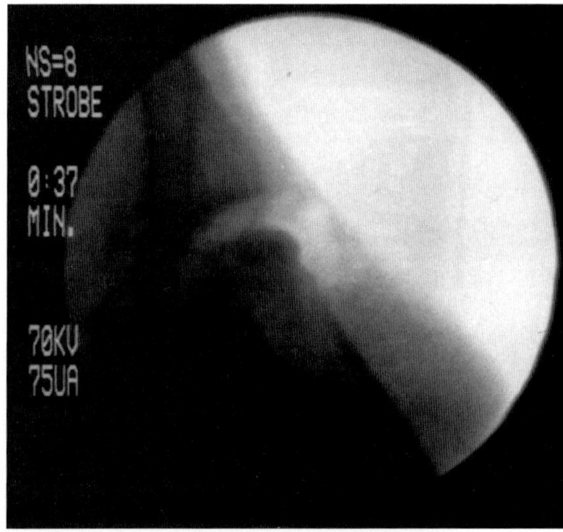

F

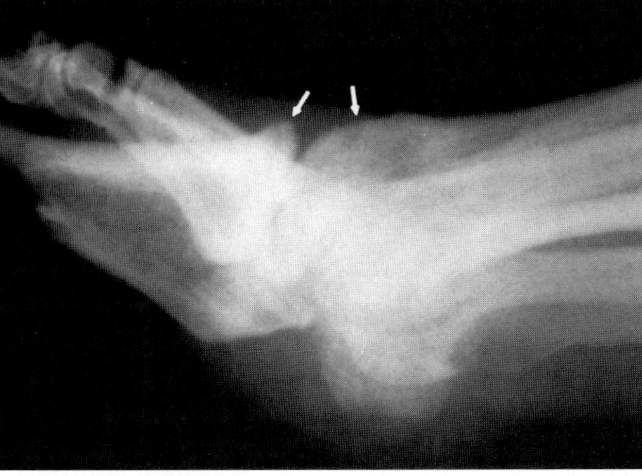

G

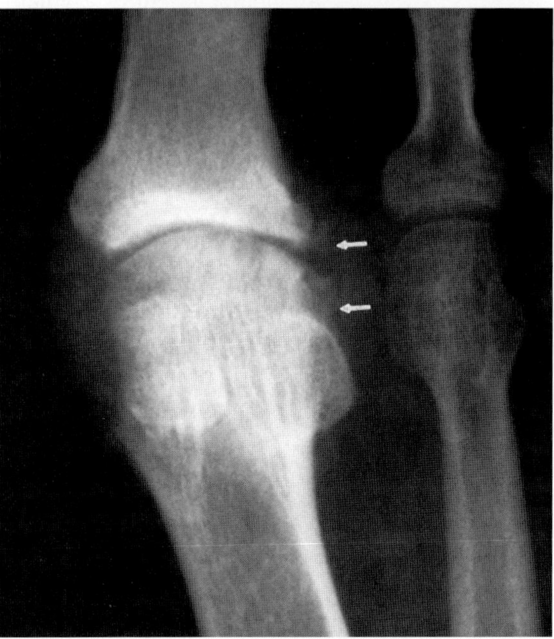

H

Figure 26. *(Continued).* **E:** The flattened dorsal metatarsal head after osteophyte removal. Large *arrowheads,* dorsal first metatarsal head; *small arrows,* MTPJ. **F:** Fluoroscopic view after dorsal osteophyte removal. **G:** Postoperative lateral radiograph showing removal of dorsal MTPJ osteophytes (*arrows*). **H:** Postoperative AP radiograph showing removal of lateral MTPJ osteophytes (*arrows*).

resisted exercises and weight bearing as outlined in Table 1. After 11 cases, we have seen an average 40 degree increase in MTPJ range of motion and return to professional level athletics in 3 of 3 cases. Open synovectomy and/or cheilectomy is performed when the bony osteophytes are too large or when arthroscopic visualization is inadequate.

SUMMARY

In summary, athletic injuries of the MTPJ can be painful and very functionally disabling. Even though ankle injuries outweigh great toe injuries four to one in major university studies, the lost time/lost games from MTPJ injuries is equal to that of ankle injuries, and MTPJ injuries rank third as the cause of lost-time athletic injuries! Hyperextension is by far the most common mechanism of MTPJ injury, followed by hyperflexion and valgus injuries. Although the subject is slightly controversial, several studies have shown that the harder, unyielding synthetic turfs correlate with an increase in great toe MTPJ injuries. Also correlated are the more flexible turf type shoe and increasing player age. Significant, but less well established as causative of MTPJ injuries, are preinjury MTP motion and metatarsal head shape.

Thorough evaluation of MTPJ injuries is essential. A history and physical are crucial to determine the mechanism of injury. Reduction and stability of the MTPJ must be assessed. Bony injury must be ruled out and addressed if present. The integrity of the supporting capsuloligamentous–sesamoid complex must be noted. Regular radiographs are always obtained. Special tests, such as tomograms, arthrogram, bone scan, or MRI, may be helpful in the evaluation process.

Initial treatment of most MTPJ injuries is nonoperative and Clanton and Ford's (5) grading system is helpful in guiding rehabilitation. However, joint stability, range of motion, swelling, and weight tolerance are the crucial factors in determining progression of rehabilitation. Relative rest, edema control, joint protection, and early joint mobilization are keys to the initial treatment of MTPJ injuries. Weight bearing is progressed as tolerated with progressive resisted exercises, running, and sport-specific exercises permitted as tolerated. Even with proper treatment, disability times with these injuries can range from 3 days to 3 months!

Operative intervention is less common and is reserved for cases of displaced intraarticular fractures, avulsion fractures, irreducible subluxation/dislocation of the MTPJ, intraarticular loose bodies, displaced sesamoid fractures, or separation of bipartite sesamoids. Early aggressive surgical intervention, in these cases, followed by the above rehabilitation program when healed, has produced good results. Surgery may also be indicated in chronic cases of pain/limitation of motion after MTPJ injury. New arthroscopic methods of cheilectomy and joint release are available in addition to the more traditional open surgical methods.

REFERENCES

1. Mann RA, Coughlin MJ. *Surgery of the foot and ankle,* 6th ed. St. Louis: CV Mosby–Year Book, 1993:623–636.
2. Hardy RH, Clapham JR. Observations on hallux valgus. *J Bone Joint Surg [Br]* 1951;33:516.
3. Coker TP, Arnold JA, Weber DL. Traumatic lesions of the metatarsophalangeal joint of the great toe in athletes. *Am J Sports Med* 1978;6:326.
4. Joseph J. Range of movement of the great toe in men. *J Bone Joint Surg [Br]* 1954;36:450.
5. Clanton TO, Ford JJ. Turf toe injury. *Clin Sports Med* 1994;13:731.
6. Sammarco GJ. Biomechanics of the foot. In: Nordin M, Frankel VH, eds. *Basic biomechanics of the musculoskeletal system,* 2nd ed. Philadelphia: Lea & Febiger, 1988:163–181.
7. Sarrafian SK. *Anatomy of the foot and ankle: descriptive, topographical, functional,* 2nd ed. Philadelphia: Lea & Febiger, 1993:221.
8. Gibbs RC. Tennis toe. *JAMA* 1974;228:24.
9. Hamilton WG. Foot and ankle injuries in dancers. *Clin Sports Med* 1988;7:143–173.
10. Leach RE. Leg and foot injuries in racquet sports. *Clin Sports Med* 1988;7:359–370.

11. Mata SG, Ovejero AMH, Grande MM. Dorsal dislocation of the first metatarso-phalangeal joint. *Int Orthop (SICOT)* 1988;12:237–238.
12. Mullis DL, Miller WE. A disabling sports injury of the great toe. *Foot Ankle* 1980;1:22–25.
13. Nigg BM, Segesser B. The influence of playing surfaces on the load on the locomotor system and on football and tennis injuries. *Sports Med* 1988;5:375–385.
14. Rodeo SA, O'Brien S, Warren RF, et al. Turf-toe: an analysis of metatarsophalangeal joint sprains in professional football players. *Am J Sports Med* 1990;18:280–285.
15. Rodeo SA, Warren RF, O'Brien SJ, et al. Diastasis of bipartite sesamoids of the first metatarsophalangeal joint. *Foot Ankle* 1993;14:425–434.
16. Bowers KD Jr, Martin RB. Turf-toe: a shoe-surface related football injury. *Med Sci Sports Exerc* 1976;8:81.
17. Clanton TO, Butler JE, Eggert A. Injuries to the metatarsophalangeal joints in athletes. *Foot Ankle* 1986;7:162.
18. Coker TP, Arnold JA, Weber DL. Traumatic lesions of the metatarsophalangeal joint of the great toe in athletes. *J Ark Med Soc* 1978;74:309.
19. Garrick JG. Artificial turf: pros and cons (a round table). *Phys Sports Med* 1975;3:41–50.
20. Coughlin MJ. Sesamoid pain: causes and surgical treatment. In: Coughlin M, Karpman RR, eds. *Review course 1990. Surgery of the foot and ankle.* Rosemont, IL: American Orthopaedic Foot and Ankle Society, 1990:200.
21. Richardson EG. Injuries to the hallucal sesamoids in the athlete. *Foot Ankle* 1987;7:229–244.
22. Bowers KD Jr, Martin RB. Impact absorption, new and old Astro-Turf. *WV Med Sci Sports Exerc* 1974;6:217–221.
23. Torg JS, Quendenfeld TC. Knee and ankle injuries traced to shoes and cleats. *Phys Sports Med* 1973;1:39–43.
24. Jahss MH. The sesamoids of the hallux. *Clin Orthop* 1981;157:88–97.
25. Tewes DP, Fischer DA, Fritts HM, Guanche CA. MRI findings of acute turf toe. *Clin Orthop* 1994;304:200–203.
26. Sammarco GJ. Turf toe. In: Heckman JE, ed. *Instructional course lectures,* vol 42. Chicago: American Academy of Orthopaedic Surgeons 1993:207.
27. Sammarco GJ. How I manage turf toe. *Phys Sports Med* 1988;169:113–118.
28. Salter RB, Gross A, Hall JH. Hydrocortisone arthropathy—an experimental investigation. *Can Med Assoc J* 1967;97:374–377.
29. Giannikas AC, Papachristou G, Papavasiliou N, Nikifordis P, Hartofilakidis-Garofalidis G. Dorsal dislocation of the first metatarso-phalangeal joint. *J Bone Surg [Br]* 1975;57:384–386.
30. Jahss MH. Traumatic dislocations of the first metatarsophalangeal joint. *Foot Ankle* 1980;1:15–21.
31. Hulkko A, Orava S, Pellinen, Puranen J. Stress fractures of the sesamoid bones of the first metatarsophalangeal joint in athletes. *Arch Orthop Trauma Surg* 1985;104:113–117.
32. Mann RA, Coughlin MD, DuVries HL. Hallux rigidus. *Clin Orthop* 1979;142:57–62.

EDITORIAL COMMENTS

Athletic Injuries of the Great Toe MTP Joint

Michael W. Bowman

Dr. Michael Bowman has shared with us his large experience in treating athletic injuries to the great toe. This is an area that has been devoid of attention and science over the last decade but is becoming much more important due to the significant disability and loss of game time for these injuries. It is important that we remember the intricate anatomic structures of the MTPJ, particularly the volar plate and sesamoid metatarsal phalangeal ligaments. The intimate relationship with the sesamoids must be remembered, and the sesamoids must be evaluated as part of this joint injury. In the acute dislocation, one must focus on the fact that these may be irreducible if there is entrapment of the volar plate and one should be able to identify the point of capsular failure. The capsule can fail either at the proximal phalanx base or the sesamoid attachment to the capsule, or through a sesamoid fracture. The dislocations are rather catastrophic and not difficult to diagnose, but chronic turf toe is a significant problem in diagnosis and treatment. These injuries are often more morbid than ankle injuries because their morbidity lasts longer and without the ability to push or pull off on the first metatarsal complex, the athlete usually cannot perform at an adequate level to compete.

The etiology of these chronic problems is still fairly anecdotal, and there are authors on both sides of the artificial turf controversy; it certainly is clinically apparent that with artificial turf the velocity of the game picks up and that the turf, which was introduced in the last decade, is now starting to age; the cost of replacement gives us concern about artificial turf maintenance. There has been a significant movement to revert back to natural turf, and thus we should see a reduction in these injuries. One should also be aware that in turf toe there is restriction in motion and a subconscious transfer of stress over to the lateral complex of the foot. Therefore, these patients may present with problems related to metatarsalgia or lateral foot pain as they try to decrease the force transmitted to the first metatarsal phalangeal complex.

Dr. Bowman has introduced arthroscopic treatment of the first metatarsal joint, which is an evolving technology. It is quite dependent on having proper small instruments and small scopes available, and it requires a fairly steep learning curve. Synovectomies are appropriately performed through the arthroscope in the first MTPJ, and with further practice one can develop techniques of cheilectomy. It is quite important to follow his regimen of introduction of instruments to avoid the cartilage damage that can occur during these procedures.

Robert S. Adelaar, M.D.

Complex Foot and Ankle Trauma,
edited by Robert S. Adelaar,
Lippincott–Raven Publishers, Philadelphia © 1999.

20

Guidelines for Soft Tissue Coverage of Complex Foot and Ankle Injuries

L. Scott Levin

Soft tissue deficiencies of the foot or ankle are caused by several mechanisms. These include deficiencies related to trauma, tumor, vascular disease, or diabetes. Compounding the reconstructive problem further is that soft tissue problems may often present in patients with underlying diseases such as peripheral vascular disease, diabetes, or both. For example, a 65-year-old diabetic who smoked two packs of cigarettes per day sustains an ankle fracture. He undergoes open reduction, internal fixation of his fracture, and subsequent wound dehiscence over his fibular plate. The wound edges cannot be reapproximated, and there is loss of soft tissue. What should be the treatment for this soft tissue problem? Another example is the 45-year-old rheumatoid patient on 20 mg of steroids a day who undergoes posterior tibial tendon repair. At 1 month after surgery, her wound dehisces, with exposure of tendon. What is the approach for adequate and effective soft tissue treatment? The purpose of this chapter is to address such complex problems and to provide an algorithm for soft tissue reconstruction of the foot and ankle.

GUIDING PRINCIPLES

Before discussing regional differences in foot or ankle tissue deficiencies, several principles should be stated. First and foremost, when undertaking treatment for foot

L. S. Levin: Division of Orthopaedic and Plastic and Reconstructive Surgery, Duke University Medical Center, Durham, North Carolina 27710.

and ankle wounds, a patient's vascular status must be determined (1). It is common in this author's practice to see patients who have been treated expectantly for wounds as described in the previous examples, only to discover inadequate documentation of vascular inflow and outflow. Studies such as presence or absence of pulses, auscultable Doppler examination, noninvasive vascular studies for both arterial as well as venous competence, pulse oximetry or laser Doppler cutaneous mapping, and, if necessary, arteriography must be performed before any selection of soft tissue techniques for wound closure (1). Often elderly patients with chronic refractory wounds will have vascular disease compromising inflow. Simple angio-

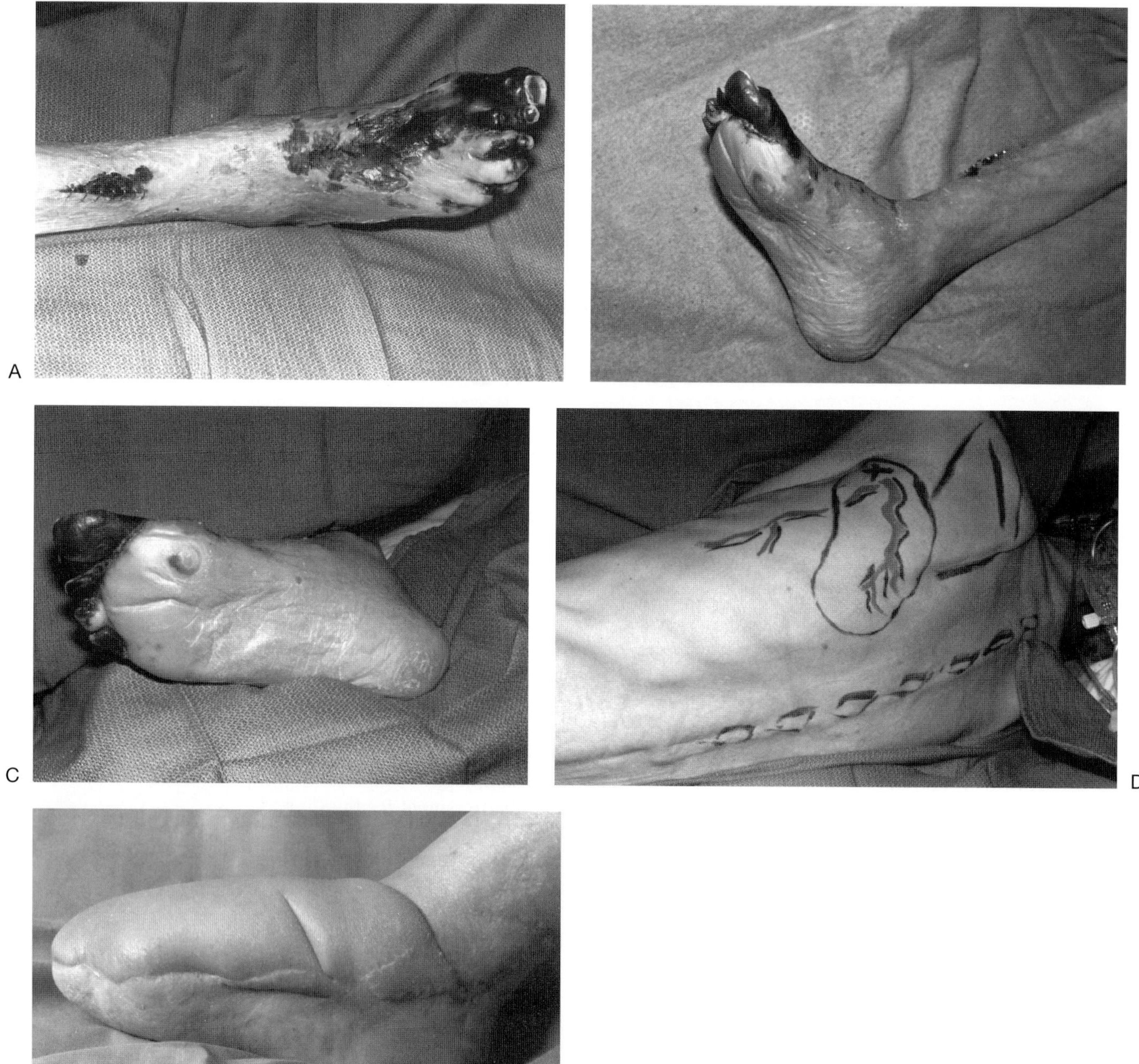

Figure 1. A–C: Patient with severe peripheral vascular disease with infarction of the entire forefoot and dorsum of the foot. **D:** The patient was treated with vascular bypass graft and scapular free flap with preservation of forefoot. **E:** Dorsal view.

plasty in these patients may allow such wounds to heal. More complex procedures such as conventional bypass grafting with autogenous vein. Gortex grafts or in situ bypass grafting may be necessary to establish a vascular ''platform'' on which to build other reconstructive procedures (Fig. 1).

Second, establishing a clean wound is paramount. All necrotic bone and soft tissue must be radically debrided. Only after debridement can the true size of the wound be determined. Subsequently, selection of coverage techniques can be made. Harold Gillies states: ''Replace like with like.'' It may even be desirable after debridement to provide immediate coverage. If a surgically clean wound cannot be established, for example in an open fracture dislocation of the ankle covered with mud, then staged debridement and later coverage should be performed. The most important principle in treatment of the open wound is that the tissues should not be allowed to desiccate. Continuous wet to wet dressings or preferentially a ''bead pouch'' can be placed that will allow exposed structures to be bathed in a physiologic medium. Any tissue desiccation results in cell death, tissue necrosis, infection, edema, and further destruction of soft tissue.

Third, the timing of wound closure should be considered. Emphasis in recent years has been on early soft tissue reconstruction following trauma. Emergency free flaps are possible and may be required. If uncertain on the night of injury regarding definitive closure, the bead pouch, or pigskin, could be used for temporary coverage depending on the size and depth of the wound. Topical materials such as Duoderm or Betadine gauze have not been helpful in promoting granulation tissue and are not used in the author's practice.

RECONSTRUCTIVE LADDER

The fourth principle in management of soft tissue injury is to establish an algorithm that is universal for wounds and applicable to acute, chronic, large, or small defects in any location. Simply stated, closure selection is based on a reconstructive ladder (2).

If possible, primary closure is performed, such as following correction of hallux valgus deformity. Small sutures are used, often with a dermal layer, and primary wound healing can be expected. Delayed primary closure may be necessary in grossly contaminated wounds that require a second look in the operating room at 48 to 72 hr after initial debridement, such as a grade II ankle fracture. Secondary intention healing can be reserved for wounds in which dermal elements are preserved. Typically these are abrasions often seen in bicycle accidents or second-degree burns. Topical care with moist dressings, Silvadene, or other antibiotic creams maintain a moist environment while epithelialization and wound contraction occur.

The next rung on the ladder is the use of skin grafts. Most wounds about the foot and ankle can be managed by skin grafting. Success or failure of grafts depends on several factors. First, preparation of the wound bed is important. If a good layer of granulation tissue is present, grafts have a better chance of inosculation. This returns us to our principle emphasizing adequate blood supply. For example, patients with marginal wounds, not candidates for free flaps or local flaps, can be treated with angioplasty. In some cases hyperbaric oxygen has been effective in stimulating capillary and fibroblast proliferation. Subsequently these patients can undergo relatively simple skin grafting to reestablish the integrity of the integument, with little morbidity compared with more complex surgical intervention.

The next rung on the reconstructive ladder is the use of local flaps, such as transposition, rotation, or advancement flaps. These are discussed separately, but they include medial plantar flaps, V-Y advancement plantar flaps, and fasciocutaneous flaps. Common muscle flaps include the abductor hallucis and flexor hallucis brevis flaps. Although these are all effective flaps for coverage, each has morbidity in terms of foot function and balance and can create secondary deformity in the foot. Several advances have been made in the understanding of vascular territories or angiosomes, as described by Taylor (3) that have expanded the armamentarium of soft tissue reconstructions available for the foot and ankle. These include island pedicle flaps such as the supramalleolar flap or peroneal artery flap (4). These new and promising techniques have obviated the need for free tissue transfer in some cases and are taking their place on the reconstructive ladder.

Finally, on the highest rung on the ladder are the techniques that are the most complex yet often required; if properly selected, these can truly answer Sir Harold Gillies' challenge to the reconstructive surgeon. Soft tissue technology exists for autologous composite tissue transplantation. For example, osteocutaneous free flaps can deliver well-vascularized bone and soft tissue to defects created by tumor or gunshot wounds. Myocutaneous flaps can use muscle components to fill dead space, while skin is transferred for surface recontouring. Innervated flaps can supply sensibility, which may prove useful in preventing ulceration, particularly on the plantar surface of the foot.

The selection of soft tissue procedures for coverage of the foot and ankle will be determined by several factors (4). These include tissue requirement (muscle, skin, bone, composite), the origin of the requirement (chronic ulcer, acute injury, unstable wound), the location (plantar, instep, forefoot, heel, dorsal–dorsum, malleoli, Achilles tendon), and the underlying architecture of the foot (sensibility, osteology, and musculoskeletal status). The soft tissue replacement procedure will often be combined with orthopaedic procedures; ignoring or not integrating soft tissue reconstruction with orthopaedic procedures for muscle balancing, fusions, and tendon balancing will lead to prolonged disability, higher costs of treatment, and ultimately treatment failure due to lack of a coordinated "orthoplastic approach."

Treatment of traumatic soft tissue deficits involving the calcaneus has been classified by Levin and Nunley (6). This classification can be applied to all regions of the foot and ankle. There are four major categories of deficit, each with its own reconstructive ladder.

CLOSED FRACTURES TREATED BY OPEN REDUCTION AND INTERNAL FIXATION

When considering surgical intervention for fractures of the foot and ankle, an important determinant for successful healing is the amount of soft tissue swelling present at the time of surgery, as well as the swelling that develops after surgery. Ice, elevation and bulky dressings will allow edema to subside within a few days. If swelling is not sufficiently decreased, problems with wound closure will occur.

Operative technique is important in preventing soft tissue complications of open treatment. Atraumatic technique, the use of skin hooks rather than self-retaining retractors, loupe magnification, hemostasis during exposure, drains, and postoperative dressings all are important contributions to uncomplicated wound healing. When primary wound closure cannot be performed, porcine allograft, Epigard (Synthes, Pennsylvania), or a split-thickness skin graft can be applied as a temporary coverage. Delayed closure can be done at a later time. The main advantage of using a skin graft is that it may remain in place as definitive treatment. If applied as a meshed graft, the graft will contract, decreasing the skin grafted area relative to the surrounding normal tissue and improving the aesthetic result. It is rarely necessary to ascend the reconstructive ladder beyond skin grafting in cases of internal fixation in which wound edges cannot be brought together without tension. Often the gap is small, with sufficient muscle or peritenon exposed that will accept a graft readily.

POSTOPERATIVE WOUND BREAKDOWN

The etiology for this soft tissue problem is usually a wound that is closed under excess skin tension. As a result, with postoperative swelling, edema causes increased ischemia at the suture line, resulting in necrosis and dehiscence. Partial thickness wound defects can be initially managed with conservative measures, such as wet to wet dressings, whirlpool, oral antibiotics, and wound debridement. If in the course of superficial debridement vital structures become exposed (such as the lateral wall of the calcaneus, or hardware), then early aggressive soft tissue reconstruction should be performed.

In cases requiring full-thickness coverage (vascularized tissue), local or distant flaps are selected, based on (a) presence of infection, (b) depth of the defect, (c) vascular supply, and (d) damage to other areas of the foot that preclude the use of local flaps. In instances of trauma, local flaps such as the abductor muscle should be used with caution for two reasons. First, the pedicles that supply these flaps may be compromised. Second, use of certain intrinsic flaps, although helpful for coverage, may disturb the architecture of the foot, leading to progressive imbalance and deformity. The use of extrinsic island pedicle flaps may be a better choice (such as the peroneal artery flap).

OPEN FRACTURES OF THE FOOT AND ANKLE

There is good evidence to suggest that early coverage of open fractures is the treatment of choice provided the wound environment is suitable (Fig. 2) (7). The type of soft tissue coverage will depend on the underlying reconstructive needs and must be tailored to them. Rather than commit patients to multiple procedures over a long period, with anticipated poor outcomes, consideration should be given to immediate amputation if bone as well as soft tissue parts are not salvageable. Poor prognosticators include dysvascular feet requiring revascularization, insensate plantar surface with nerve avulsion or defect, and absent hindfoot bone stock, such as in gunshot wounds that ablate the calcaneus or talus.

OSTEOMYELITIS OF THE FOOT AND ANKLE

Osteomyelitis usually occurs late and is frequently preceded by marginal soft tissue over implants or bone. Inflamed, reactive, or fibrotic tissues cannot be used to close defects after sequestrectomy. In this case, distant muscle flap should be imported as dead space fillers and harbingers of improved blood supply that will deliver antibiotics and combat sepsis. The Cierny (8) protocol should be applied to foot and ankle osteomyelitis, and soft tissue requirements can be fulfilled based again on the reconstructive ladder.

RECONSTRUCTIVE LADDER FOR UNSTABLE SOFT TISSUE

Unstable soft tissue usually results from repetitive mechanical irritation (medial midfoot plantar ulcer from Charcot foot) or traumatic injury in which soft tissue is lost (an avulsion injury of the calcaneus). The specialized fat pad may initially be replaced with a reconstruction such as a skin graft (Fig. 3). Over time, despite graft hypertrophy, dystrophic local changes occur, leading to ulceration, pain, and infection. In such cases, composite tissue transfer is the treatment of choice, to provide padding and bulk (9). Because of continued shear and tangential stress, orthotics are often required in conjunction with soft tissue replacement, to maintain balance of forces during the gait cycle (9).

FLAP SELECTION FOR FOOT AND ANKLE RECONSTRUCTION

Assuming that skin grafting is not adequate for soft tissue coverage, the reconstructive ladder leads to the use of local flaps. Simple fasciocutaneous flaps on the dorsum of the foot or plantar surface (such as the V-Y advancement flap) can be used for very small defects. The advantages is that the dissection is confined to local areas. The disadvantage is that these are reserved for small defects [i.e., the medialis pedis flap described by Masquelet (4)]. Figure 4 gives an example of a flap based on a single cutaneous perforator. The difficulty with these flaps is that the dissection is often tedious, particularly in an area of the foot that has been damaged, and the vascular supply to the flaps may be unreliable.

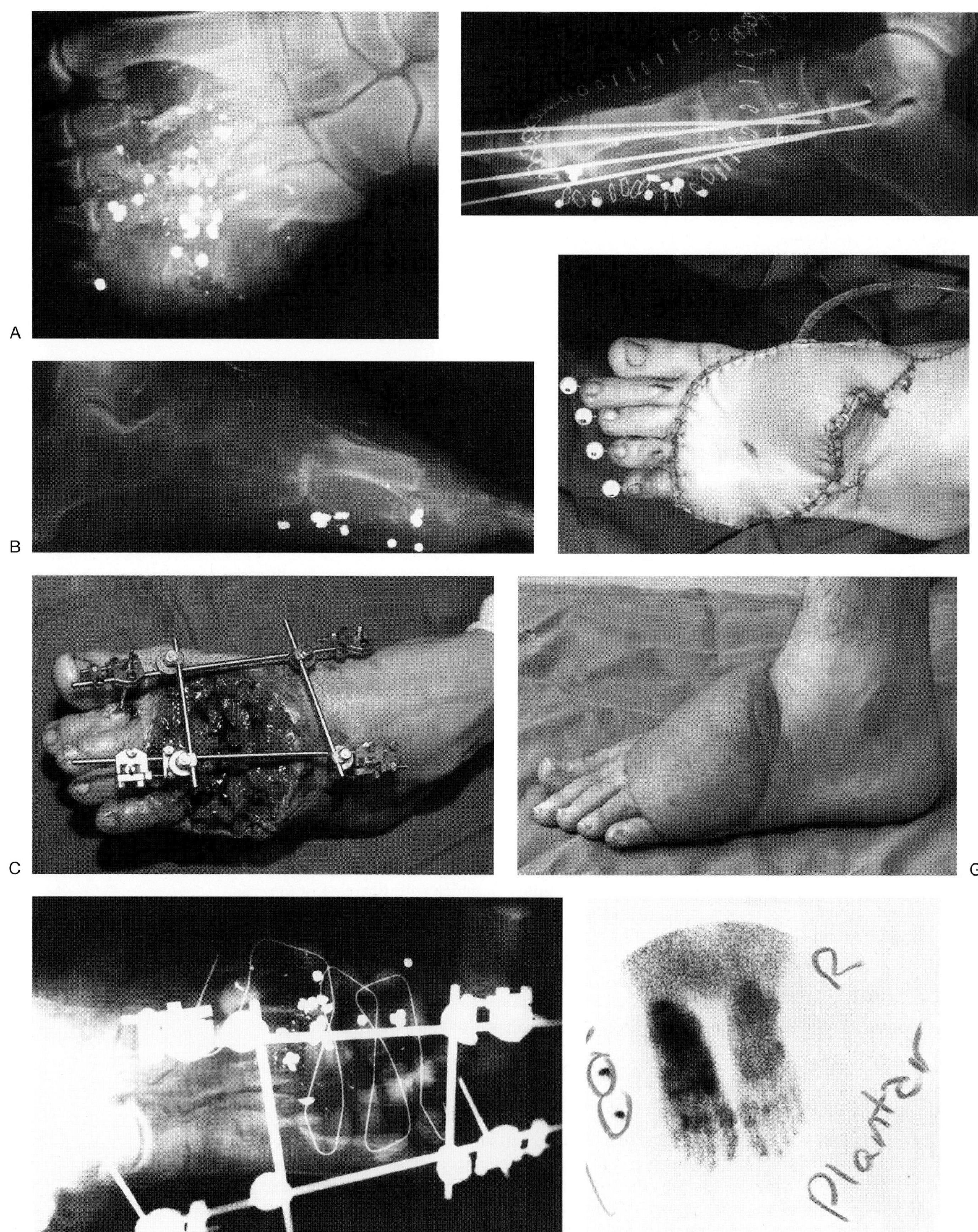

Figure 2. A,B: Radiograph of gunshot wound to the foot with bone and soft tissue destruction. **C–F:** After debridement and placement of an external fixator, a scapular flap was used with conventional iliac crest bone graft. **G:** The patient had incorporation of the bone graft at 1 year postoperatively, with a normal foot. **H:** Bone scan demonstrating good uptake.

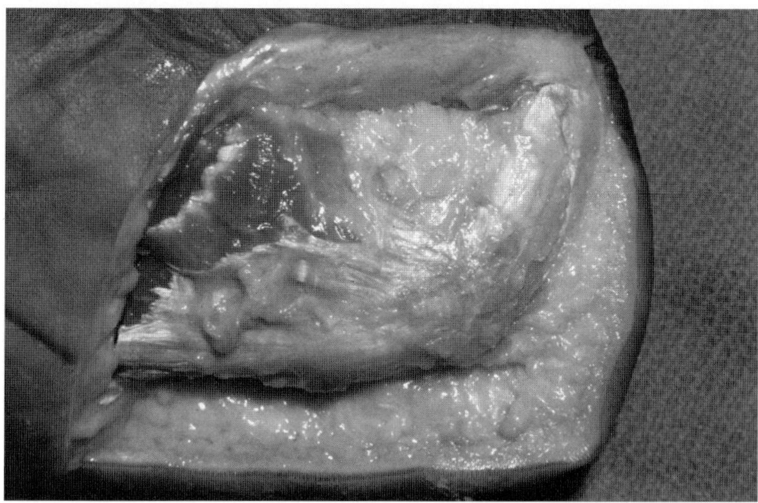

Figure 3. Cadaver dissection of heel. Lateral view showing plantar musculature, calcaneal tuberosity, thickened dermis, and specialized fat cells and septi. This tissue is quite unique and is difficult to replace with any kind of local or free tissue transfer.

A 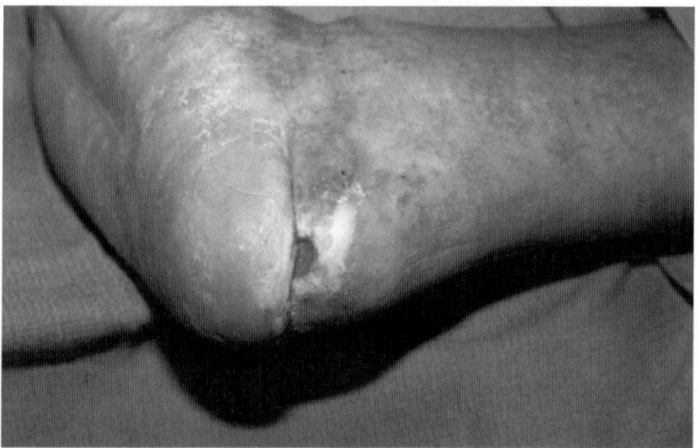

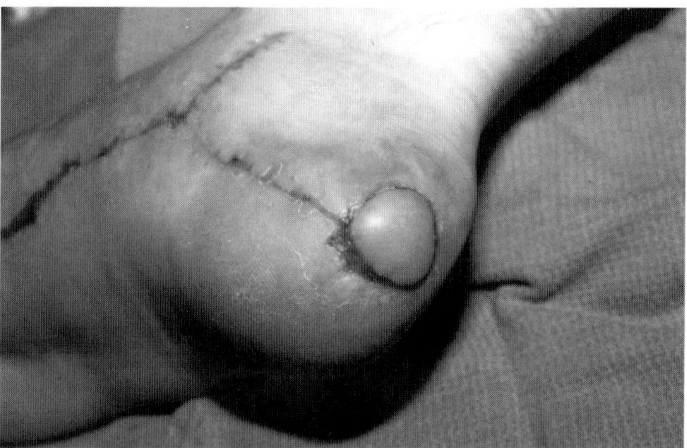 B

Figure 4. A: Posterior wound breakdown after excision of pump bump. The calcaneus is exposed as well as the insertion of heel cord. **B:** Using a medialis pedis flap, a transposition is made and an island pedicle flap is raised and used to close the defect.

Other options for local flap selections are local muscle flaps such as the flexor hallucis brevis, abductor hallucis longus, or extensor digitorum brevis muscles (11). Dissection of these muscles is more straightforward, but the arc of rotation and the amount of muscle actually delivered to the deficit may be small relative to the amount of dissection required. In my practice these are reserved for small defects. Furthermore, flaps such as these local muscle flaps intrinsic to the foot will lead to some degree of musculotendinous imbalance over time, which is one of the relative disadvantages that can be avoided by using tissue from other sites.

There has been a resurgence of interest in fasciocutaneous flaps, and several of these have been developed for ankle and hindfoot, as well as forefoot, coverage. The fascial subcutaneous turndown flap can be useful for the exposed heel cord or calcaneus, and the anterior tibial fasciocutaneous flap can be used for forefoot and dorsal foot defects (Fig. 5). Disadvantages of the anterior tibial turndown flap include the need to take the anterior tibial artery as well as occasional interference with function of the deep peroneal nerve. Nevertheless, the flaps can provide a large surface area for foot and ankle coverage without the use of microsurgical techniques.

Assuming that local foot flaps, fasciocutaneous flaps, or extrinsic fasciocutaneous flaps are not selected, free tissue transfer is now considered. In terms of the selection of free flaps for the foot and ankle, flap choice depends on tissue deficit. A study by Levin and Serafin (9) showed no evidence that the muscle, compared with the skin,

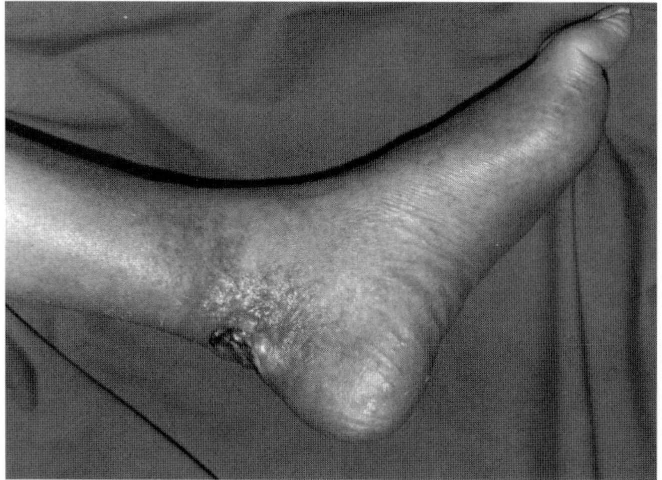

A

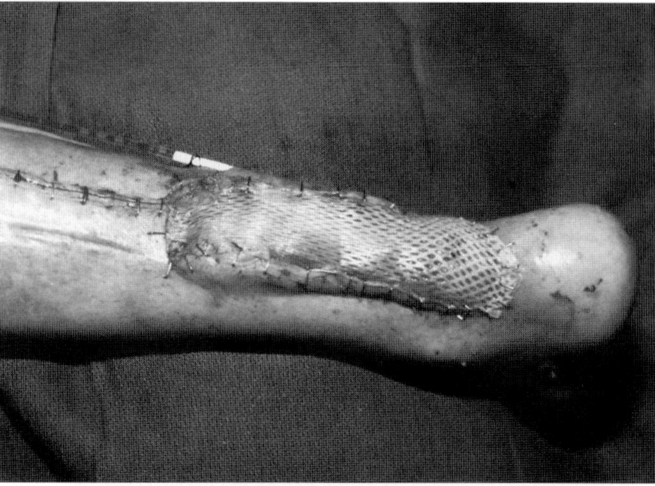

C

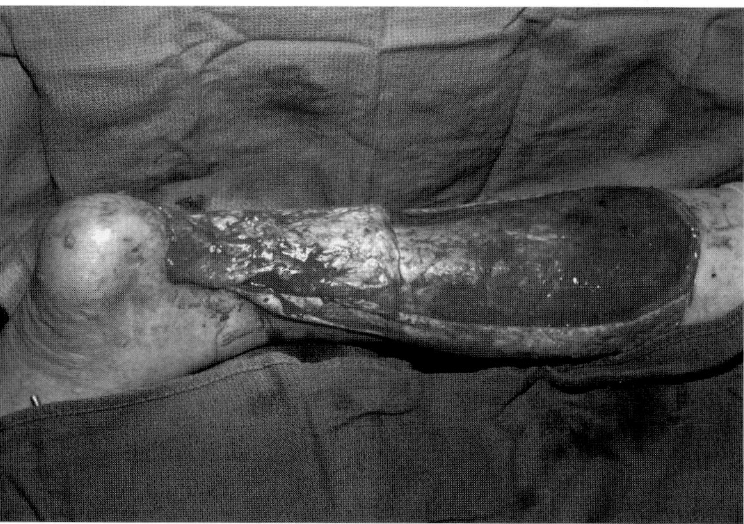

B

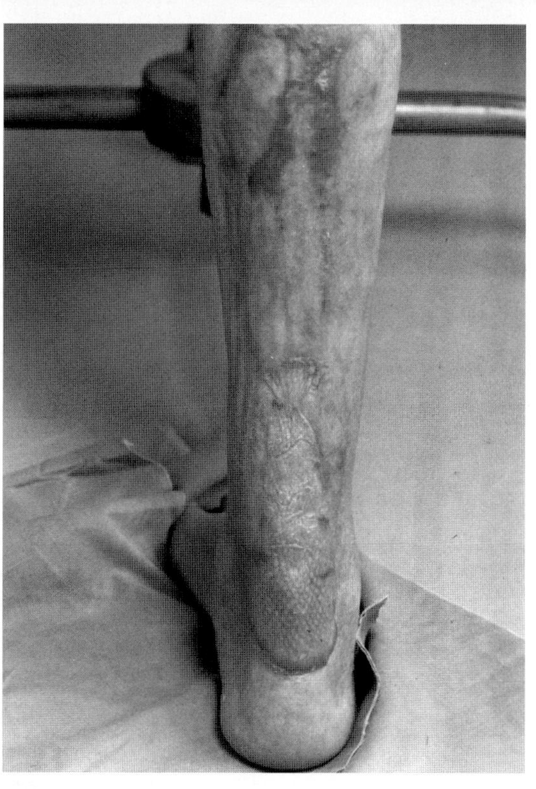

D

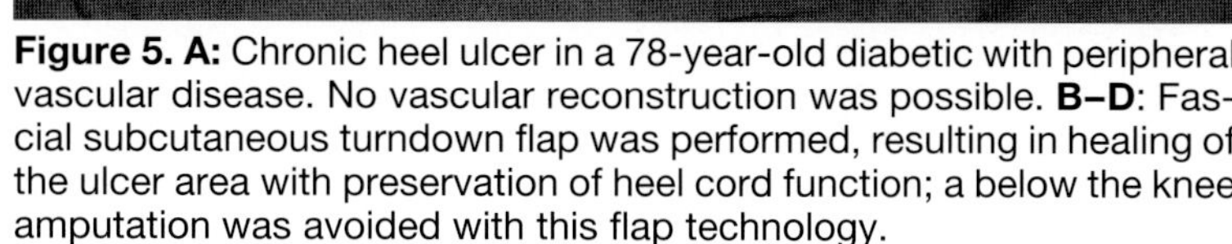

Figure 5. A: Chronic heel ulcer in a 78-year-old diabetic with peripheral vascular disease. No vascular reconstruction was possible. **B–D**: Fascial subcutaneous turndown flap was performed, resulting in healing of the ulcer area with preservation of heel cord function; a below the knee amputation was avoided with this flap technology.

flap is any better for use in the foot (particularly on the plantar surface) in terms of incidence of breakdown. All patients have some degree of difficulty following free flap transfer to the foot and ankle. These include factors such as contour, interface healing, callous formation, shear of flaps, and the need for ongoing orthotics and balancing procedures (Fig. 5A,B).

→

Figure 6. A: Chronic heel ulcer of 2 years' duration in a 55-year-old diabetic clergyman. **B:** Closeup view of granulation tissue. The patient has not walked in 2 years. Arteriogram demonstrated poor vascular inflow to the foot. **C,D:** The patient required bypass grafting and simultaneous free radial innervated forearm flap. **E,F:** Postoperative view shows donor site and healing of the flap. The flap developed protective sensibility and is durable coverage for gait. **G:** Extrinsic bracing was required to counterbalance intrinsic muscle deficiencies.

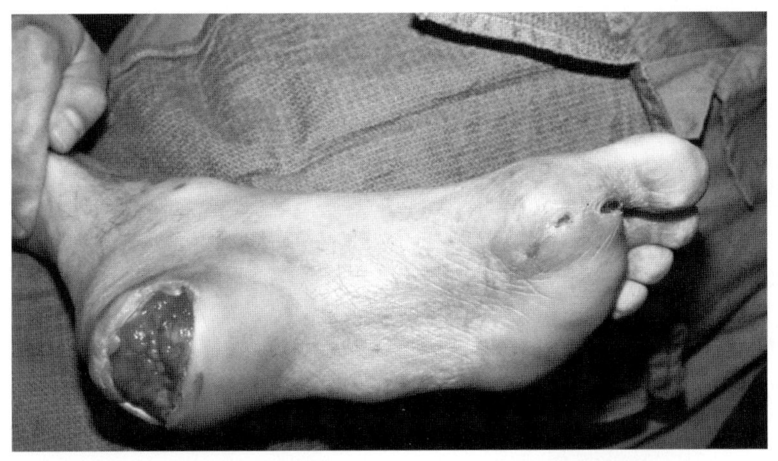
A

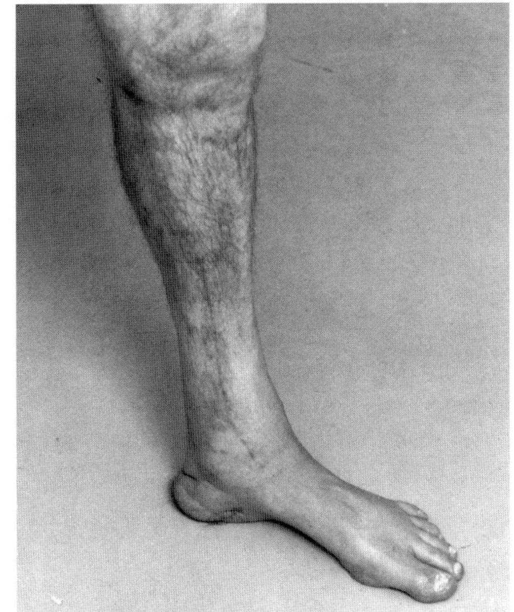
E

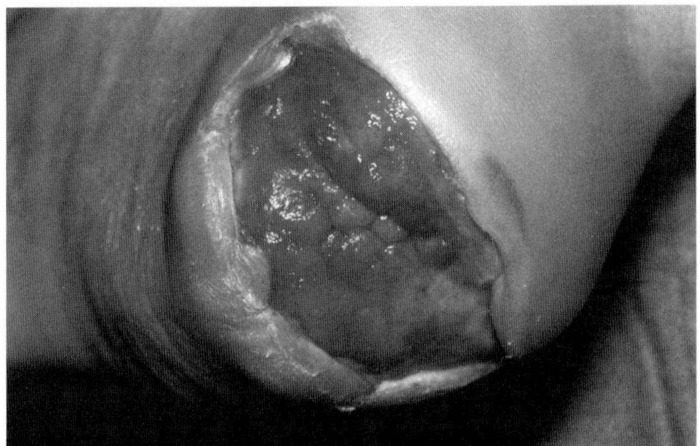
B

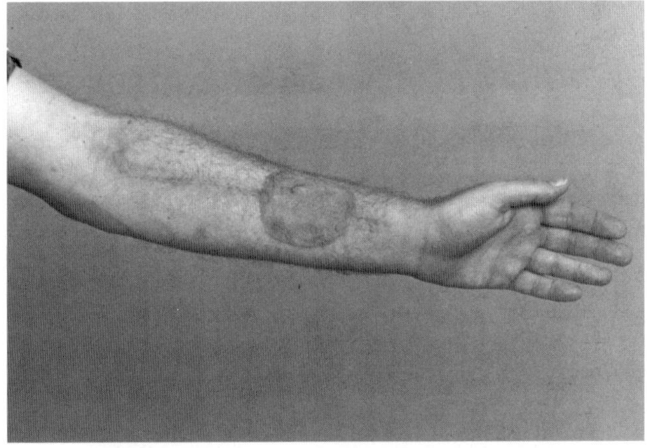
F

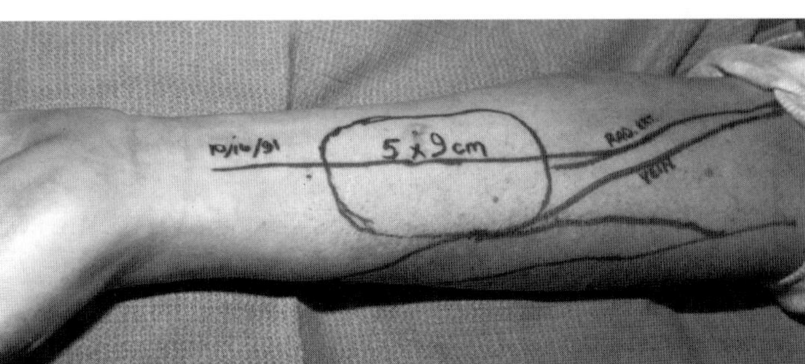

C

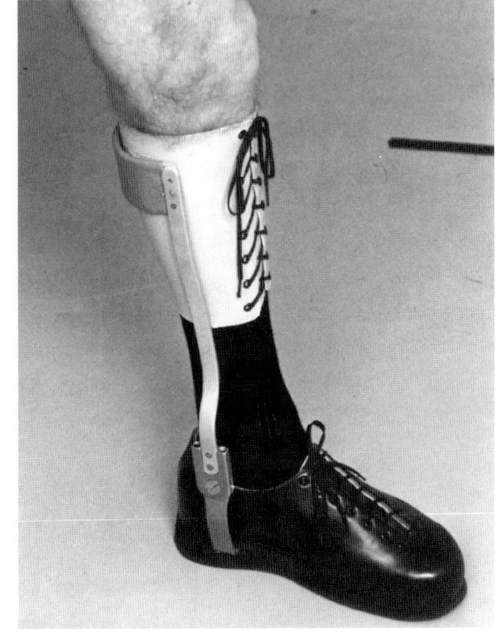
G

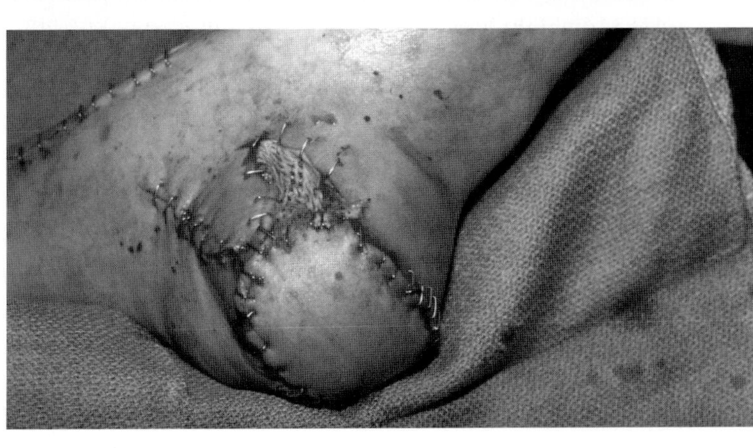
D

A

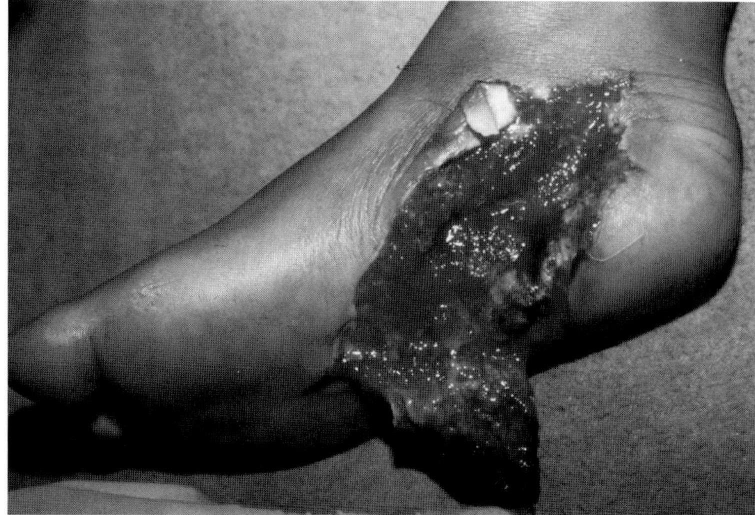

B

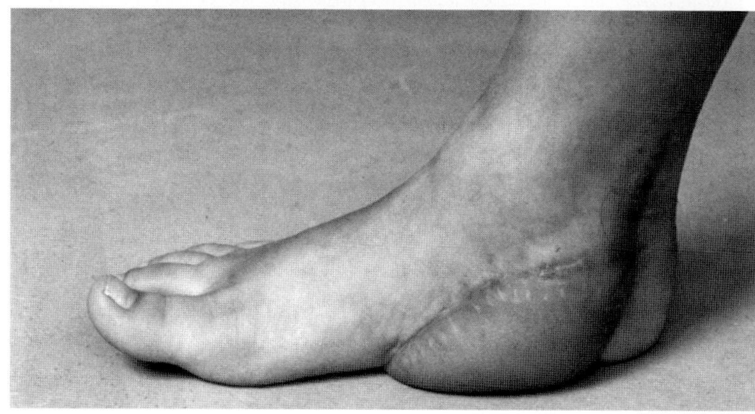

Figure 7. A: Six-year-old child with lawnmower injury with unstable plantar and medial soft tissue. **B:** Patient at 6 months. Due to the fat content, the flap required debulking and recontouring but did provide stable plantar coverage.

Skin Flaps

The lateral arm flap can be used for small defects such as the instep. Advantages include remote harvest site, and disadvantages include donor site morbidity such as the aesthetic result from resultant flap harvest if the skin graft is needed for closure.

Another cutaneous choice from the upper extremity is the radial forearm flap. Again, this donor cosmetic problem is not insignificant if the deficit can be closed primarily. It provides some innervation potential, as does the lateral arm flap. A long vascular pedicle can be used for anastomosis out of the zone of injury (Fig. 6).

The free scapular flap is reserved for large cutaneous defects. The advantage is that the donor site has a low associated morbidity. The disadvantage is that in particularly obese patients, the thickness of the flap may lead to excessive bulk precluding normal shoe wear and the flap itself may have to be debulked (Fig. 7).

Fascial flaps include lateral arm, radial forearm, scapular, and temporalis fascia. The temporalis fascia has been used for dorsal coverage, particularly of exposed tendons. The disadvantages are that it is very thin. It has been our observation that skin graft healing of these flaps has some degree of hypertrophy that may be unacceptable. In addition, donor site allopecia occurs infrequently.

Muscle Flaps

Several choices exist for muscle flaps, and tailoring and custom design of all potential donor sites is possible. These include the gracilis muscle if one chooses to remain in the same extremity. The gracilis can supply adequate muscle coverage and may be harvested from the same extremity, allowing the procedure to be done under epidural anesthesia. The rectus abdominis muscle is particularly suitable if the patient requires supine positioning. The serratus anterior and latissimus dorsi are excellent sources for muscle flaps. The serratus is more suitable than the latissimus in that the muscle is thinner and can be tailored to a smaller flap. The latissimus dorsi harvest usually provides more muscle than is required. Morbidity of muscle flaps is least for the gracilis and probably potentially the most for the rectus abdominus in that some times these patients can develop abdominal wall hernias.

Osteocutaneous Flaps

Osteocutaneous flaps may be required for treatment of composite defects such as bone and soft tissue. Both the lateral arm and radial forearm flaps can be harvested with bone from the humerus or radius. Disadvantages, particularly in the radius, are that this may lead to stress fracture and that the amount of bone provided is usually of insufficient quality and cancellous content to be structurally beneficial, particularly if dealing with large defects of the foot and ankle. Although it is acceptable to perform conventional iliac crest grafting (Fig. 7) with free tissue transfer coverage, other benefits of composite flaps (such as the osteocutaneous scapular flap) would allow import of vascularized bone as well as healthy soft tissue for reconstruction.

The osteocutaneous fibular flap can be used, for example, to replace the medial ray of the foot or the first metatarsal due to tumor or infection and simultaneously provide a skin paddle over the vascularized bone. Donor site morbidity of the osteocutaneous fibula is more significant and usually involves harvest from an opposite unimpaired extremity; this flap would not necessarily be the author's first choice for replacement of bone and soft tissue defects around the foot and ankle.

SUMMARY

More important than specific flap selection is the execution of free flap transfer with maximum cosmetic and functional reconstruction. The ability to transplant living tissue from other sites in the body to the foot and ankle is not considered successful if patients cannot wear shoes, cannot ambulate without impaired gait, and have repetitive breakdown of their transfers. Sometimes debulking, recontouring, and reinsetting will be necessary, but these can be kept to a minimum with proper planning and execution.

REFERENCES

1. Serafin D. Microsurgical composite tissue transplantation. *Prob Plast Reconstr Surg* 1991;1–24.
2. Levin LS. The reconstructive ladder. *Orthop Clin North Am* 1993;24:393–409.
3. Taylor GI. The vascular territories (angiosomes) of the body: experimental study and clinical applications. *Br J Plast Surg* 1987:40:113–141.
4. Masquelet AC, Romana MC. The medialis pedis flap: a new fasiocutaneous flap. *Plast Reconstr Surg* 1990;85:765–772.
5. Levin LS. Microsurgical autologous tissue transplantation for orthopaedic reconstruction. *J Am Acad Orthop Surg* 1995;10:134–144.
6. Levin LS, Nunley JA. Management of soft tissue problems associated with calcaneus fractures. *Clin Orthop* 1993;290:151–156.
7. Godina M. Early microsurgical reconstruction of complex trauma of extremities. *Plast Reconstr Surg* 1986;78:285–292.
8. Cierny G, Maderr JT. Approach to adult osteomyelitis. *Orthop Rev* 1987;16:259–270.
9. Shaw WW. Lower extremity trauma and reconstruction. *Clin Plast Surg* 1986;13:4.
10. Levin LS, Serafin D. Plantar skin coverage. *Prob Plast Reconst Surg* 1991;1:156–184.
11. Mathes SJ, Nahai F. *Clinical applications for muscle and musculocutaneous flaps.* St. Louis: CV Mosby, 1982.

EDITORIAL COMMENTS

Guidelines for Soft Tissue Coverage of Complex Foot and Ankle Injuries

L. Scott Levin

Dr. Scott Levin has given us an excellent treatment approach to soft tissue injuries around the foot and ankle secondary to trauma. Possible wound complications should be addressed after the initial assessment. Complicating factors such as age (with poor nutritional status, bone defects, and osteopenia), peripheral vascular disease, diabetes mellitus, and degree of trauma to tissue are important in making a treatment assessment. The timing of surgical intervention, particularly around the ankle and calcaneus, is critical to the prevention of soft tissue defects. The degree of force of trauma and suspected future swelling and shear injuries to tissue should help one to determine whether immediate open treatment would be appropriate. At the Medical College of Virginia, when we are in doubt, we use the following techniques to aid in decision making: judicious debridement of open wounds; careful tension-free closures around joints, bone, and tendon structures; and delay for a period appropriate to allow safe reduction techniques with their accompanying tissue trauma. To decrease swelling, we use elevation, foot pump intermittent pressure on plantar surface, and frequent assessment. Skin blisters indicate increased shear and are treated until they pop spontaneously. These would be an appropriate cause for delay in surgery. Judgment and experience are vital in making the proper decision; we use degree of swelling and whether the tissue wrinkles appropriately to help us make that decision. Proper tension-free closure and allowance for drainage of hematoma and tissue fluid are also important.

When our efforts result in a coverage problem, then it is important that the tissue not be allowed to dessicate, as Dr. Levin has stressed. Timely coverage depends on the degree of contamination and lost blood supply. Proper nutritional status as determined by serum albumin and a total lymphocyte count can be used as an index. It is important that caustic agents such as betadine and peroxide not be used; biologic dressings are most appropriate. When in doubt, wet to dry dressing with fine mesh gauze will lead to development of appropriate granulation response if the host is capable. We should also remember that the use of skin that is devitalized at the time of initial debridement, such as a split-thickness skin graft, is appropriate. When nonviable tissue requires skin coverage, that tissue should never be discarded but used to help the physiologic coverage. Dr. Levin has given an excellent program, with appropriate wound care, then skin graft and the more difficult local flap, and finally appropriate free flap coverage. We must remember that the flap should be as physiologic as possible and allow for stress directed to that area. The flap should be able to accommodate the natural contours of the foot and ankle, conventional shoewear, and orthotics. The key in soft tissue problems about the foot and ankle is prevention and planning. One must be aware of the danger signs and poor host factors for coverage, in addition to planning for the rigid biomechanical fixation of fractures.

Robert S. Adelaar, M.D.

Subject Index

A
Abductor digiti quinti, fifth metatarsal insertion of, 219, 220f
Abductor hallucis, 236, 236f
Abductor hallucis longus flap, 263
Achilles tendon, lengthening of, for calcaneal malunion, 141
Adductor hallucis, 236, 236f
  oblique head of, 236, 236f
  transverse head of, 236, 236f
Age, in great toe metatarsophalangeal joint injury, 244
Aminoglycosides, for wound infection, in open ankle fracture, 32
Ankle
  complex fracture dislocations of, syndesmotic diastasis with, 9–19
    complications of, risk factors for, 19
    late results in, 17
    management of
      clinical, 12–13, 12f
      operative, 15–17, 16f
      postoperative, 17
    radiographic considerations in, 13–15, 13f–15f
  dorsiflexion of, in great toe metatarsophalangeal joint injury, 244
  fractures of
    classification of, 3, 4f
    closed, open reduction and internal fixation for, soft tissue management in, 260
    open, 31–37
      classification of, 33t
      late skeletal reconstruction in, 36
      management of
        antimicrobial, 31–32, 37
        emergency, 32
        presurgical planning in, 33
        surgical, 33–34, 33f, 34f
      neurovascular injury in, 37
      soft tissue management in, 261
      transverse medial wound in, 33, 33f
      wound reconstruction in
        complex, 35–36, 35f, 36f
        delayed, 34–35
  injury to
    complex, soft tissue coverage of, guidelines for, 257–268
    incidence of, 1, 2f
    pronation external rotation, 4, 5f
    supination external, 3–4, 5f
  instability of, assessment of, Cotton test in, 12–13, 12f
  osteomyelitis of, soft tissue management in, 261
  range of motion of, 1
  reconstruction of, flaps in
    muscle, 266–267
    osteocutaneous, 267
    selection of, 261–267, 263f–266f
    skin, 266, 265f, 266f
  stability of
    deltoid ligament in, 6
    lateral malleolus in, 4–6
    posterior malleolus in, 22
  syndesmosis of
    anatomy of, 10–12, 10f, 11f
    biomechanics of, 1–7, 2f–6f, 40
    function of, 10
    ligaments of, function of, 11
    in pilon fracture, 48
    stabilization of
      in deltoid tear, 7
      indications for, 7
    structures of, 1–2, 2f
    treatment of
      data summary of, 42–43
      historical review of, 39–44
Ankle block, in crush/soft tissue injuries of foot, 178, 180
Anterior tibial fasciocutaneous flap, 263
Anterior tibial margin, in pilon fracture, 47, 47f
Anterior tibialis artery, 163
  distribution of, 46f
  in talus circulation, 66, 68f
Anterior tibialis tendon, entrapment of, in tarsometatarsal injuries, 172
Anterior tibiofibular ligament, 1, 2f
  anatomy of, 39
Anterior–inferior tibiofibular ligament, anatomy of, 10, 11f
Antibiotics, for open ankle fracture, 37
Antimicrobials, for open ankle fracture, 31–32
AO classification, of distal tibial fracture, 48f
Apophysis, of fifth metatarsal, 219–221, 220f
  fracture vs., 219
Artery(ies). *See also* names of specific arteries
  cutaneous, of pilon fracture, 47
  of great toe, 236, 237f
Arthritis
  after pilon fracture, 62
  after subtalar dislocation, 112
  after talar fracture, 92
  subtalar
    after displaced intraarticular calcaneal fracture, 131
    after talar neck fracture, 81, 82f
Arthrodesis
  calcaneocuboid, for cuboid fracture, 159
  for navicular body fracture, 154
  primary, of tibiotalar joint, in pilon fracture, 61
  of proximal interphalangeal joint, in compartment syndrome of foot, 203
  tibiocalcaneal, for talar body fracture, 88, 90f, 91f
  triple, for calcaneal malunion, 140
Arthroscopic cheilectomy, 252f, 253–254, 253f
Arthroscopy
  of great toe metatarsophalangeal joint injury, 250, 250f
  of osteochondral talar lesions, 104, 106f
Arthrosis, after talar fracture, 92

NOTE: Page numbers followed by "f" indicate figures. Page numbers followed by "t" indicate tables.

Artificial turf, and great toe metatarsophalangeal joint injuries, 243–244
AV Impulse foot pump, 179, 179f
  for compartment syndrome, 196
    with calcaneal fracture, 197
Aviator astralagus, 65
Avulsion fracture, of proximal fifth metatarsal, mechanism of, 223–224
Axial compression, in pilon fracture, 48

B

Benirschke incision, 116, 117f
Bimalleolar fracture, treatment of, results of, 41
Blair fusion, for talar body fracture, 88, 90f, 91f
Blood supply
  of fifth metatarsal
    extraosseous, 220, 221f, 222
    intraosseous, 222, 222f
  of great toe, 236, 237f
Bohler's angle, after displaced intraarticular calcaneal fracture reduction, 133
Bone grafting
  for intraarticular calcaneal fracture, 124–125
    displaced, 134
  for proximal fifth metatarsal fracture, 227f, 228
Bone scan, of talar posterior process fracture, 97f, 98
Bony hallux limitus, 241, 242f
  after great toe metatarsophalangeal joint injury, 252–253
Broden view, of intraarticular calcaneal fracture, 124, 124f
"Buddy taping"
  for great toe metatarsophalangeal joint injury, 249
  for phalangeal fractures, 213

C

Calcaneal compartment, of foot
  anatomy of, 192, 192f
  pressure measurement in, 195
Calcaneal fracture(s)
  with compartment syndrome of foot
    clinical presentation of, 193
    fasciotomy for, 200, 200f
    treatment of, 196–197
  intraarticular, 115–126
    classification of, 121–123, 122f
    clinical correlations with, 123
    displaced
      classification of, 128, 129f
      complications of, 131
      historical perspective on, 127–128
      prognosis in, 132
        with closed treatment, 132
        with operative treatment, 132–133
      treatment of, 127–136
        lateral approach to, 130, 133
        medial approach to, 133
        nonoperative, 130
        primary fusion in, 130–131
        results of, 131–133
    joint depression, 118–119, 119f
    mechanism of, 118–121, 118f–121f
    natural history of, 121
    pathoanatomy of, 118–121, 118f–121f
    primary fracture line in, 119–120, 119f
    surgical treatment of, 123–125, 124f
    tongue, 118–119, 119f
    wound complications after, 116
  malunion of, 137–143
    clinical examination in, 137–138, 138f, 139f
    surgical treatment of, 140–141
      incisions in, 140
      results of, 141–142
    type I, 138, 138f
      surgical treatment of, 140
        results of, 141
    type II, 138, 139f
      surgical treatment of, 140–141
        results of, 141–142
    type III, 138, 139f
      surgical treatment of, 141
        results of, 142
  treatment of, nonoperative, complications of, 137
Calcaneal pin traction, for pilon fracture, 54–55
  selection criteria for, 52–53, 53f
Calcaneocuboid arthrodesis, for cuboid fracture, 159
Calcaneus
  anatomy of, 115–118, 116f–118f
    cortical, 116, 118f
    trabecular, 116, 117f
  facets of, 116, 116f
  relationship of, to talus, 120
Capsulitis, adhesive, after great toe metatarsophalangeal joint injury, 251f, 252–253
  management of, 251f, 253
Capsulo–ligamentous–sesamoid complex, of great toe, 234–235, 234f, 235f
Carbon fiber plate, for athletic shoe, 248, 248f
Cartilaginous hallux limitus, 239, 241f
Cast, short leg
  for fracture of base of fifth metatarsal, 210, 212
  for metatarsal fractures
    displaced, 208
    undisplaced, 207
  for phalangeal fractures, 213
  for subtalar dislocation, 113
Cefazolin, for wound infection, in open ankle fracture, 32
Central compartment, of foot
  anatomy of, 192, 192f
  pressure measurement in, 194, 194f
Cephalosporin, for wound infection, in open ankle fracture, 32
Cephamandole, for wound infection, in open ankle fracture, 32
Chaput tubercle, in pilon fracture, 47f, 48
Cheilectomy, arthroscopic, 252f, 253–254, 253f
Chinese finger traps, for displaced metatarsal fractures, 208
Circulation
  to navicular, 146, 146f
  to talus, 66–68, 68f
Clanton grading system, for turf toe, 247t, 248
Claw toes, compartment syndrome and, 201f, 202
Closed fracture
  of foot/ankle, open reduction and internal fixation for, soft tissue management in, 260
  undisplaced, of metatarsals, treatment of, 207
Clostridium perfringens, and wound infection, in open ankle fracture, 32
Compartment pressures, of foot, measurement of, 194–195, 194f, 195f
Compartment syndrome(s)
  of foot. *See* Foot, compartment syndromes of
  in tarsometatarsal injuries, 168
Complex fracture dislocations, of ankle. *See* Ankle, complex fracture dislocations of
Complex fractures, of talus, 65–93
  outcome in, 92
Compression, axial, in pilon fracture, 48
Computed tomography (CT)
  of calcaneal malunion, 138
  of cuboid fracture, 157, 158f
  of intraarticular calcaneal fracture, 121, 122f
    displaced, 128, 129f
  of posterior malleolus fracture, 23, 24f
  of talar body fracture, 85, 85f
Cortisone, for great toe metatarsophalangeal joint injury, 250
Cotton test, 12–13, 12f
Crista, 235, 235f
Crush injury
  of foot. *See* Foot, crush/soft tissue injuries of
  of talar body, 84f, 85, 85f
CT. *See* Computed tomography (CT)
Cuboid
  anatomy of
    osseous, 145–146, 146f
    variants in, 147, 147f
    vascular, 146, 146f
  fractures of, 145–160
    mechanism of, 148, 157
    patterns of, 157
    radiography of, 157, 158f
    treatment of, 158–159, 159f
Cuneiform ligaments, of navicular, 145–146
Cuneiforms, in tarsometatarsal anatomy, 161–163

D

Danis–Weber classification, of ankle fractures, 3, 4f
Deep peroneal nerve, 237, 238f
Deltoid artery, in talus circulation, 66–68, 68f
Deltoid ligament, 3, 3f
  in ankle stability, 6
  deep, 3, 3f
    in ankle syndesmosis biomechanics, 40
    components of, 40
  superficial, components of, 39–40
  tear of
    in complex ankle fracture dislocation, screw fixation of, 19
    syndesmosis stabilization in, 7
Diaphyseal fracture, of proximal fifth metatarsal, 222, 224–225
  acute, 225
  chronic, 225
  delayed union of, 225
  nonunion of, 225
Diastasis
  interosseous, 41
  syndesmotic. *See* Syndesmotic diastasis
Dislocation
  subtalar. *See* Subtalar joint, dislocation of
  talonavicular, in talar neck fractures, 73, 73f

Distractor, femoral
  for talar body fracture, 88, 89f
  for talar neck fracture, 80, 80f
Dorsal lip fracture, of navicular, 148, 148f
Dorsiflexion
  active
    of interphalangeal joint, 234
    of metatarsophalangeal joint, 232
  of ankle, in great toe metatarsophalangeal joint injury, 244
  passive
    of interphalangeal joint, 234
    of metatarsophalangeal joint, 232
Drilling, of osteochondral talar lesions, 104, 106f
Dual pin redresser, 59
Dwyer osteotomy, for calcaneal malunion, 141

E

Elastic fixation, of syndesmosis screw, 12
Epiphysis, of fifth metatarsal, 220f
Exercises, for great toe metatarsophalangeal joint injury, 249
Exostectomy, lateral, for calcaneal malunion, 140, 141
Explosion fracture. *See* Pilon fracture
Extensor digitorum brevis flap, 263
Extensor hallucis brevis, 235, 235f, 236f
Extensor hallucis longus, 235, 235f, 236f
Extensor tendons, blockage of, by subtalar dislocation, 111f, 112
External fixation
  of navicular body fracture, 151f, 154
  of open ankle fracture, 34
  of pilon fracture, 54f, 59–61
    hybrid, 54f, 61
    temporary, 53
  of talar body fracture, 88, 89f
External fixator
  for skeletal stabilization, in crush/soft tissue injuries of foot, 187
  for tarsometatarsal injuries, 172, 172f
  temporary, for pilon fracture, 56, 57f

F

Fascial flaps, 266
Fascial subcutaneous turndown flap, 263, 264f
Fasciocutaneous flap, 261, 263f
  anterior tibial, 263
Fasciotomy, for compartment syndromes of foot, 197–201, 197f–200f
  with calcaneal fracture, 200, 200f
  dorsal approach to, 197f, 198–200, 198f, 199f
  incisions for, 197f, 198
  indications for, 196
  medial approach to, 199f, 200
Femoral distractor
  for talar body fracture, 88, 89f
  for talar neck fracture, 80, 80f
Fibula
  fixation of
    in pilon fracture, 56
    plate, in complex ankle fracture dislocation, with syndesmotic diastasis, 16, 16f
  fracture of
    in pilon fracture, 47
    in pronation external rotation injury, 4
    in supination external injury, 4
  short, in syndesmotic diastasis, 6f
Fibular plantar marginal artery, 220, 220f
Fifth metatarsal
  anatomy of, 218–222, 219f, 220f, 222f
    vascular, 221–222, 221f, 222f
  base of, fractures of, 210–212, 211f
    classification of, 210
  growth/development of, 219–221, 220f, 221f
  ligaments of, 218, 219f
  ossification of, centers of, 219, 220f
  osteology of, 218–222, 218f–220f
  proximal, fractures of, 217–230
    algorithm for, 228f
    classification of, 222–223
    diaphyseal, 224–225
    historical overview of, 217–218
    mechanism of, 223–226, 223f
    postoperative care in, 228
    stress, 225–226
    treatment of, 223–226
      immobilization vs. screw fixation in, 229–230
      surgical, 226f, 227–228, 227f
    tuberosity, 223–224
  tendon insertions on, 218, 220f
Figure-of-eight taping, for great toe metatarsophalangeal joint injury, 249
First dorsal metacarpal artery, 163
First dorsal metatarsal artery, 236, 237f
First plantar metacarpal artery, 163
Fixation
  elastic, of syndesmosis screw, 12
  external. *See* External fixation
  internal. *See* Internal fixation
  pin. *See* Pin fixation
  plate
    of fibula, in complex ankle fracture dislocation, with syndesmotic diastasis, 16, 16f
    of intraarticular calcaneal fracture, 124, 126
    of pilon fracture, 57–60, 60f
    of talar body fracture, 85–88, 87f, 88f
Fixator, external
  for skeletal stabilization, in crush/soft tissue injuries of foot, 187
  for tarsometatarsal injuries, 172, 172f
  temporary, for pilon fracture, 56, 57f
Flap(s)
  abductor hallucis longus, 263
  extensor digitorum brevis, 263
  fascial, 266
  fascial subcutaneous turndown, 263, 264f
  fasciocutaneous, 261, 263f
    anterior tibial, 263
  flexor hallucis brevis, 263
  gracilis, 266–267
  lateral arm, 264
  latissimus dorsi, 267
    in open ankle fracture, 36, 36f
  local, in complex foot/ankle injuries, 259–260
  medialis pedis, 261, 263f
  osteocutaneous, fibular, 267
  radial forearm, 264–266, 265f
  rectus abdominis, 267
  scapular, 262f
    free, 266, 266f
  serratus anterior, 267
  temporalis fascia, 266
  in wound reconstruction, in open ankle fracture, 36, 36f, 37
Flexor digitorum longus tendon, contracture of, in compartment syndrome of foot, 202
Flexor hallucis brevis, 234f, 235–236, 236f
Flexor hallucis brevis flap, 263
Flexor hallucis longus, 192f, 200f, 234f, 235, 235f
  entrapment of, in talar fracture, 97–98
Flexor hallucis tendon, contracture of, in compartment syndrome of foot, 202
Fluorescein, in viable tissue identification, in crush/soft tissue injuries of foot, 182–183
Foot
  compartment syndromes of, 191–204
    anatomy of, 191–193, 192f
    with calcaneus fractures, treatment of, 196–197
    chronic, 201–203, 201f
      complications of, 201–202
      and myoneural ischemia, 202
      toe deformities in
        claw, 201f, 202
        correction of, 203
        hyperflexed, 202
    clinical presentation of, 193
    diagnosis of, 194–195, 194f, 195f
    pathogenesis of, 193
    postoperative care in, 201
    treatment of, 195–201
      fasciotomy in, 197–201, 197f–200f
      principles of, 195–196
  complex injuries of, soft tissue coverage of, guidelines for, 257–268
  crush/soft tissue injuries of
    bursting, 176, 177f
    compartment syndrome with, 193
    compressive, 176, 176f
    contamination of
      dirt/gravel in, 182
      oil/grease in, 182
    coverage of, timing of, 180–185, 180f, 181f, 183f, 184f
    debridement of, 180–181
    initial evaluation of, 178–180
    injury zone in, 180–185
    management of, 175–190
      principles of, 178–180, 179f
    mangling, 176, 177f
    mechanism of, 175–176, 176f–178f
    results in, 187–188
    shear (degloving), 176, 178f
    skeletal stabilization in, 185–187, 187f
    viable tissue identification in, 182–185
    wound contamination in, 185–187, 186f
  fracture of
    closed, open reduction and internal fixation for, soft tissue management in, 260
    open, soft tissue management in, 261, 262f
  osteomyelitis of, soft tissue management in, 261
  reconstruction of, flaps in
    muscle, 266–267
    osteocutaneous, 267
    selection of, 261–267, 263f–266f
    skin, 264–266, 265f, 266f
Foot pump
  for compartment syndrome, 196
    with calcaneal fracture, 197
  for crush/soft tissue injuries of foot, 179, 179f
Forceps, reduction, in posterior malleolus fracture repair, 27, 28f
Forefoot
  complex injuries of, treatment of, 205–216
  disruption of, navicular fracture with, 156f, 157

Fracture. *See* specific site or type of fracture
Fracture dislocations, complex, of ankle. *See* Ankle, complex fracture dislocations of
Free scapular flap, 266, 266f
Free tissue transfer, in complex foot/ankle injuries, 263–264
Fusion
  Blair, of talar body fracture, 88, 90f, 91f
  of subtalar joint
    for calcaneal malunion, 140, 141
    primary, for displaced intraarticular calcaneal fractures, 130–131
  talonavicular, of talar head fracture, 70, 71f

G
Gissane's angle, after displaced intraarticular calcaneal fracture reduction, 133
"Glide hole first" technique, in posterior malleolus fracture repair, 26
Gracilis muscle flap, 266–267
Grafting
  bone
    for intraarticular calcaneal fracture, 124–125
      displaced, 134
    for proximal fifth metatarsal fracture, 227f, 228
  skin
    in complex foot/ankle injuries, 259
    in open reduction and internal fixation, of closed fractures, 260
    split-thickness, in viable tissue identification, in crush/soft tissue injuries of foot, 183–185, 184f
Great toe. *See also* Hallux
  capsulo–ligamentous–sesamoid complex of, 234–235, 234f, 235f
  metatarsophalangeal joint of. *See* Metatarsophalangeal joint (MTPJ), of great toe
  neurovascular supply to, 236–237, 237f, 238f
Guidewire, in proximal fifth metatarsal fracture repair, 226f, 227

H
Hallux. *See also* Great toe
  phalanges of, fractures of, treatment of, 213
Hallux limitus
  after great toe metatarsophalangeal joint injury, 244, 252–253
  bony, 239–241, 242f
    after great toe metatarsophalangeal joint injury, 252–253
  cartilaginous, 239, 241f
Hallux rigidus, after great toe metatarsophalangeal joint injury, management of, 252f, 253–254, 253f
  surgical, 250
Hallux valgus, metatarsophalangeal joint injury and, surgical treatment of, 250, 251f
Hardcastle classification, of tarsometatarsal injuries, 166–167, 166f
Hawkins classification, of talar neck fractures, 73, 73f
Hawkins sign, 77, 79f, 81
Henry, posterolateral approach of, in posterior malleolus fracture repair, 26, 26f
Hindfoot
  in intraarticular calcaneal fractures, restoration of, 126
  in tarsometatarsal injuries
    pronation of, 168
    supination of, 168
Hybrid external fixation, of pilon fracture, 54f, 61
Hyperextension, and great toe metatarsophalangeal joint injury, 239, 239f, 240f
Hyperflexion, and great toe metatarsophalangeal joint injury, 241, 242f

I
Iliac crest bone block, for calcaneal malunion, 141
Ilizarov frame
  for calcaneal malunion, 141
  for open ankle fracture, 34
    pin placement in, 35f, 36
Immobilization
  for displaced metatarsal fractures, 207–210, 208f, 209f
  for navicular stress fracture, 156
  for phalangeal fractures, 213
  for proximal fifth metatarsal fracture, screw fixation vs., 229–230
Incision(s)
  Benirschke, 116, 117f
  for calcaneal malunion, 140
  for fasciotomy, in compartment syndromes of foot, 197f, 198
  for open reduction and internal fixation, of tarsometatarsal injuries, 170, 170f
Infection
  in crush/soft tissue injuries of foot, prevention of, 181–182
  wound, in open ankle fractures, antimicrobial management of, 31–32
Inferior transverse ligament, anatomy of, 39
Intercuneiform joints, stabilization of, in navicular fracture with forefoot disruption, 157
Internal fixation
  of fracture of base of fifth metatarsal, 210, 211f
  of great toe metatarsophalangeal joint injury, 250
  of navicular fracture
    Sangeorzan, 149f, 154
    tuberosity, 149f, 150
  of open ankle fracture, 34
  open reduction with. *See* Open reduction and internal fixation
Interosseous compartment, of foot
  anatomy of, 192, 192f
  pressure measurement in, 195, 195f
Interosseous diastasis, 41
Interosseous ligament, 1, 2f
  anatomy of, 39
  in ankle syndesmosis biomechanics, 40
Interphalangeal joint (IPJ), of great toe, 232f
  dorsiflexion of
    active, 234
    passive, 234
  plantar flexion of, active, 234
  range of motion of, 232–234
Intersesamoidal ligament, 234f, 235
  damage to, in metatarsophalangeal joint dislocation, 212
Inversion, and lateral tubercle fracture, 101, 101f
IPJ. *See* Interphalangeal joint (IPJ)
Ischemia, myoneural, compartment syndrome of foot and, 202

J
Joint depression fracture, of calcaneus, 118–119, 119f
Jones fracture, 210, 217

K
Kocher approach, to calcaneal malunion, 140
K-wires
  for displaced metatarsal fractures, 208–210
  for phalangeal fractures, 213
    of lesser toes, 214
  for talar head fractures, 70, 70f
  for talar neck fractures, class I, 75–76
  for tarsometatarsal injuries, 168, 169f

L
Lateral arm flap, 264
Lateral capsular ligament (LCL), 234
Lateral compartment, of foot, anatomy of, 192, 192f
Lateral malleolus
  in ankle stability, 4–6
  osteotomy of, for talar body fracture, 86f, 88
Lateral plantar artery, 220, 220f
  distribution of, 46f
Lateral plantar hallucial artery, 236, 237f
Lateral plantar hallucial nerve, 237, 238f
Lateral posterior process, of talus, fractures of, 95, 96f, 97f
Lateral tubercle, of talus, fractures of, 84f, 85, 100f–102f, 101
  mechanism of, 100f, 101
Latissimus dorsi flap, 267
  in open ankle fracture, 36, 36f
Lauge-Hansen classification, of ankle fractures, 3
LCL (lateral capsular ligament), 234
Ligament(s). *See also* names of specific ligaments
  of ankle syndesmosis, function of, 11
  of fifth metatarsal, 218, 219f
  tibiofibular, 1, 2f
Lisfranc fracture, 157
Lisfranc's joint, 218, 218f
Lisfranc's ligament, 163
  avulsion fracture of, 162f, 167
Long plantar ligament, 219f
Lumbar sympathetic block, for chronic pain, after crush/soft tissue injuries of foot, 188

M
Magnetic resonance imaging (MRI)
  of navicular stress fracture, 155f, 156
  of osteochondral talar lesions, 104, 105f
  of osteonecrosis, after talar neck fracture, 81–85, 83f
Malleolus
  lateral
    in ankle stability, 4–6
    osteotomy of, for talar body fracture, 86f, 88
  medial
    fracture of, in complex ankle fracture dislocation, repair of, 15
    in pilon fracture, 47, 47f
  posterior. *See* Posterior malleolus

Malunion
of calcaneal fractures. *See* Calcaneal fracture(s), malunion of
of phalangeal fractures, 214f
of talar fractures, 92
MCL (medial capsular ligament), 234, 234f
repair of, in hallux valgus, 250, 251f
Medial capsular ligament (MCL), 234, 234f
repair of, in hallux valgus, 250, 251f
Medial clear space
measurement of, 40
radiographic assessment of, 13f, 14, 14f
in syndesmotic diastasis, 6f
Medial compartment, of foot
anatomy of, 191–192, 192f
pressure measurement in, 194, 194f
Medial malleolus
fracture of, in complex ankle fracture dislocation, repair of, 15
in pilon fracture, 47, 47f
Medial plantar artery, distribution of, 46f
Medial plantar hallucial artery, 236, 237f
Medial plantar hallucial nerve, 237, 238f
Medial tubercle, of talus, fracture of, 101, 102f
Medialis pedis flap, 261, 263f
Metatarsal head, flat, and great toe metatarsophalangeal joint injury, 244
Metatarsal(s)
fifth. *See* Fifth metatarsal
fractures of, 205–210
clinical manifestations of, 206
closed, undisplaced, treatment of, 207
displaced, treatment of, 207–210, 208f, 209f
functional anatomy of, 205–206
incidence of, 206
mechanism of, 206
open, treatment of, 207
radiographic evaluation of, 206–207
treatment of, 207–210, 208f, 209f
second, anatomy of, 161
traction on, for tarsometatarsal injuries, 168, 169f
Metatarsophalangeal joint (MTPJ)
dislocations of, 212
types of, 212
of great toe
anatomy of, 231–237, 232f–238f
athletic injuries of, 231–256
classification of, 237–243, 238t
etiology of, 243–244
evaluation of, 244–245
radiographic, 245, 246f
hyperextension, 239, 239f, 240f
hyperflexion, 241, 242f
mechanism of, 237–243, 239f–243f
sequelae of, 252–254, 252f, 253f
treatment of, 246–250, 247f–249f, 247t
algorithm for, 246–248, 247f
surgical, 250, 250f, 251f
valgus force, 241–243, 243f
varus stress, 243
biomechanics of, 231–237, 233f
dorsiflexion of
active, 232
passive, 232
flattened, 231, 233f
muscular attachments of, 235–236, 237f
plantar flexion of, active, 232
range of motion of, 232, 233f
in turf toe injury, 244
spherical, 231, 233f
lesser, dislocation of, 212
Metatarsosesamoid ligaments, 234f, 235
MRI (magnetic resonance imaging)
of navicular stress fracture, 155f, 156
of osteochondral talar lesions, 104, 105f
of osteonecrosis, after talar neck fracture, 82–85, 83f
MTPJ. *See* Metatarsophalangeal joint (MTPJ)
Muscle flap, for foot/ankle reconstruction, selection of, 266–267
Myoneural ischemia, compartment syndrome of foot and, 202

N

Navicular
anatomy of
osseous, 145–146, 146f
variants in, 147, 147f
vascular, 146, 146f
body of, fractures of, 149f–153f, 150–154
displaced, 154
nondisplaced, 154
type I, treatment of, 149f, 154
type II, treatment of, 150f, 151f, 154
type III, treatment of, 152f, 153f, 154
fractures of, 145–160
dorsal lip, 148, 148f
forefoot disruption with, 156f, 157
mechanism of, 148
stress, 154–156, 155f
treatment of, 156
tuberosity, 149–150, 149f
ligaments of
cuneiform, 145–146
talonavicular, 145–146
Nerve(s). *See also* names of specific nerves
of great toe, 236–237, 238f
injury to, in open ankle fracture, 37
Neuritis, sural, after displaced intraarticular calcaneal fracture, 131
Night-walker fracture, 212

O

Ollier incision, for calcaneal malunion, 140
Open fractures
of ankle. *See* Ankle, fractures of, open
of foot, soft tissue management in, 261
of metatarsals, 207
of talus, 92
Open reduction and internal fixation
of closed fracture, soft tissue management in, 260
of cuboid fracture, 158f, 159
of displaced metatarsal fracture, 208–210, 209f
of displaced navicular body fracture, 151f, 153f, 154
of great toe metatarsophalangeal joint injury, 250
of phalangeal fracture, 213
of pilon fracture, 55–59, 57f–60f
of tarsometatarsal injuries, 170–172, 170f–172f
incisions for, 170, 170f
Orthoplast splint, 249, 249f
Orthosis, short leg, after complex ankle fracture dislocation, with syndesmotic diastasis, 17
Os calcis, pin fixation of, for talar neck fracture, 79f, 80
Os tibiale externum, 147, 147f
Os vesalianum, 219–221
fracture vs., 219, 218f
Ossification, of fifth metatarsal, centers of, 219, 220f
Osteochondral fracture, of talar body, 84f, 85
Osteochondral fragment, in subtalar dislocation, management of, 112, 113f
Osteochondral lesions, of talus. *See* Talus, osteochondral lesions of
Osteocutaneous flap
fibular, 267
for foot/ankle reconstruction, selection of, 267
Osteology, of proximal fifth metatarsal, 218–219, 219f, 220f, 222f
Osteomyelitis
after displaced intraarticular calcaneal fracture, 131
soft tissue management in, 261
Osteonecrosis
after subtalar dislocation, 112
after talar fracture, 92
of neck, 81–85, 83f
magnetic resonance imaging of, 81–85, 83f
Osteophytes, in hallux rigidus, after great toe metatarsophalangeal joint injury, debridement of, 252f, 253, 253f
Osteoporosis, in complex ankle fracture dislocations, with syndesmotic diastasis, 12
Osteotomy
for calcaneal malunion, 141
of lateral malleolus, for talar body fracture, 86f, 88

P

Pain
after crush/soft tissue injuries of foot, 188
in compartment syndrome of foot, 194
in intraarticular calcaneal fractures, 121
Penicillin, for wound infection, in open ankle fracture, 32
Peroneal artery
distribution of, 46f
in talus circulation, 66, 68f
Peroneal tenolysis, for calcaneal malunion, 140, 141
Peroneus brevis, fifth metatarsal insertion of, 219, 220f
Peroneus longus, fifth metatarsal insertion of, 219, 220f
Peroneus tertius, fifth metatarsal insertion of, 219, 220f
Phalanges
fractures of, 212–214
clinical diagnosis of, 213
functional anatomy of, 213
malunion of, 214f
treatment of, 213, 214f
of lesser toes, fractures of, 214
Picot's incision, for calcaneal malunion, 140
Pilon fracture, 45–63
classification of, 48–53, 48f
complications of, 62
cutaneous arterial distribution of, 47
displaced
reconstructible, 51, 51f
unreconstructible, 49, 50f
evaluation of, soft tissue assessment in, 52, 52f
mechanism of, 48

Pilon fracture (*contd.*)
  pathologic anatomy of, 47–48, 47f
  postoperative care in, 61–62
  treatment of
    calcaneal pin traction in, 54–55
    decisions in, 48–53, 49f–53f
    external fixation in, 54f, 59–61
    modalities of, 53–61
    open reduction and internal fixation in, 55–59, 57f–60f
    tibiotalar joint arthrodesis in, 61
  types of, 45
Pin fixation
  of displaced metatarsal fractures, 208
  of open ankle fracture, 34, 34f
  of os calcis, for talar neck fracture, 79f, 80
  of osteochondral talar lesions, 104
  for skeletal stabilization, in crush/soft tissue injuries of foot, 186–187, 187f
  of tarsometatarsal injuries, 168, 169f
Pin traction, calcaneal, for pilon fracture, 54–55
  selection criteria for, 52–53, 53f
Plafond, tibial, anatomy of, 45, 46f
Plantar compartments, of foot, anatomy of, 192
Plantar fascia, 219f
Plantar flexion, active
  of interphalangeal joint, 234
  of metatarsophalangeal joint, 232
Plantar metatarsal artery, 220, 220f
Plantar metatarsal ligament, 218, 219f
Plantar tarsometatarsal ligament, 218, 219f
Plate fixation
  of fibula, in complex ankle fracture dislocation, with syndesmotic diastasis, 16, 16f
  of intraarticular calcaneal fracture, 124, 126
  of pilon fracture, 57–60, 60f
Posterior facet, displacement of, in intraarticular calcaneal fracture, 121–123, 122f
  prognotic implications of, 123
  reduction of, 124, 124f
Posterior malleolus
  anatomy of
    functional, 22
    gross, 21, 22f
    pathologic, 23, 23f
  fracture of, 21–29
    in complex ankle fracture dislocation, repair of, 15
    mechanism of, 23
    radiology of, 23, 24f
    size of, estimation of, 23, 24f
    treatment of, 25, 25f
      surgical, 26–27, 26f–28f
        posterior approach of Henry in, 26, 26f
        posterior to anterior technique in, 26–27, 27f
        posteromedial technique in, 27
    types of, 23, 23f
  in pilon fracture, 47f, 48
Posterior process
  lateral, of talus, fractures of, 95, 96f, 97f
  of talus, fractures of, 84f, 85, 95–99, 96f–99f
    posterior lateral approach to, 97f–99f, 99
Posterior tibial artery
  distribution of, 46f
  in talus circulation, 66, 68f
Posterior tibial nerve, injury to, in open ankle fracture, 37
Posterior tibialis tendon
  blockage of, by subtalar dislocation, 111f, 112
  contracture of, in compartment syndrome of foot, 202
Posterior tibiofibular ligament, 1, 2f
  anatomy of, 39
Posterior–inferior tibiofibular ligament, anatomy of, 10, 11f
Posterolateral approach of Henry, in posterior malleolus fracture repair, 26, 26f
Pronation, of hindfoot, in tarsometatarsal injuries, 168
Pronation-external rotation injury, of ankle, 4, 5f
  repair of, late results after, 17
Propionobacterium acnes, and wound infection, in open ankle fracture, 32
Proximal interphalangeal joint, arthrodesis of, in compartment syndrome of foot, 203
Pseudomonas aeruginosa, and wound infection, in open ankle fracture, 32
Pulse, absence of, in compartment syndrome of foot, 194

R

Radial forearm flap, 264–266, 265f
Radiography
  of calcaneal malunion, 138
  of cuboid fracture, 157, 158f
  of metatarsal fractures, 206–207
  of metatarsophalangeal joint of great toe, 245, 246f
  of posterior malleolus fracture, 23, 24f
  of syndesmotic diastasis, 4, 6f, 40
  of tarsometatarsal injuries, 167–168, 167f
Range of motion exercises, for great toe metatarsophalangeal joint injury, 249
Rectus abdominis muscle flap, 267
Reduction
  open, internal fixation with. *See* Open reduction and internal fixation
  of subtalar dislocation, 111
Reduction forceps, in posterior malleolus fracture repair, 27, 28f
Reflex sympathetic dystrophy, after crush/soft tissue injuries of foot, 188
  treatment of, 190
''Road burn'' injury, 182
Rotation, in pilon fracture, 48

S

Sanders classification, of intraarticular calcaneal fractures, 121, 122f
  displaced, 128, 129f
Sangeorzan fracture, of navicular, 149f–153f, 154
  internal fixation of, 149f, 154
Scapular flap, 262f
Screw fixation
  of calcaneal malunion, 141
  of displaced metatarsal fractures, 210
  of intraarticular calcaneal fracture, 124, 126
  of proximal fifth metatarsal fractures, 226f, 227–228, 228f
    immobilization vs., 229–230
    stress, 226
  of Sangeorzan navicular fracture, 149f, 154
  of tarsometatarsal injuries, 168, 169f, 170, 171f
Screw(s)
  anterior–posterior, for posterior malleolus fracture, 26
  cancellous, for talar body fracture, 88, 91f
  cannulated, for talar neck fracture, class I, 76–77, 76f–78f
  posterior–anterior, for posterior malleolus fracture, 26–27, 27f
  subarticular, for talar head fracture, 70, 70f
  syndesmosis. *See* Syndesmosis screw
Sensation, lack of, in compartment syndrome of foot, 194
Serratus anterior muscle flap, 267
Sesamoids
  disruption of, in metatarsophalangeal joint dislocation, 212
  fracture of, nonunion of, surgical treatment of, 250
  injury to, in great toe metatarsophalangeal joint injury, radiographic evaluation of, 245, 246f
  lateral, 235
  medial, 235
Shenton's line, 45
Shoe
  athletic, carbon fiber plate for, 248, 248f
  type of, in great toe metatarsophalangeal joint injuries, 244
Short leg cast
  for fracture of base of fifth metatarsal, 210, 212
  for metatarsal fractures
    displaced, 208
    undisplaced, 207
  for phalangeal fractures, 213
  for subtalar dislocation, 113
Short leg orthosis, after complex ankle fracture dislocation, with syndesmotic diastasis, 17
Skeletal stabilization, in crush/soft tissue injuries of foot, 185–187, 187f
Skin flap, for foot/ankle reconstruction, selection of, 264–266, 265f, 266f
Skin grafting
  in complex foot/ankle injuries, 259
  in open reduction and internal fixation, of closed fractures, 260
  split-thickness, in viable tissue identification, in crush/soft tissue injuries of foot, 183–185, 184f
Soft tissue
  assessment of, in pilon fracture, 52, 52f
  of foot, injury of. *See* Foot, crush/soft tissue injuries of
  injury to, in subtalar dislocation, 109, 110f
  management of
    in complex foot/ankle injuries
      guidelines for, 257–268
      principles of, 257–259, 258f
      reconstructive ladder in, 259–260
      vascular status assessment in, 258–259, 258f
      wound cleanliness in, 259
      wound closure in, timing of, 259
    in open fracture, 261, 262f
      of ankle, 35–36
    in open reduction and internal fixation, of closed fracture, 260
    in osteomyelitis, 261
    in pilon fracture
      intraoperative, 55–56
      postoperative, 56–60
      preoperative, 55
    in postoperative wound breakdown, 260–261

full thickness, 261
partial thickness, 260–261
unstable, reconstructive ladder for, 261, 263f
Splint, orthoplast, 249, 249f
Split-thickness skin excision (STSE), in viable tissue identification, in crush/soft tissue injuries of foot, 183–185, 184f
Staphylococcus aureus, and wound infection, in open ankle fracture, 32
Staphylococcus epidermidis, and wound infection, in open ankle fracture, 31
Stress fractures
of navicular, 154–156, 155f
treatment of, 156
of proximal fifth metatarsal, 225–226
Stress test, after complex ankle fracture dislocation repair, with syndesmotic diastasis, 19
STSE (split-thickness skin excision), in viable tissue identification, in crush/soft tissue injuries of foot, 183–185, 184f
Styloid, fracture of, in proximal fifth metatarsal fracture, 222
Subarticular screw, for talar head fracture, 70, 70f
Subluxation
subtalar, in talar neck fractures, 73, 73f
talar
radiographic assessment of, 13f, 14–15, 14f
in syndesmotic diastasis, 6f
Subtalar joint
arthritis of
after displaced intraarticular calcaneal fracture, 131
after talar neck fracture, 81, 82f
dislocation of, 109–114, 110f, 111f
irreducible, 111f–113f, 112
lateral, 109
mechanism of, 109
medial, 109, 110f
open, 112
osteochondral fragments with, management of, 112, 113f
reduction of, 111
soft tissue damage with, 109, 110f
treatment of, 113
fusion of
for calcaneal malunion, 140, 141
primary, for displaced intraarticular calcaneal fractures, 130–131
subluxation of, in talar neck fractures, 73, 73f
Superficial peroneal nerve, medial dorsal cutaneous branch of, 237, 238f
Superomedial fragment, reduction of, in intraarticular calcaneal fracture, 124
Supination, of hindfoot, in tarsometatarsal injuries, 168
Supination external injury, of ankle, 3–4, 5f
Supination-external rotation type IV injury, 9
Sural neuritis, after displaced intraarticular calcaneal fracture, 131
Synchondritic fracture, 147, 147f
Syndesmosis, of ankle. *See* Ankle, syndesmosis of
Syndesmosis A, radiographic assessment of, 13f, 14, 14f
Syndesmosis B, radiographic assessment of, 13f, 14, 14f
Syndesmosis screw, 7
for complex ankle fracture dislocation, with syndesmotic diastasis, 16–17
removal of, 17, 19
for deltoid injury, in complex ankle fracture dislocation, 19
elastic fixation of, 12
functional effects of, 11
indications for, 42
results of, 41–42
for talar subluxation, 14–15
use of, technique of, 42
Syndesmotic diastasis
complex ankle fracture dislocations with, 9–19
late results in, 17
management of
clinical, 12–13, 12f
operative, 15–17, 16f
postoperative, 17
radiographic considerations in, 13–15, 13f–15f
radiographic criteria for, 4, 6f, 40
Syndesmotic ligament, rupture of, 6–7

T

Talar head, fractures of, 69f–71f, 70–71
complications of, 70
stabilization of, 70, 70f
Talar neck
anatomy of, 66
fractures of, 71–73, 72f
anteromedial approach to, 75–76, 75f, 76f
classification of, 73, 73f, 74f
complications of, 81–85, 81f, 82f, 83f
malunion after, 81, 81f
mechanism of, 71, 72f
nonunion after, 81, 82f
posterolateral approach to, 76, 77f, 78f
injury of
class I, treatment of, 75–77, 75f–78f
class II, treatment of, 77, 79f
class III, treatment of, 79f, 80, 80f
malalignments of, 74–85
Talar shift
lateral, 6
measurement of, 40
Talar subluxation
radiographic assessment of, 13f, 14–15, 14f
in syndesmotic diastasis, 6f
Talar tilt
radiographic assessment of, 13f, 14, 14f
in syndesmotic diastasis, 6f
Talectomy, for talar body fracture, 88
Talocalcaneal ligament, disruption of, in talar neck fracture, 74f, 77
Talocrural angle
measurement of, 40
radiographic assessment of, 13, 13f
in syndesmotic diastasis, 6f
Talonavicular dislocation, in talar neck fractures, 73, 73f
Talonavicular fusion, for talar head fracture, 70, 71f
Talonavicular ligaments, 145–146
Talus
anatomy of, 66, 67f
body of, fractures of, 85–88, 85f–88f
classification of, 84f, 85, 95, 96f
fixation of, 87f, 88, 88f
talar salvage in, 88, 89f–91f
circulation of, 66–68, 68f
fractures of
complex, 65–93
outcome in, 92
open, 92
injury of
history of, 65–66
occult, 95–106
lateral tubercle of, fractures of, 84f, 85, 100f–102f, 101
mechanism of, 100f, 101
medial tubercle of, fracture of, 101, 102f
osteochondral lesions of, 101–104, 103f–106f
arthroscopy of, 104, 106f
lateral, 102, 103f
mechanism of, 102–104, 104f
medial, 101–102, 103f, 105f
mechanism of, 102, 104f
soft lesion with, 104
stages of, 102, 103f
posterior process of
fractures of, 84f, 85, 95–99, 96f–99f
posterior lateral approach to, 97f–99f, 99
lateral, fractures of, 95, 96f, 97f
relationship of, to calcaneus, 120
Taping
"buddy," for phalangeal fractures, 213
for great toe metatarsophalangeal joint injury, 249
Tarsal canal artery, in talus circulation, 66, 68f
Tarsal sinus artery, in talus circulation, 66, 68f
Tarsometatarsal joint
anatomy of, 161–166, 162f, 163f
dislocation of, 162f
dorsal, 163, 163f
injuries of
classification of, 166–167, 166f
mechanism of, 164f, 165f, 166
occult, 173
radiologic criteria for, 167–168, 167f
treatment of, 161–173, 169f–172f
closed, 168, 169f
open, 170–172, 170f–172f
criteria for, 170
postoperative care in, 172
results of, 172–173
Temporalis fascia flap, 266
Tendon(s). *See also* names of specific tendons
insertion of, on fifth metatarsal, 218, 220f
Tenolysis, peroneal, for calcaneal malunion, 140, 141
Tetanus toxoid, for wound infection, in open ankle fracture, 32
Tibia
distal, fracture of, AO classification of, 48f
reconstruction of, in pilon fracture, 57, 58f
Tibial plafond, anatomy of, 45, 46f
Tibiocalcaneal arthrodesis, for talar body fracture, 88, 90f, 91f
Tibiofibular clear space
measurement of, 40
radiographic assessment of, 14
in syndesmotic diastasis, 4, 6f
Tibiofibular joint, reduction of, in complex ankle fracture dislocation, with syndesmotic diastasis, 17
Tibiofibular ligaments, 1, 2f, 10, 11f
interosseous, anatomy of, 10, 11f

Tibiofibular overlap
measurement of, 40
radiographic assessment of, 14
in syndesmotic diastasis, 6f
Tibiotalar angle, in syndesmotic diastasis, 4
Tibiotalar clear space, in syndesmotic diastasis, 4, 6f
Tibiotalar joint, primary arthrodesis of, in pilon fracture, 61
Tissue, viable, identification of, in crush/soft tissue injuries of foot, 182–185
Tissue transplantation, in complex foot/ankle injuries, 260
Tobramycin, for wound infection, in open ankle fracture, 32
Toe spacer, for great toe metatarsophalangeal joint injury, 249
Toe(s)
claw, compartment syndrome and, 201f, 202
deformities of, in compartment syndrome of foot, correction of, 203
great. *See* Great toe
hyperflexed, compartment syndrome and, 202
lesser, phalangeal fractures of, 214
turf. *See* Turf toe
Tongue fracture, of calcaneus, 118–119, 119f
Traction
pin, calcaneal, for pilon fracture, 54–55
selection criteria for, 52–53, 53f
for tarsometatarsal injuries, 168, 169f
Transplantation, tissue, in complex foot/ankle injuries, 260
Transverse tibiofibular ligament, 1, 2f
anatomy of, 10, 11f, 39
Triangular external fixator, for open ankle fracture, 34, 34f
Trimalleolar fracture, treatment of, results of, 41
Tuberosity fracture
of navicular, 149–150, 149f
of proximal fifth metatarsal, 222, 223–224
nonunion of, 223–224
Turf, artificial, and great toe metatarsophalangeal joint injuries, 243–244
Turf toe
grading of, 247t, 248
hyperextension in, 239, 239f, 240f
hyperflexion in, 241, 242f
metatarsophalangeal joint range of motion in, 244
valgus in, 241–243, 243f

V

Valgus, and great toe metatarsophalangeal joint injury, 241–243, 243f
Varus, and great toe metatarsophalangeal joint injury, 243
Volkman's triangle, 21

W

Weber B fracture, syndesmosis screw for, indications for, 42
Weber C fracture
syndesmosis screw for, indications for, 42
treatment of, results of, 42
Weight, in great toe metatarsophalangeal joint injury, 244
Weight bearing
after closed undisplaced metatarsal fractures, 207
after complex ankle fracture dislocation, with syndesmotic diastasis, 17
after great toe metatarsophalangeal joint injury, 248
after proximal fifth metatarsal fracture, 228
after talar neck fracture, 81–85
Wound(s)
in calcaneal fracture
complications of, 116
intraarticular, displaced, dehiscence of, 131
in complex foot/ankle injuries
closure of, timing of, 259
management of, cleanliness in, 259
in crush/soft tissue injuries of foot, contamination of, 185–187, 186f
in open ankle fracture
infection of, antimicrobial management of, 31–32
reconstruction of
complex, 35–36, 35f, 36f
delayed, 34–35
postoperative breakdown of, soft tissue management in, 260–261

Z

Zone I fracture, of proximal fifth metatarsal, treatment of, 223–224
Zone II fracture, of proximal fifth metatarsal, treatment of, 224
Zone III fracture, of proximal fifth metatarsal, treatment of, 224